# CLINICAL REASONING
## FOR MEDICAL STUDENTS
### Bridge the Gap

# CLINICAL REASONING
## FOR MEDICAL STUDENTS
## Bridge the Gap

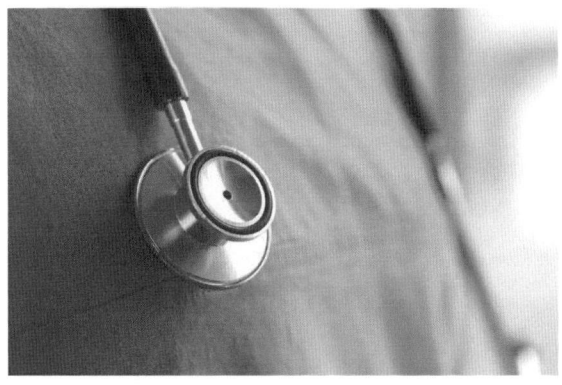

## Lasith Ranasinghe
Imperial College Healthcare NHS Trust, UK

**World Scientific**

NEW JERSEY · LONDON · SINGAPORE · BEIJING · SHANGHAI · HONG KONG · TAIPEI · CHENNAI · TOKYO

*Published by*

World Scientific Publishing Europe Ltd.

57 Shelton Street, Covent Garden, London WC2H 9HE

*Head office:* 5 Toh Tuck Link, Singapore 596224

*USA office:* 27 Warren Street, Suite 401-402, Hackensack, NJ 07601

**Library of Congress Cataloging-in-Publication Data**

Names: Ranasinghe, Lasith, author.

Title: Clinical reasoning for medical students : bridge the gap /
   Lasith Ranasinghe, Imperial College Healthcare NHS Trust, UK.

Description: New Jersey : World Scientific, [2024] | Includes index.

Identifiers: LCCN 2023031769 | ISBN 9781800614567 (hardcover) |
   ISBN 9781800614659 (paperback) | ISBN 9781800614574 (ebook) |
   ISBN 9781800614581 (ebook other)

Subjects: MESH: Clinical Reasoning | Diagnosis, Differential | Handbook

Classification: LCC RC71.3 | NLM WB 39 | DDC 616.07/5--dc23/eng/20230929

LC record available at https://lccn.loc.gov/2023031769

**British Library Cataloguing-in-Publication Data**

A catalogue record for this book is available from the British Library.

For any available supplementary material, please visit
https://www.worldscientific.com/worldscibooks/10.1142/Q0430#t=suppl

Desk Editors: Balasubramanian Shanmugam/Rosie Williamson/Shi Ying Koe

Typeset by Stallion Press
Email: enquiries@stallionpress.com

Printed in Singapore

# Foreword

Even as a relatively new doctor, I've seen first-hand the incredible relationship we can have with our patients. The deeply personal moments we share, the conversations that bring you to tears and the lasting impact that we can have when treating debilitating health issues. We are more than a service provider, more than an algorithm and more than a cog in a machine. We really do make a difference and we do truly leave an impression on patients that will often last a lifetime.

Being in a position of such privilege comes with responsibility. The responsibility to advocate for our patients, provide them with up-to-date information and empower them to make decisions about their health. We can only do this because of the vast knowledge we've acquired through hundreds of hours spent sitting at a desk, in cadaver labs, in lecture halls, in hospital corridors, in operating rooms and by the patient's bedside. It is this time, this labour and this sacrifice we have made that puts us in a unique position to be able to call ourselves *Doctors*.

Remember that every moment you spend studying is a moment spent honing your knowledge and preparing yourself for future scenarios that you can scarcely imagine as a medical student. All so that, when you show up on the day and someone's life is in your hands, you're able to think clearly and make the right decisions to improve their outcomes.

Becoming a doctor has lived up to every expectation that I had of it and more. Every day I'm surrounded by incredibly intelligent people, all pushing each other to do better. No two days are the same, and every patient brings with them a sense of excitement and intrigue as we gain a small yet valuable insight into their lives.

Resources, like this book, help lay the foundation upon which our clinical practice is built. Case studies, treatment algorithms, acronyms and questions are essential in retaining all the information doctors use on a daily basis. Lasith is a wonderful teacher, inspired and practical with his knowledge and deeply caring about his students. I have no doubt this resource will be irreplaceable to any aspiring doctor and will be a staple on their bookshelves for years to come.

Dr. Nasir Kharma
*Junior Doctor & Content Creator*

# About the Author

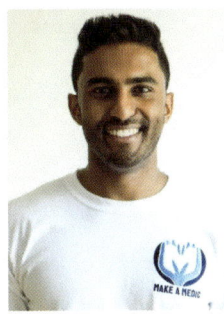 **Lasith Ranasinghe** is a junior doctor based in London who has a keen interest in Anaesthetics and Intensive Care Medicine. Since medical school, he has maintained an exceptional academic standard having frequently ranked in the top 3 in his cohort at Imperial College London, received 25 prizes for academic excellence and ranked within the top 3% and 1% of candidates in the MRCP Part 1 and Part 2 exams, respectively. In his spare time, he runs a charity called *Make a Medic* that produces high-quality medical educational resources for students and uses the funds raised to create grants for education and public health initiatives in low- and middle-income countries. Before this publication, he authored the highly rated RevMED series.

# The Contributors

Dr. Syra Dhillon
University Hospitals Sussex NHS Foundation Trust

Dr. Adam Graham
Lewisham and Greenwich NHS Trust

Aleksandra Dunin-Borkowska
Imperial College School of Medicine

Ghavin Kuganesan
Imperial College School of Medicine

Alexandra M. Cardoso Pinto
Imperial College School of Medicine

Justyna Gromala
Imperial College School of Medicine

# Acknowledgements

The author and illustrators would like to express their gratitude to several individuals who reviewed our content and helped shape it into the book that you are holding with your hands in front of you. We collected feedback from both junior doctors and medical students to ensure that the resource is both user-friendly and clinically sound.

Dr. Sarah Kelly
Guy's and St Thomas' NHS Foundation Trust

Dr. Jessica Muirhead
London Northwest University Healthcare NHS Trust

Dr. Katharine Alder
Imperial College Healthcare NHS Trust

Dr. Nicholas Ubhi
University Hospitals Sussex NHS Foundation Trust

Dr. Jaya Chawla
London Northwest University Healthcare NHS Trust

Sujil James
University of Cambridge School of Clinical Medicine

Muhammad Aniq
University of Cambridge School of Clinical Medicine

Shubham Gupta
Imperial College School of Medicine

Abhishek Viswanath
King's College London School of Medical Education

Eu Fang Foo
Cardiff University School of Medicine

Aroosa Malik
Medical University of Sofia

Max Fogelman
University of St Andrews School of Medicine

Rhea E Patel
Imperial College School of Medicine

Abigail Merison
Imperial College School of Medicine

Ioanna Voyatzaki
King's College London School of Medical Education

Pippa Whitaker
Bart's and the London School of Medicine and Dentistry

# Contents

# Introduction

The worst advice I ever got as a young doctor readying myself to start my career was

*Working is nothing like medical school. The things you learnt at medical school will not help you.*

My initial reaction to hearing such a daring statement was one of bewilderment. Why had I just sat through dozens of medical school exams over the course of 6 years if none of it is going to be useful?

Three years and several rotations later, I feel that I have accumulated enough experience at this early stage in my career to confidently declare that the statement could not be further from the truth. There are, of course, plenty of aspects of working as a doctor that cannot be simulated or tested under controlled conditions, however, medical schools have existed for hundreds of years and have constantly been iterating through curricula to prepare us as best as possible.

We have a pretty good idea of how the body works and maintaining a decent understanding of preclinical subjects (anatomy, physiology and biochemistry) will undoubtedly help you in your career. As you begin your clinical training at medical school, you are brimming with knowledge that you may not quite know how to apply. This gap between the preclinical and clinical realms is what this book aims to bridge.

This book will take you through the thought processes that should be going through your head as you have a conversation with a patient about whatever is bothering them. It will teach you how to think both critically and clinically, in order to arrive at a sensible diagnosis and management plan. We sincerely hope that this book will aid you in your clinical development and help smoothen the transition into your clinical career!

# How to Use This Book

The **main flow chart** at the start of the chapter will provide an overview of the thought processes that should be going through your mind when you assess a patient with a given presentation.

The ***Patient Background*** box allows you to build an image of the patient in your mind's eye. It will contain important demographic information and details about their past medical, drug, social and family histories. The **boxes in the midline** follow the main components of a conversation between the doctor (**red** circle) and patient (**blue** circle). To conserve space, we have sometimes included multiple questions though it is worth noting that this is generally advised against in the context of OSCEs!

The **arrows extending to the side** demonstrate the additional questions that you should ask at that point in a history (e.g. red flags and SOCRATES). In clinical practice, a history is often followed by an assessment which will be listed in the form of ***Observations*** and ***Examination*** findings. The information provided will culminate in a **diagnosis**, shown at the bottom of the page. Each chapter will go through each of these sections in turn to ensure that you have a robust understanding of why certain questions are asked.

Once you have made a diagnosis, you will likely have to explain what the condition is, any additional investigations that are required to facilitate the diagnosis and the subsequent management plan. To keep the information concise, we have only listed the key investigations and aspects of management — it is by no means an exhaustive list but should be more than enough to enable you to answer viva questions.

We would also like to draw your attention to the *Classical Presentations* tables that are available in each chapter. It can sometimes be difficult to tease apart various differentials as, in list form, the associated symptoms can be very similar. We have, therefore, written a 'classical presentation' of each condition so that you can visualise how it typically presents. This will be useful for both your OSCEs and for interpreting single-best-answer questions in your written exams.

Given that you are likely early on in your clinical development, some of the differentials may be unfamiliar to you and it may seem as though there are a lot of differentials to keep in mind for a single presenting complaint. To address this, we have designed *Bridge Boxes* which illustrate an important concept that features in the chapter or provide a visual summary of the differentials.

If you want to learn more about the key differentials for each presentation, please refer to the *Differentials in Detail* section towards the back of this book.

# Chapter 1

# Headache

Most people will experience headaches at some point in their lives and, most of the time, it can be managed effectively with simple analgesia and lifestyle changes. A headache, however, could also be the presenting symptom of several sinister underlying conditions.

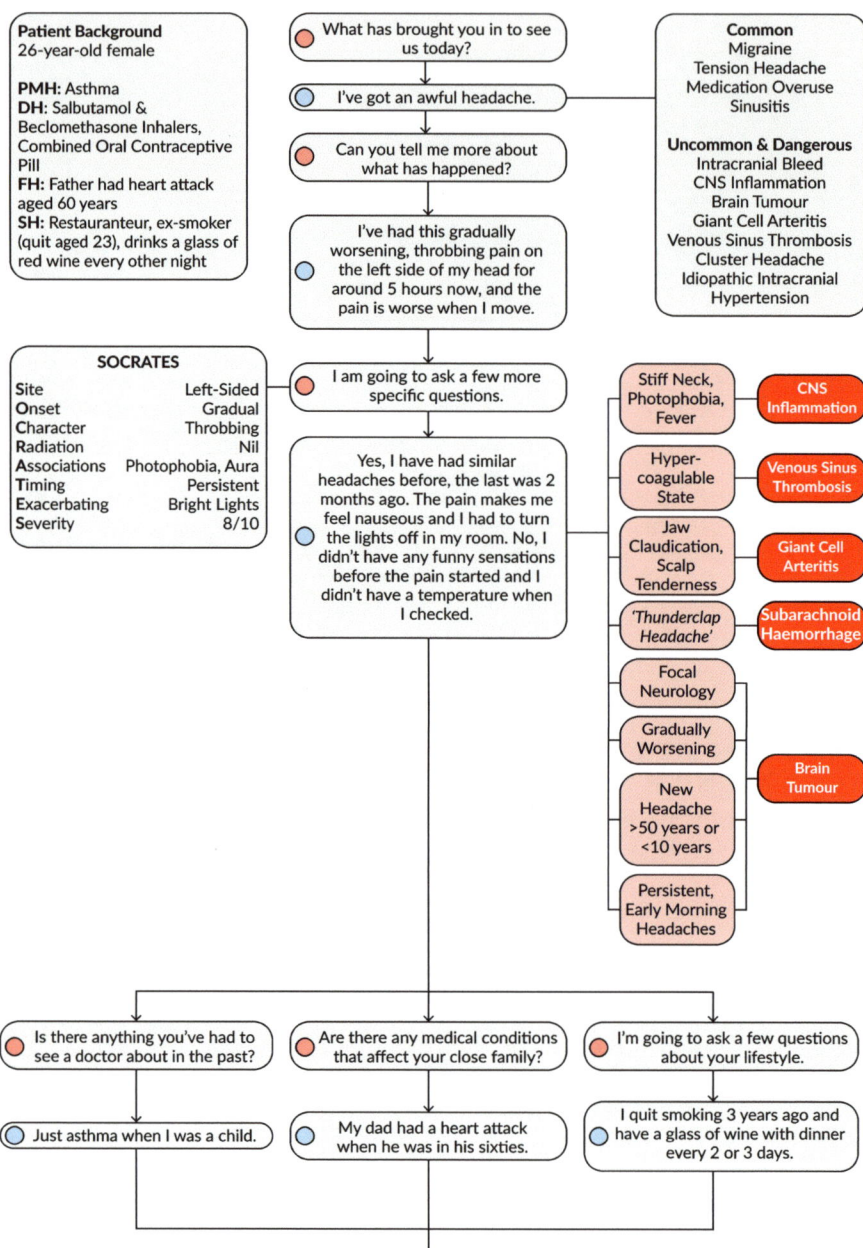

**Patient Background**
26-year-old female

**PMH:** Asthma
**DH:** Salbutamol &
Beclomethasone Inhalers,
Combined Oral Contraceptive
Pill
**FH:** Father had heart attack
aged 60 years
**SH:** Restauranteur, ex-smoker
(quit aged 23), drinks a glass of
red wine every other night

What has brought you in to see us today?

**Common**
Migraine
Tension Headache
Medication Overuse
Sinusitis

**Uncommon & Dangerous**
Intracranial Bleed
CNS Inflammation
Brain Tumour
Giant Cell Arteritis
Venous Sinus Thrombosis
Cluster Headache
Idiopathic Intracranial
Hypertension

I've got an awful headache.

Can you tell me more about what has happened?

I've had this gradually worsening, throbbing pain on the left side of my head for around 5 hours now, and the pain is worse when I move.

**SOCRATES**

| | |
|---|---|
| Site | Left-Sided |
| Onset | Gradual |
| Character | Throbbing |
| Radiation | Nil |
| Associations | Photophobia, Aura |
| Timing | Persistent |
| Exacerbating | Bright Lights |
| Severity | 8/10 |

I am going to ask a few more specific questions.

Yes, I have had similar headaches before, the last was 2 months ago. The pain makes me feel nauseous and I had to turn the lights off in my room. No, I didn't have any funny sensations before the pain started and I didn't have a temperature when I checked.

Stiff Neck, Photophobia, Fever → **CNS Inflammation**

Hyper-coagulable State → **Venous Sinus Thrombosis**

Jaw Claudication, Scalp Tenderness → **Giant Cell Arteritis**

'Thunderclap Headache' → **Subarachnoid Haemorrhage**

Focal Neurology

Gradually Worsening

New Headache >50 years or <10 years

Persistent, Early Morning Headaches

→ **Brain Tumour**

Is there anything you've had to see a doctor about in the past?

Just asthma when I was a child.

Are there any medical conditions that affect your close family?

My dad had a heart attack when he was in his sixties.

I'm going to ask a few questions about your lifestyle.

I quit smoking 3 years ago and have a glass of wine with dinner every 2 or 3 days.

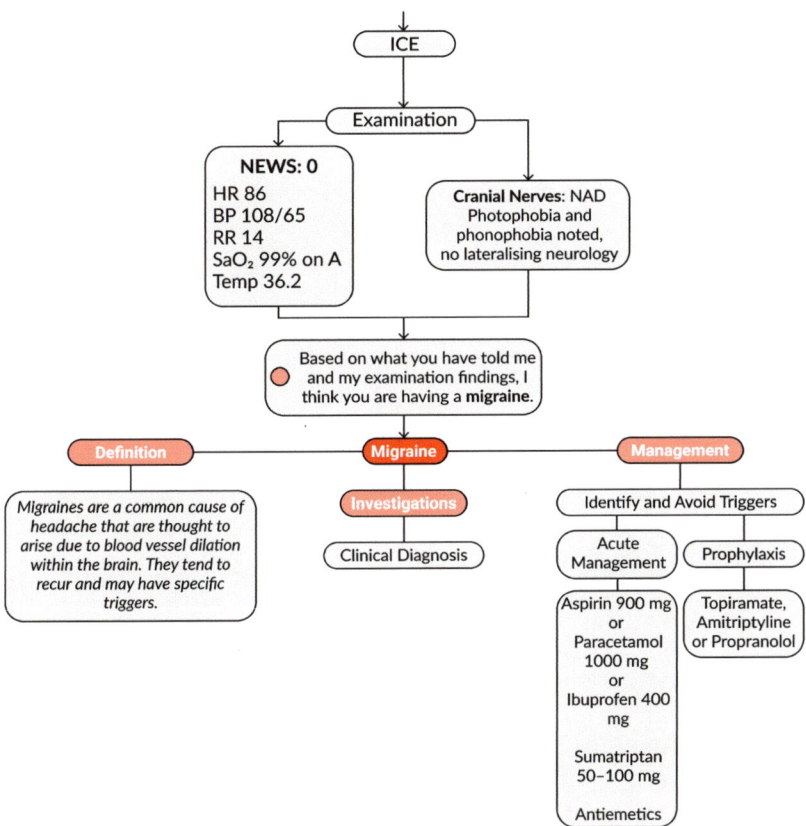

ICE

Examination

**NEWS: 0**
HR 86
BP 108/65
RR 14
SaO₂ 99% on A
Temp 36.2

**Cranial Nerves**: NAD
Photophobia and
phonophobia noted,
no lateralising neurology

Based on what you have told me
and my examination findings, I
think you are having a **migraine**.

**Definition**

**Migraine**

**Management**

Migraines are a common cause of
headache that are thought to
arise due to blood vessel dilation
within the brain. They tend to
recur and may have specific
triggers.

**Investigations**

Clinical Diagnosis

Identify and Avoid Triggers

Acute
Management

Prophylaxis

Aspirin 900 mg
or
Paracetamol
1000 mg
or
Ibuprofen 400
mg

Sumatriptan
50–100 mg

Antiemetics

Topiramate,
Amitriptyline
or Propranolol

# Patient Background

**Patient Background**
26-year-old female

**PMH:** Asthma
**DH:** Salbutamol &
Beclomethasone Inhalers,
Combined Oral Contraceptive
Pill
**FH:** Father had heart attack
aged 60 years
**SH:** Restauranteur, ex-smoker
(quit aged 23), drinks a glass of
red wine every other night

The **age** of a patient presenting for the first time with a headache can help point you towards the likely causes. Tension headaches and migraines are more likely to present for the first time in younger patients, whereas intracranial bleeds and giant cell arteritis (GCA) typically present in older patients. Venous sinus thrombosis is a serious cause of a headache that is associated with **hypercoagulability**, so the patient's background should be screened to determine if there are any factors that may make their blood hypercoagulable (e.g. combined oral contraceptive pill, pregnancy and cancer). It is also important to consider the patient's **body habitus** — idiopathic intracranial hypertension (IIH) is a rare but important cause of a persistent headache that responds poorly to analgesia and is about 20 times more common in obese patients.

## Differential Diagnosis

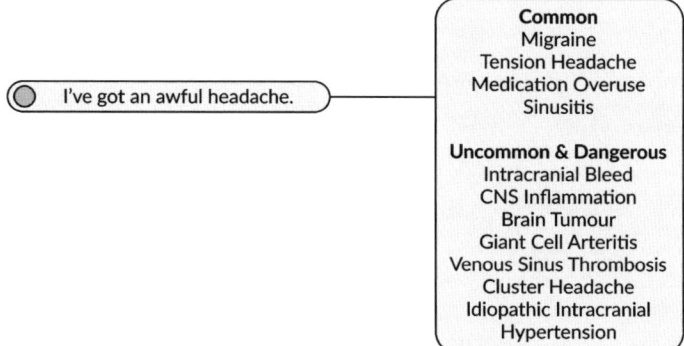

I've got an awful headache.

**Common**
Migraine
Tension Headache
Medication Overuse
Sinusitis

**Uncommon & Dangerous**
Intracranial Bleed
CNS Inflammation
Brain Tumour
Giant Cell Arteritis
Venous Sinus Thrombosis
Cluster Headache
Idiopathic Intracranial
Hypertension

**Common** causes of headaches, such as migraines, tension headaches and medication overuse headaches, can be managed effectively in primary care with careful counselling and appropriate use of medication. These headaches can be severe, but they tend to have a chronic history. There are some features of migraine (e.g. neck stiffness and photophobia) that can be difficult to distinguish from more serious causes of a headache.

**Uncommon** causes of a headache that are *not* usually an acute cause for concern include cluster headaches and IIH. These headaches can be severe and are known to respond poorly to conventional analgesia.

**Dangerous** causes of headaches include intracranial bleeds, central nervous system (CNS) inflammation (e.g. encephalitis and meningitis), brain tumours, GCA and venous sinus thrombosis. Brain tumours are likely to present with a chronic history, whereas GCA and CNS inflammation are likely to present with a subacute history of a headache developing over the course of several days. Intracranial bleeds and venous sinus thrombosis tend to present acutely, though it is worth noting that subdural haemorrhages can present with worsening confusion and neurological sequelae over days and weeks following a head injury.

## SOCRATES

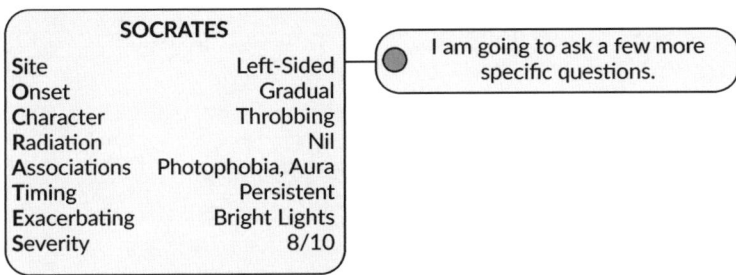

There are a few patterns of symptoms that are worth keeping at the back of your mind while you explore SOCRATES in a patient presenting with a headache:

- **Site**
  - ○ **Unilateral**: Migraine, GCA, venous sinus thrombosis and cluster headache
  - ○ **Generalised**: Tension headache, medication overuse headache, sinusitis, CNS inflammation, brain tumour, IIH and intracranial bleeds
- **Onset**
  - ○ **Rapid Onset**: Migraine, venous sinus thrombosis, cluster headache and intracranial bleed
  - ○ **Gradual Onset**: Tension headache, medication overuse headache, sinusitis, GCA, CNS inflammation, brain tumours and subdural haemorrhage
- **Character**
  - ○ **Intense and Throbbing**: Cluster headache, migraine and venous sinus thrombosis. A subarachnoid haemorrhage will cause a sudden onset worst headache ever that reaches maximum intensity within seconds of onset.

- ○ **Aching and Persistent**: Tension headache, medication over-use headache, sinusitis, brain tumours, CNS inflammation and IIH
- **Radiation**
  - ○ **Neck Stiffness**: Migraine, subarachnoid haemorrhage and CNS inflammation
  - ○ **Eye**: Cluster headache and venous sinus thrombosis
- **Associated Symptoms**
  - ○ **Photophobia**: Migraine and meningitis
  - ○ **Seizures**: CNS inflammation, intracranial bleeds and brain tumour
  - ○ **Lacrimation**: Cluster headache
- **Timing**
  - ○ **Stress**: Migraine and tension headaches
  - ○ **Specific Triggers (e.g. Chocolate)**: Migraine
  - ○ **Specific Time Every Day**: Cluster headache
  - ○ **Worse in the Morning**: Brain tumour
- **Exacerbating**
  - ○ **Bright Lights and Loud Noises**: Migraine, subarachnoid haemorrhage and CNS inflammation
  - ○ **Lying Down**: Brain tumour and IIH
- **Severity**: Though each type of headache can be severe in its own right, the headaches that are *typically* associated with being very severe are cluster headaches, migraines, subarachnoid haemorrhage and venous sinus thrombosis.

Read through the classical presentations table in the following section to develop an understanding of how the main differentials are classically present.

## Classical Presentations

| Differential | Classical Presentation |
|---|---|
| **Migraine** | Acute onset unilateral throbbing headache associated with photophobia and phonophobia. Patients may feel nauseous, and some may experience an aura before the onset of the headache. |

| Tension Headache | Relatively mild bitemporal headache with a *band*-like distribution across the forehead. May be associated with stress, poor sleep or ill health. |
|---|---|
| Medication Overuse | Recurrent headaches in patients who frequently use painkillers (e.g. paracetamol). |
| Sinusitis | Gradual onset headache associated with coryzal symptoms. Patients may complain of the pain worsening when leaning forward and when tapping their forehead. |
| Intracranial Bleed | **Extradural**: Head injury with initial loss of consciousness followed by a lucid interval and, later, a rapid deterioration in consciousness. **Subdural**: May or may not have a clear history of preceding head injury. Gradually worsening confusion, headache and drowsiness. More common in the elderly. **Subarachnoid**: Sudden onset worst headache ever (maximum intensity within seconds), often occipital and associated with nausea, vomiting, photophobia and neck stiffness. |
| CNS Inflammation | Generally unwell with a fever, generalised headache, photophobia and neck stiffness. Some patients may have a rash. Patients with *encephalitis* may develop seizures and reduced consciousness. |
| Brain Tumour | Persistent headaches that are worse when lying down and in the mornings. May be associated with nausea and vomiting. |
| Giant Cell Arteritis | Unilateral headache associated with temporal artery tenderness, scalp tenderness and jaw claudication. Visual impairment is a serious sign suggestive of retinal artery involvement. |
| Venous Sinus Thrombosis | Acute onset severe headache that does not respond well to analgesia. May be associated with lateralising neurology and seizures. |

| | |
|---|---|
| **Cluster Headache** | Intense unilateral headache that occurs at roughly the same time every day and may occur for weeks or months. Often associated with lacrimation. |
| **Idiopathic Intracranial Hypertension** | Persistent generalised headache that is worse when lying down. Associated with obesity. |

## Red Flags

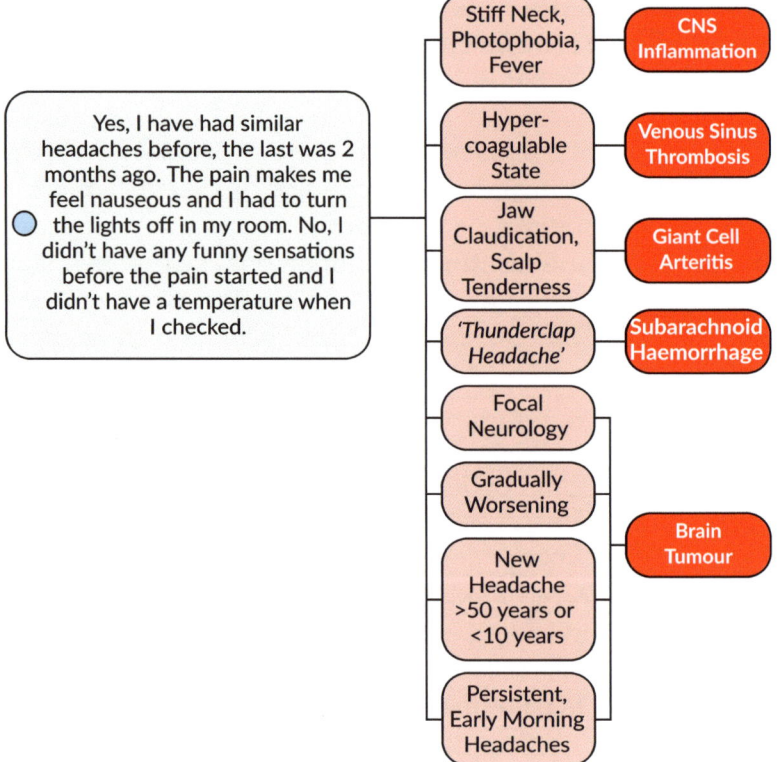

Though headaches are common, it is vital that you screen appropriately for dangerous causes of a headache as they could be catastrophic if missed.

Patients who are unwell with a fever secondary to a simple viral infection often complain of a headache, however, it is important to screen for a constellation of symptoms that are classically associated with meningitis and encephalitis: **neck stiffness** and **photophobia**. **Risk factors for venous thromboembolism** (e.g. pregnancy) should raise suspicion of a venous sinus thrombosis. GCA usually presents in older patients and may be associated with **jaw claudication**, **scalp tenderness** and, most worryingly, **visual changes**. Several causes of a headache can be extremely severe and debilitating but subarachnoid haemorrhages are associated with causing a **sudden onset worst headache ever** (*thunderclap*) that reaches maximal intensity within seconds of onset.

Brain tumours tend to present insidiously with persistent headaches that usually fail to respond to simple analgesia. Other important features include the headaches being **worse in the morning**, **progressive worsening** over several weeks or months and, in particular, the presence of **focal neurology**. It should also be considered as a differential in anyone **under the age of 10 years or over the age of 50 years** presenting for the first time with a headache.

## Assessment

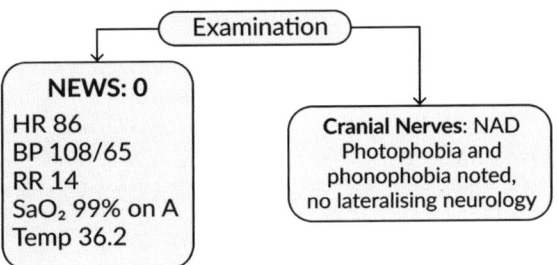

## *Observations*

In most cases, the observations of a patient presenting with a head-ache will be normal. Patients with intracranial infections may have a **fever** and other features of systemic upset (e.g. tachycardia and hypotension). If patients present acutely with an intracranial bleed, it is important to monitor for **Cushing's reflex** (hypertension and bradycardia) which is a feature of raised intracranial pressure that requires urgent neurosurgical attention.

## Examination

Patients with space-occupying lesions, such as brain tumours and intracranial bleeds, can develop focal neurological features (e.g. **lateralising weakness** and **visual field defects**). Similarly, venous sinus thromboses can cause **cranial nerve defects**. Patients with GCA classically have a **tender temporal artery with an impalpable pulse** and may demonstrate scalp tenderness. In severe cases of meningococcal septicaemia, patients may develop a **non-blanching rash** secondary to coagulopathy and damage to blood vessels.

# Migraine

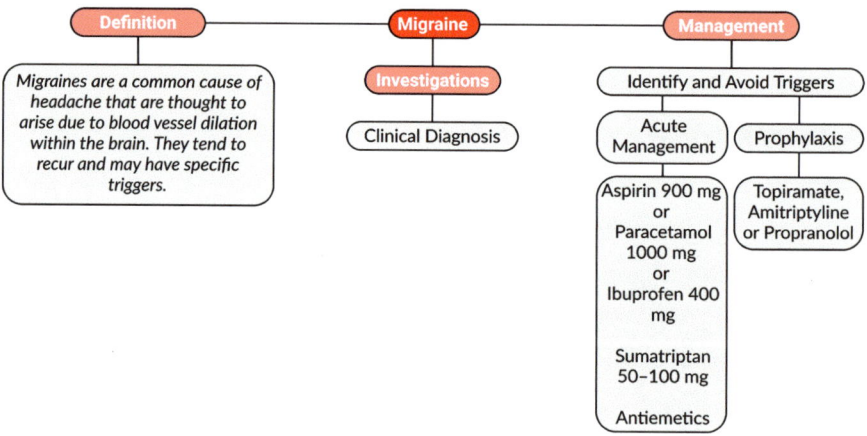

## Definition

Migraines are a very common cause of headache, and they are thought to arise due to issues with blood vessel dilation within the brain. They tend to recur and may have specific triggers (e.g. chocolate, stress and lack of sleep). Some patients may experience abnormal sensory phenomena immediately before a migraine (e.g. zig-zag patterns in their field of vision); this is referred to as an aura.

## *Investigations*

Migraines are primarily a clinical diagnosis and do not usually require further investigation. A headache diary may be recommended to help identify potential triggers.

## *Management*

The **acute** management of a migraine involves managing the pain as best as possible. If taken early, **triptans** (e.g. sumatriptan) can help terminate the migraine. It can be administered orally, intranasally or subcutaneously. Once a migraine is established, the analgesic options that are generally recommended are **Aspirin 900 mg**, **Paracetamol 1000 mg** or **Ibuprofen 400 mg**. Sometimes, migraines are associated with nausea, and this can be managed with **antiemetics** (e.g. prochlorperazine).

Patients who experience frequent migraines may be started on **topiramate**, **amitriptyline** or **propranolol** which can reduce the frequency of migraine attacks. Patients should also be advised to attempt to identify and avoid any triggers.

# Bridge Box

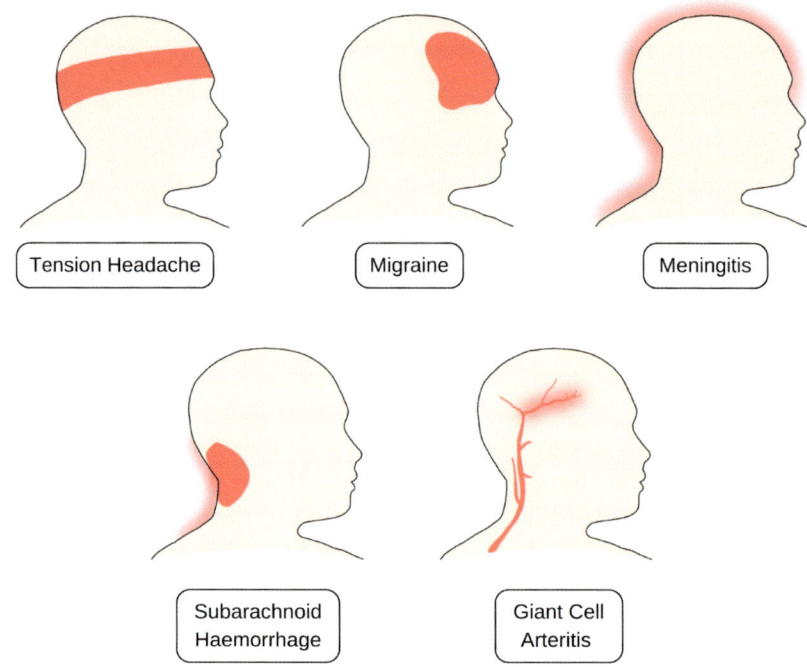

Differentials for headache.

# Chapter 2

# Confusion

Confusion is a relatively common presentation among elderly patients presenting to A&E and primary care services. A thorough clinical assessment as well as a collateral history are necessary to determine the underlying cause.

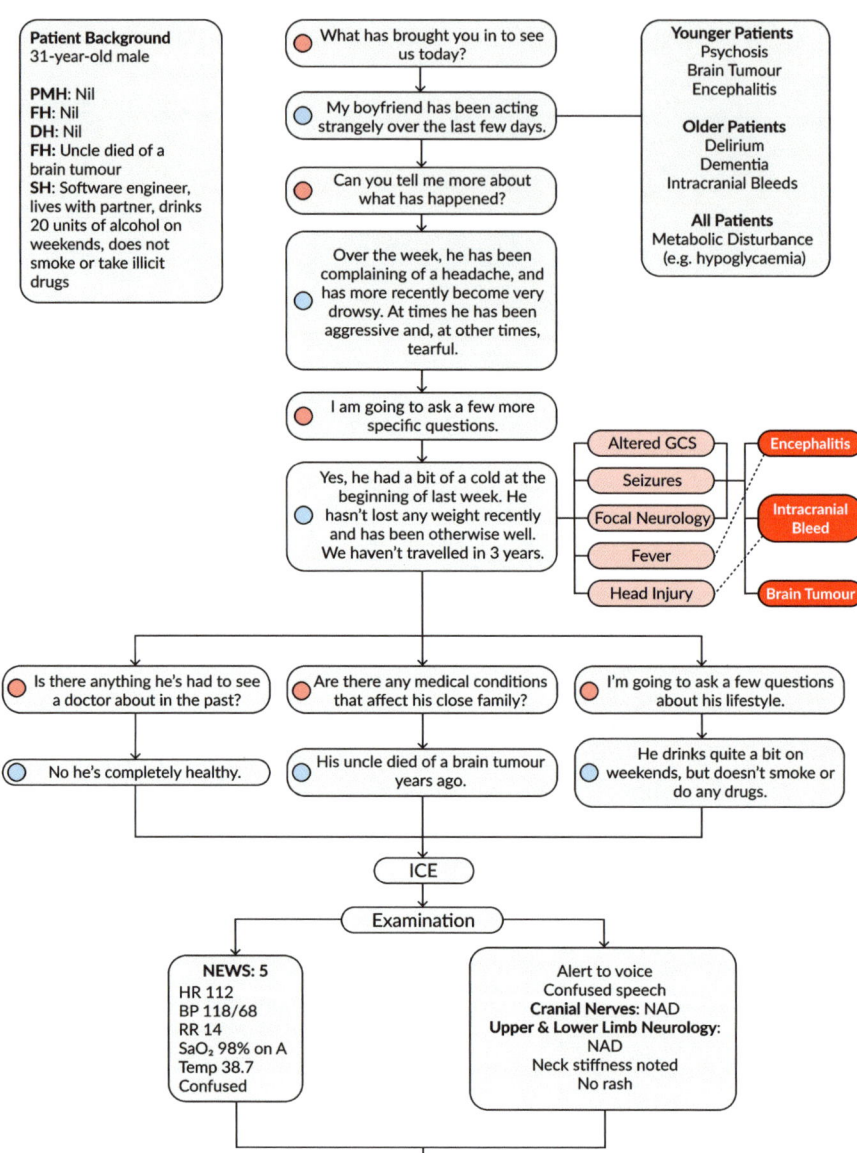

**Patient Background**
31-year-old male

**PMH:** Nil
**FH:** Nil
**DH:** Nil
**FH:** Uncle died of a brain tumour
**SH:** Software engineer, lives with partner, drinks 20 units of alcohol on weekends, does not smoke or take illicit drugs

What has brought you in to see us today?

My boyfriend has been acting strangely over the last few days.

Can you tell me more about what has happened?

Over the week, he has been complaining of a headache, and has more recently become very drowsy. At times he has been aggressive and, at other times, tearful.

I am going to ask a few more specific questions.

Yes, he had a bit of a cold at the beginning of last week. He hasn't lost any weight recently and has been otherwise well. We haven't travelled in 3 years.

**Younger Patients**
Psychosis
Brain Tumour
Encephalitis

**Older Patients**
Delirium
Dementia
Intracranial Bleeds

**All Patients**
Metabolic Disturbance
(e.g. hypoglycaemia)

Altered GCS
Seizures
Focal Neurology
Fever
Head Injury

Encephalitis
Intracranial Bleed
Brain Tumour

Is there anything he's had to see a doctor about in the past?

No he's completely healthy.

Are there any medical conditions that affect his close family?

His uncle died of a brain tumour years ago.

I'm going to ask a few questions about his lifestyle.

He drinks quite a bit on weekends, but doesn't smoke or do any drugs.

ICE

Examination

**NEWS: 5**
HR 112
BP 118/68
RR 14
$SaO_2$ 98% on A
Temp 38.7
Confused

Alert to voice
Confused speech
**Cranial Nerves:** NAD
**Upper & Lower Limb Neurology:**
NAD
Neck stiffness noted
No rash

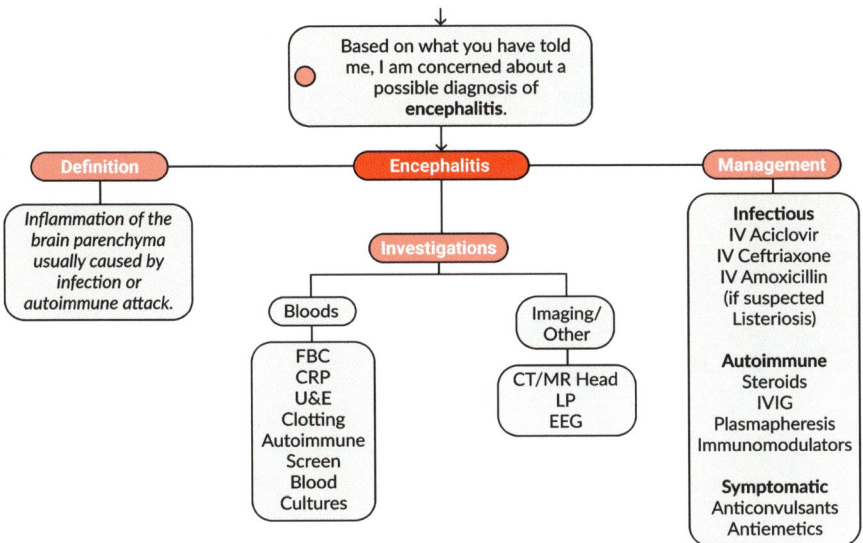

# Patient Background

**Patient Background**
31-year-old male

**PMH:** Nil
**FH:** Nil
**DH:** Nil
**FH:** Uncle died of a brain tumour
**SH:** Software engineer, lives with partner, drinks 20 units of alcohol on weekends, does not smoke or take illicit drugs

The patient's **age** is of particular importance in patients presenting with confusion as the differentials vary considerably between older and younger patients. Older patients generally have lower physiological and cognitive reserves and so are more susceptible to becoming confused as a result of relatively minor insults (e.g. urinary tract infections). Younger patients are more likely to abuse illicit drugs and present for the first time with psychotic disorders.

In older patients who have a background of cognitive impairment (e.g. dementia), a detailed collateral history should be taken to identify their **baseline cognitive and functional state**, thereby enabling you to determine whether the patient is off their baseline. The patient's social setting and baseline mobility should also be noted as they provide an idea of the degree of their **frailty** and the risk of them having potentially sustained an unwitnessed head injury (e.g. an elderly patient with Parkinson's disease who mobilises with a Zimmer frame and lives alone is at high risk of having an unwitnessed fall).

In the social history, a background of **alcohol excess** means that the patient is at risk of developing **Wernicke's encephalopathy** and **subdural haemorrhages** (because of cerebral atrophy and the risk of falling while intoxicated). A history of **illicit drug use** could alert you to the possibility of intoxication being the cause of the confusion.

## Differential Diagnosis

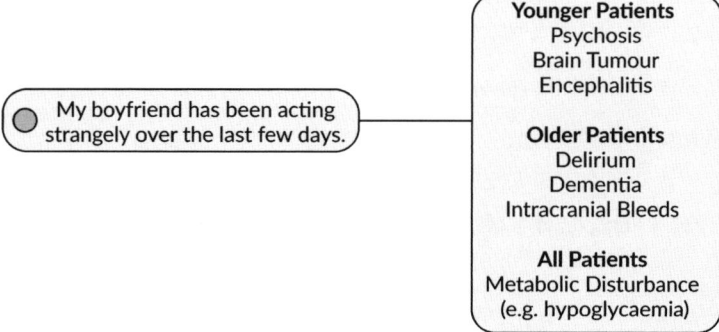

As discussed above, though there is a degree of overlap, the age of the patient can immediately help narrow the differential diagnosis.

The most common cause of acute confusion in older patients is **delirium**, which is defined as an acute confusional state caused by an underlying physical health problem (e.g. infection). Elderly patients with a chronic history of cognitive decline may be developing **dementia** — the patterns of decline can be useful in helping delineate the different types (e.g. stepwise in vascular dementia vs gradual in Alzheimer's disease). Intracranial bleeds (in particular, **subdural haemorrhages**) should always be considered in elderly patients presenting with confusion where there is no other obvious cause of the confusion or where there has been a history of recent head injury.

In younger patients, acute confusion is rare and very concerning as it may be the presenting symptom of serious intracranial pathology. In any first presentation, it is important to ask probing questions about recreational drug use as **intoxication** can manifest with confusion and some drugs can precipitate **psychotic episodes**. CNS inflammation (i.e. encephalitis) is an important cause that must be treated empirically as it can progress rapidly and lead to other troublesome complications, such as seizures and reduced GCS. In patients with a subacute history of confusion or personality changes, **brain tumours** should be considered as a possible cause. In all patients, **metabolic disturbances** such as hypoglycaemia, hyponatraemia and hypercalcaemia can cause confusion.

Clinicians should do their best to resist developing tunnel vision when focusing on any one differential as they can exist in tandem. For example, a patient can have a background of a psychotic disorder but also present intoxicated and having sustained a head injury.

Read through the classical presentations table in the following section to develop an understanding of how the main differentials are classically present.

## Classical Presentations

| Differential | Classical Presentation |
|---|---|
| **Psychosis** | Characterised by abnormal thought patterns and delusions (false, fixed beliefs that are held despite the presence of conflicting evidence). May be associated with visual or auditory hallucinations. |
| **Brain Tumour** | Persistent headaches that are worse when lying down or in the mornings. May be associated with nausea and vomiting. |
| **Encephalitis** | Generally unwell with a fever, generalised headache, photophobia and neck stiffness. Some patients may have a rash. Patients may develop seizures and reduced GCS. |

| | |
|---|---|
| **Delirium** | Acute deterioration in cognitive function. Can be described as *hypoactive* (associated with reduced engagement with others) or *hyperactive* (associated with more noticeable symptoms, such as agitation and aggression). |
| **Dementia** | **Alzheimer's Disease**: Gradual deterioration in short-term memory and cognitive function. **Vascular Dementia**: Stepwise decline in cognitive function. **Dementia with Lewy Bodies**: Progressive deterioration in cognitive function associated with hallucinations and Parkinsonian symptoms. **Frontotemporal Dementia**: Characterised by impairments in executive function (e.g. sexually inappropriate, offensive and aggressive behaviour). Often occurs at a younger age compared to other forms of dementia. |
| **Intracranial Bleed** | **Extradural**: Head injury with initial loss of consciousness followed by a lucid interval and then a later, rapid deterioration in consciousness. **Subdural**: May or may not have a clear history of preceding head injury. Gradually worsening confusion, headache and drowsiness. More common in the elderly. **Subarachnoid**: Sudden onset worst headache ever (maximum intensity within seconds), often occipital and associated with nausea, vomiting, photophobia and neck stiffness. |
| **Metabolic Disturbances** | Depends on the underlying pathology. Patients with diabetes who take hypoglycaemic drugs (e.g. insulin) may develop drowsiness, sweating and anxiety. |

# Red Flags

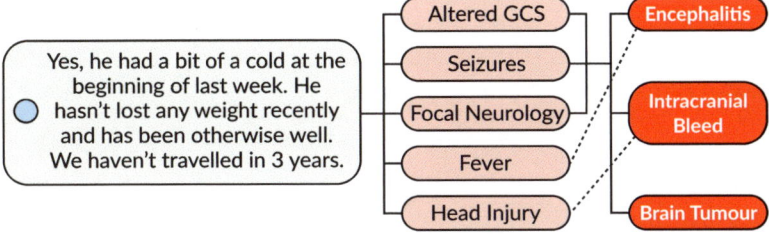

Several manifestations such as **altered GCS**, **seizures**, **focal neurology** and **loss of consciousness** can arise due to different underlying diagnoses. Altered GCS and seizures are of particular concern as patients may lose the ability to maintain their airway and require additional support (e.g., intensive care unit (ICU)). Features of sepsis (e.g. **fever**) in young people with confusion are highly suggestive of intracranial infection. In older patients, it is more likely that the source of sepsis is chest or urinary and that the confusion is due to delirium. A recent history of **head injury** should be explored further to determine the temporal relationship between the head injury and the onset of confusion.

# Assessment

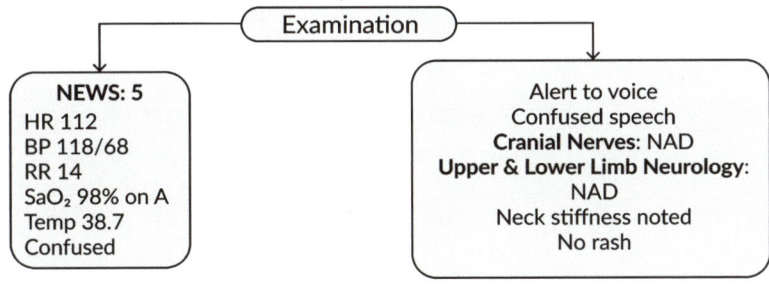

## *Observations*

As mentioned earlier, a **fever** may be suggestive of intracranial infection in younger patients presenting with confusion, whereas it is more likely to be due to an infection elsewhere driving delirium in older patients. In cases of intracranial bleeds, an increase in intracranial pressure can manifest with **Cushing's triad** (hypertension, bradycardia and irregular breathing). This is a deeply concerning feature that requires urgent cross-sectional brain imaging and discussion with the neurosurgical team.

## *Examination*

A neurological examination is a vital part of the assessment of a patient with confusion. **Lateralising neurology** (e.g. unequal pupils) is highly suggestive of an intracranial abnormality such as a bleed. Features of meningeal irritation may also be identifiable upon examination (e.g. **Brudzinski** and **Kernig's signs**). In younger patients, features of drug toxidromes may also be noted (e.g. restlessness and agitation in patients who have taken MDMA).

# Encephalitis

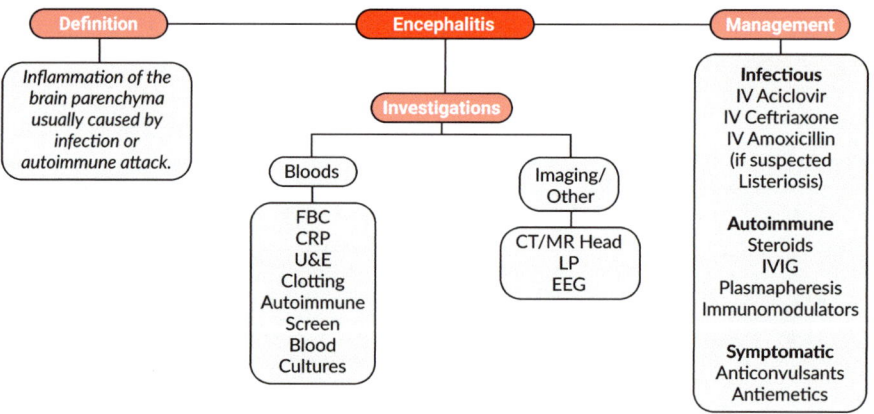

## *Definition*

Encephalitis is inflammation of the brain resulting in manifestations of brain dysfunction (e.g. confusion, seizures and drowsiness). It is most commonly caused by a viral infection (usually Herpes Simplex Virus) but can also be autoimmune.

## *Investigations*

At the bedside, non-invasive assessments of consciousness (using the **Glasgow Coma Scale**) and mental state (using the **mini-mental state examination**) should be considered. This requires close monitoring.

In patients with evidence of sepsis, a **venous blood gas** is an appropriate initial investigation to perform as it allows rapid measurement of pH and serum lactate concentration, which is used to determine the severity of sepsis. Similarly, a **full blood count** and **CRP** may demonstrate raised inflammatory markers in keeping with an infectious cause. **Blood cultures** should also be taken, ideally before commencing antimicrobial treatments.

A **CT head** scan is often normal in the early stages of encephalitis but, in some cases, may reveal low density within the temporal lobe. If the CT scan is inconclusive, an **MRI head** may be requested. A **lumbar puncture** is essential as the diagnosis can be confirmed based on the pattern noted on cerebrospinal fluid (CSF) analysis. It can also help identify the causative organism (e.g. HSV PCR). An **electroencephalogram (EEG)** may be performed to demonstrate seizure activity.

## *Management*

Infection is the most common cause of encephalitis. It is usually caused by Herpes Simplex Virus, so patients should be promptly commenced on treatment with **IV Aciclovir**. Bacteria such as *Streptococcus pneumoniae*, *Neisseria meningitidis* and *Listeria monocytogenes* can cause serious intracranial infections so empirical antibiotics (usually **ceftriaxone** with or without **amoxicillin**) are often started to cover bacterial infections. The results of blood cultures and CSF analysis can help guide antimicrobial treatment.

Autoimmune encephalitis is a much rarer yet very important diagnosis that can be successfully treated using approaches that aim to reduce the levels of the causative autoantibodies. This includes **steroids**, **IVIG**, **plasmapheresis** and **immuno-modulating drugs**.

Seizures are a concerning manifestation of encephalitis that can put the patient at risk of injury and airway compromise so symptomatic treatment with **anticonvulsants** should be considered in patients with encephalitis who are experiencing seizures.

# Bridge Box

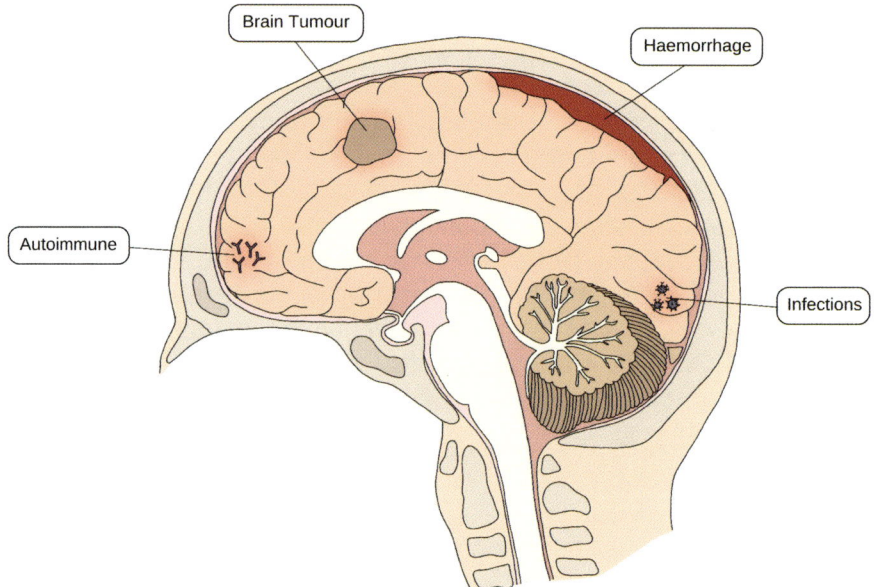

Intracranial causes of confusion.

# Chapter 3

# Collapse

A collapse can be a dramatic and concerning presentation in the emergency department. A detailed history that explores the events immediately before, during and after the collapse is vital in identifying the underlying cause.

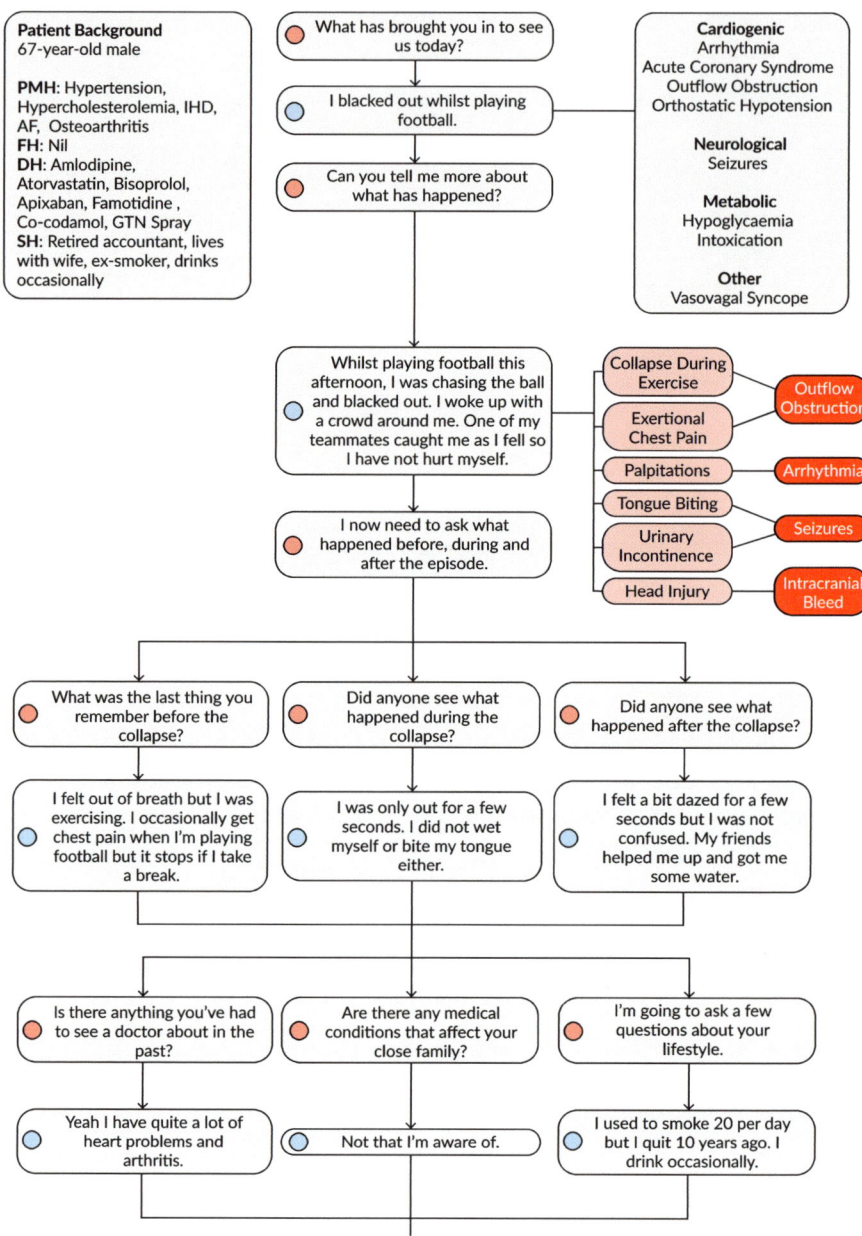

**Patient Background**
67-year-old male

**PMH:** Hypertension, Hypercholesterolemia, IHD, AF, Osteoarthritis
**FH:** Nil
**DH:** Amlodipine, Atorvastatin, Bisoprolol, Apixaban, Famotidine, Co-codamol, GTN Spray
**SH:** Retired accountant, lives with wife, ex-smoker, drinks occasionally

What has brought you in to see us today?

I blacked out whilst playing football.

Can you tell me more about what has happened?

**Cardiogenic**
Arrhythmia
Acute Coronary Syndrome
Outflow Obstruction
Orthostatic Hypotension

**Neurological**
Seizures

**Metabolic**
Hypoglycaemia
Intoxication

**Other**
Vasovagal Syncope

Whilst playing football this afternoon, I was chasing the ball and blacked out. I woke up with a crowd around me. One of my teammates caught me as I fell so I have not hurt myself.

Collapse During Exercise → Outflow Obstruction
Exertional Chest Pain
Palpitations → Arrhythmia
Tongue Biting
Urinary Incontinence → Seizures
Head Injury → Intracranial Bleed

I now need to ask what happened before, during and after the episode.

What was the last thing you remember before the collapse?

Did anyone see what happened during the collapse?

Did anyone see what happened after the collapse?

I felt out of breath but I was exercising. I occasionally get chest pain when I'm playing football but it stops if I take a break.

I was only out for a few seconds. I did not wet myself or bite my tongue either.

I felt a bit dazed for a few seconds but I was not confused. My friends helped me up and got me some water.

Is there anything you've had to see a doctor about in the past?

Are there any medical conditions that affect your close family?

I'm going to ask a few questions about your lifestyle.

Yeah I have quite a lot of heart problems and arthritis.

Not that I'm aware of.

I used to smoke 20 per day but I quit 10 years ago. I drink occasionally.

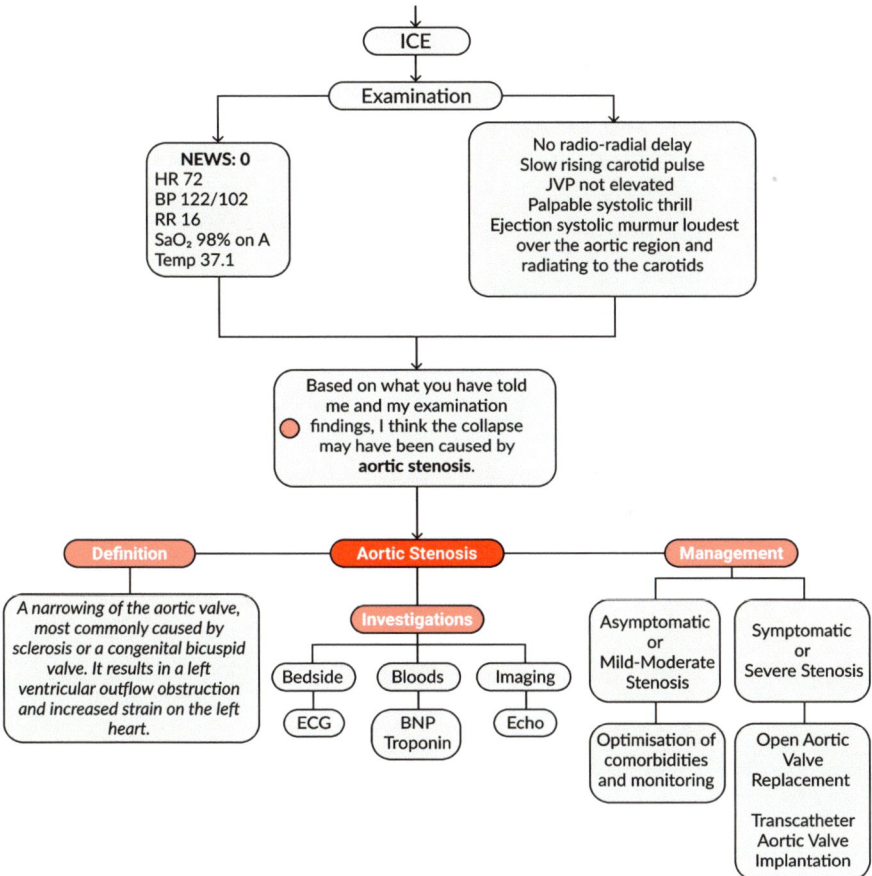

# Patient Background

**Patient Background**
67-year-old male

**PMH:** Hypertension, Hypercholesterolemia, IHD, AF, Osteoarthritis
**FH:** Nil
**DH:** Amlodipine, Atorvastatin, Bisoprolol, Apixaban, Famotidine , Co-codamol, GTN Spray
**SH:** Retired accountant, lives with wife, ex-smoker, drinks occasionally

Several different organs and organ systems can be responsible for a patient collapsing (e.g. cardiac, neurological and metabolic). Patients with a background of **cardiovascular disease** or those with **multiple cardiac risk factors** are at greater risk of developing cardiogenic syncope (e.g. arrhythmia and valvular disease). It is also important to enquire about whether the patient has **diabetes**

**mellitus** and how it is treated. Those who take **hypoglycaemic agents** (e.g. insulin and sulfonylureas) are at risk of developing hypoglycaemia which can lead to collapse. The drug history should also be screened for drugs that have an **antihypertensive effect** (e.g. calcium channel blockers, beta-blockers and diuretics). These can impair the body's ability to maintain its blood pressure when standing from a seated position (orthostatic hypotension).

# Differential Diagnosis

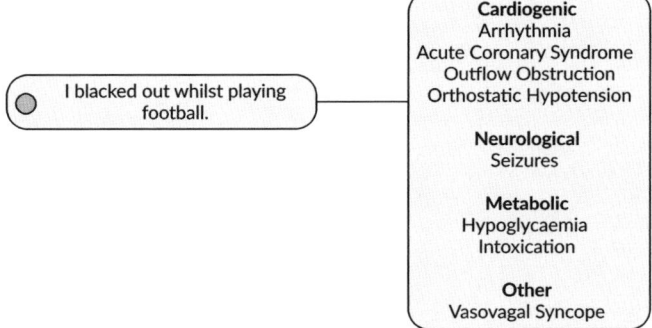

The causes of collapse can be categorised based on the system affected.

## *Cardiogenic*

This relates to the various ways in which impaired heart function can lead to a **reduction in cardiac output** and, hence, perfusion of the brain. Abnormalities in the rhythm, outflow obstruction (e.g. aortic stenosis and hypertrophic obstructive cardiomyopathy (HOCM)) and acute ischaemic events can all lead to a decline in cardiac output resulting in collapse.

## *Neurological*

Seizures are defined as excessive and abnormal brain activity that can first present with an episode of collapse. If presenting for the first time with a seizure, it is important to consider possible precipitants (e.g. tumour, intracranial bleed and intracranial infection).

## *Metabolic*

Patients with a background of diabetes mellitus which is treated with hypoglycaemic agents (e.g. insulin and sulfonylureas) are at risk of developing **hypoglycaemia** which can lead to collapse. Patients with liver failure are another subgroup who are at risk of developing hypoglycaemia due to depleted hepatic glycogen stores. **Intoxication** with drugs and alcohol is a very common cause of collapse in patients brought in by ambulance to A&E.

Read through the classical presentations table in the following section to develop an understanding of how the main differentials are classically present.

# Classical Presentations

| Differential | Classical Presentation |
|---|---|
| **Arrhythmia** | Patients may describe feeling palpitations before collapsing for a short period of time with rapid, full recovery afterwards. Sometimes associated with chest discomfort and, at other times, there may be no warning at all. |
| **Acute Coronary Syndrome** | Classically presents with central crushing chest pain that radiates to the jaw. Associated with sweating, anxiety and nausea. Patients may describe a prior history of experiencing chest pain on exertion that is relieved by rest (stable angina). |
| **Outflow Obstruction** | Sudden onset loss of consciousness that occurs without warning. Patients may mention previously experiencing chest pain on exertion and shortness of breath. Aortic stenosis is more common in older patients, whereas HOCM typically is present in active, young patients. |
| **Orthostatic Hypotension** | Dizziness and/or collapse that occurs when standing up from a sitting or lying position. More common in elderly patients who are on medications that affect their blood pressure. |

| | |
|---|---|
| **Seizures** | Patients may experience a sensory aura before collapsing. May be associated with stiffness and shaking of the limbs, tongue biting and urinary incontinence. Patients will often be drowsy or confused for hours after the episodes (postictal phase). |
| **Hypoglycaemia** | Characterised by drowsiness, sweating and anxiety though some patients may lack hypoglycaemia awareness. There may be a precipitant, such as inappropriate insulin use or nausea and vomiting. |
| **Intoxication** | Depends largely on the drug that is consumed. May be associated with nausea and vomiting. |
| **Vasovagal Syncope** | Very common cause of collapse. Patients will describe feeling dizzy and lightheaded before collapsing for a matter of seconds with rapid recovery. May be precipitated by heat or strong emotions (e.g. fear). |

## Red Flags

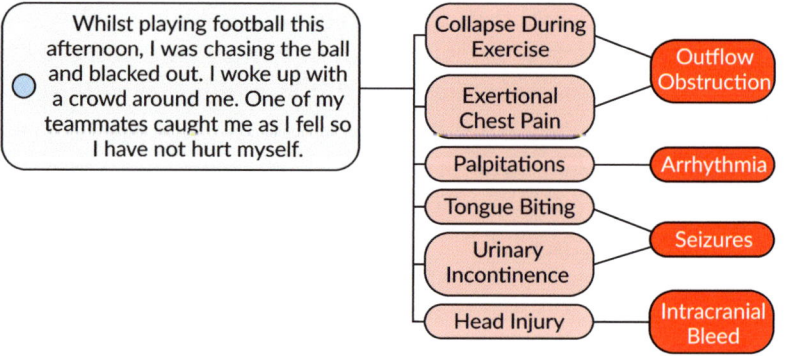

Of the various potential causes of syncope, neurological and cardiac causes are particularly concerning as the issue could recur resulting in further injury or death.

## *Cardiac Outflow Obstruction*

HOCM and aortic stenosis are two potential causes of cardiac outflow obstruction that can be fatal. Both conditions can lead to myocardial ischaemia, heart failure and complete outflow obstruction resulting in cardiac arrest.

The presence of an outflow tract obstruction can impair the heart's ability to increase output to match demand during periods of increased activity (e.g. exercise). Therefore, **collapse during exercise** can be a manifestation of both HOCM and aortic stenosis. These patients may also comment that they sometimes experience **chest pain when they exert themselves**.

## *Neurogenic*

A collateral history from a bystander can be useful to assess for features suggestive of a neurogenic cause of collapse. These include limb jerking, **tongue biting**, **urinary incontinence** and postictal confusion. If patients have an unwitnessed seizure, they may present in the postictal phase, and it may be difficult to establish a clear history.

## *Head Injury*

Enquiring or assessing a patient for a potential **head injury** is essential as it could be the cause or consequence of collapse. A head injury followed by a lucid interval or acute cognitive decline prior to collapse may be suggestive of an **intracranial bleed** (extradural or subdural). On the other hand, a collapse caused by cardiogenic or neurogenic causes can lead to a head injury, so it is important to consider cross-sectional brain imaging for patients with collapse.

# Before, During and After

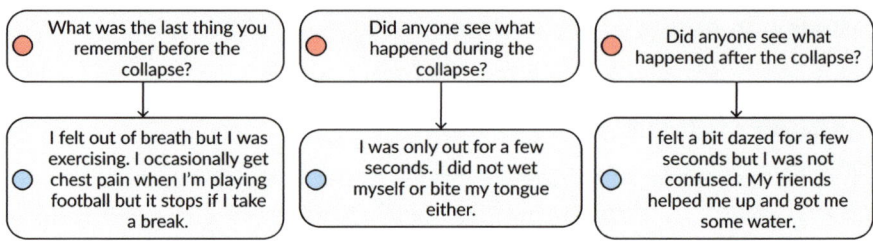

A useful structure to follow when taking a history from a patient presenting with collapse is to ask what happened before, during and after the episode.

## *Before*

Patients with cardiogenic syncope due to outflow tract obstruction or arrhythmia often have no warning at all before losing consciousness. In some cases, however, they may experience some preceding **chest pain** or **palpitations**.

Patients with neurogenic syncope due to seizures may mention that they felt some form of **aura**. This could take the form of perceptual changes (e.g. visual, olfactory and sensory) that arise before the collapse. It is key that patients are asked specifically about **recent head injury** as the collapse may be a manifestation of a traumatic intracranial bleed.

The activities of the patient at the time of the collapse should also be established. A sudden change from a **seated or lying to a standing** position can be suggestive of orthostatic hypotension. Patients who have been standing for a prolonged period or exposed to frightening stimuli may develop vasovagal syncope.

## *During*

This part of the history may need to be established by taking a collateral history from a witness.

The **duration** of time that the patient was unconscious can indicate the likely system affected. Generally, cardiogenic syncope is short-lived and lasts a matter of seconds, whereas seizures can last longer. Patients and those giving a collateral history should also be asked about **limb jerking, tongue biting** and **urinary incontinence** — these features would be in keeping with a seizure. Assessing for **potential head injury** at the time of the collapse is also essential as the patient may require cross-sectional brain imaging to rule out an intracranial bleed.

## *After*

Patients with cardiogenic syncope usually **recover fully within seconds**. They may feel dazed and startled by the collapse, however, they will likely be coherent and be able to make sense of what has just happened to them. Patients who have had a seizure, on the other hand, are often **drowsy and confused** for several hours after the collapse.

# Assessment

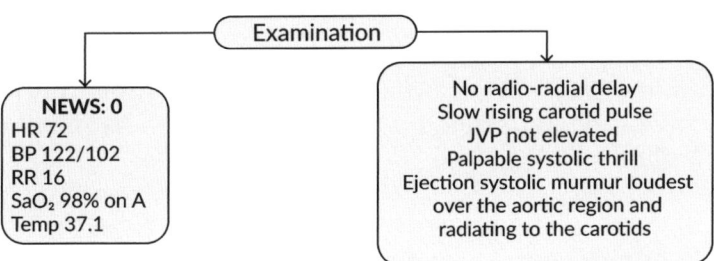

Examination

NEWS: 0
HR 72
BP 122/102
RR 16
SaO₂ 98% on A
Temp 37.1

No radio-radial delay
Slow rising carotid pulse
JVP not elevated
Palpable systolic thrill
Ejection systolic murmur loudest over the aortic region and radiating to the carotids

## *Observations*

The **heart rate** may indicate whether the patient has an arrhythmia that precipitated their fall. This could both be tachyarrhythmias (e.g. atrial fibrillation) or bradyarrhythmias (e.g. complete heart block). Furthermore, the **blood pressure** can reveal evidence of valvular abnormalities (e.g. narrow pulse pressure in aortic stenosis). **Lying–standing blood pressure** should also be measured to check for orthostatic hypotension.

## *Examination*

A cardiovascular and neurological assessment should be carried out to check for the likely cause of collapse as well as performing an external assessment to check for injuries that may have been sustained from the collapse.

- **Cardiovascular**: The rate, rhythm and character of the **pulse** can alert you to the possibility of an underlying arrhythmia. **Murmurs** upon auscultation (in particular, an ejection systolic murmur at the left sternal edge suggestive of aortic stenosis) will provide some evidence of underlying valvular abnormalities that may have caused an outflow obstruction. In HOCM and aortic stenosis with left ventricular hypertrophy, a **heave** may be palpable.
- **Neurological**: The presence of **focal neurology** (e.g. lateralising weakness and cranial nerve palsies) may be suggestive of a stroke or an intracranial bleed. The **consciousness** should also be assessed as it could be suggestive of a patient being in the postictal phase or of metabolic or intracranial pathology.
- **External Assessment**: A collapse can cause serious damage, especially in frail older patients. It is, therefore, important to perform a thorough assessment to check for **other injuries** that may have been sustained when they fell, such as fractures and lacerations.

# Aortic Stenosis

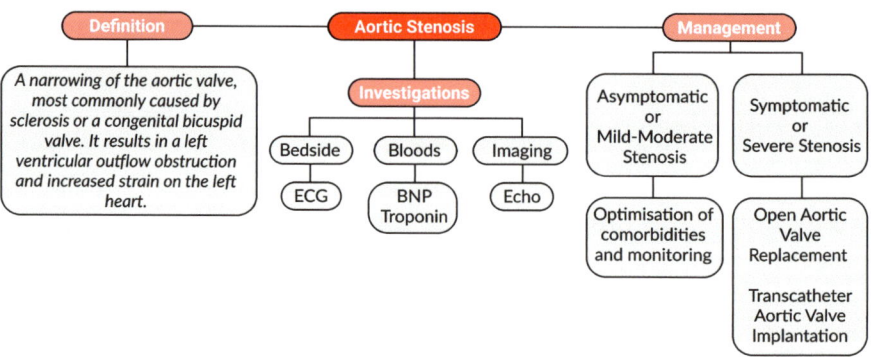

## Definition

Aortic stenosis refers to narrowing of the aortic valve that can result in a cardiac outflow obstruction. Its clinical manifestations include chest pain (due to impaired coronary blood flow and the increased demand of a hypertrophic left heart), shortness of breath (due to left heart failure leading to pulmonary oedema) and syncope (due to a brief reduction in cardiac output due to the obstruction).

## Investigations

At the bedside, an **ECG** can demonstrate arrhythmias and show evidence of left ventricular hypertrophy (increased R wave amplitude in left-sided leads and increased S wave depth in right-sided leads). A **BNP** can provide evidence of heart failure and a **troponin** will demonstrate evidence of myocardial ischaemia, both of which could result from aortic stenosis. Ultimately, an **echocardiogram** is required to visualise the valvular abnormality and determine its severity.

## Management

If asymptomatic or mild, conservative measures may be taken, such as monitoring the condition and optimising relevant comorbidities. If severe or symptomatic (as it would be in a patient that has collapsed), the patient may be considered for valve replacement which can either be achieved using an **open approach** or **transcatheter aortic valve implantation (TAVI)**.

# Bridge Box

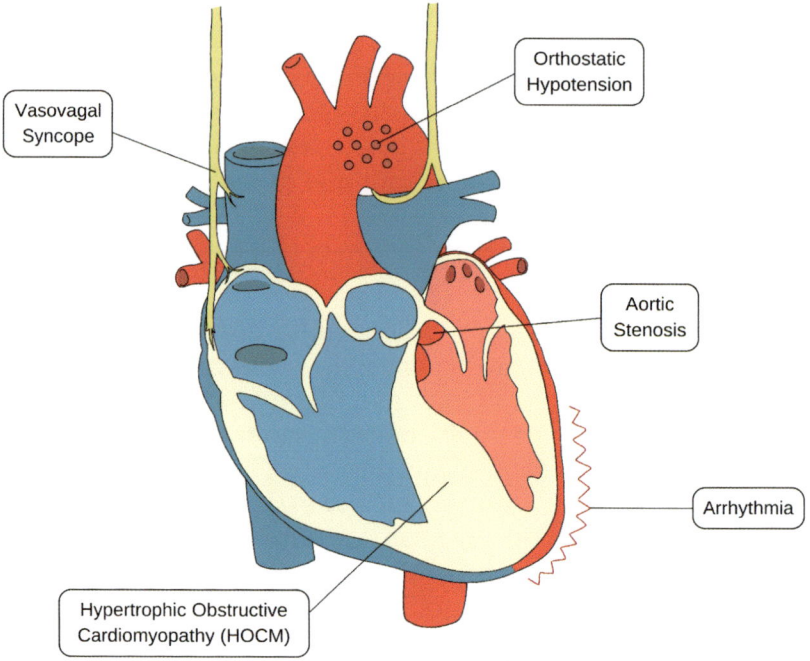

Cardiogenic causes of collapse.

# Chapter 4

# Dysphagia

Dysphagia is a serious symptom that can be the first presentation of an underlying oesophageal malignancy. Even if the cause is benign, dysphagia can lead to significant weight loss and dehydration so must be promptly investigated and managed.

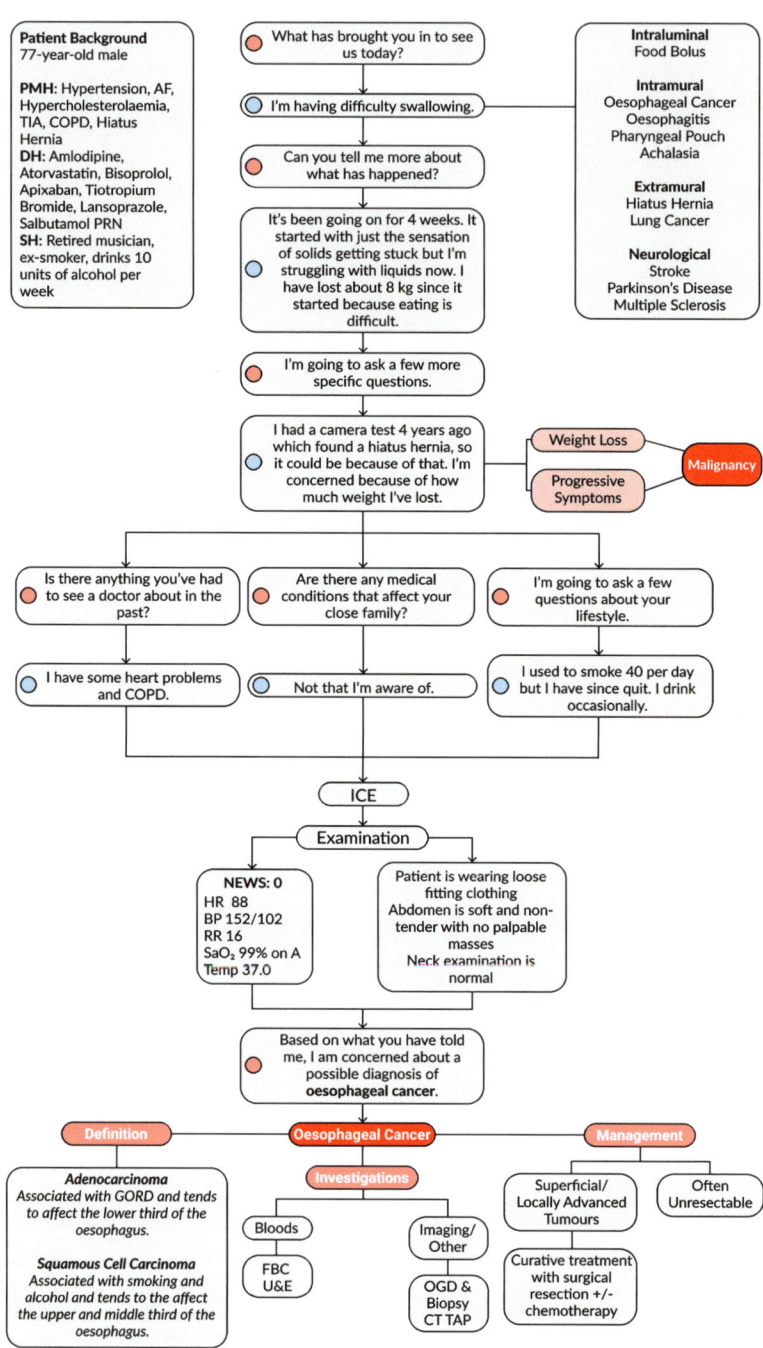

**Patient Background**
77-year-old male

**PMH:** Hypertension, AF, Hypercholesterolaemia, TIA, COPD, Hiatus Hernia
**DH:** Amlodipine, Atorvastatin, Bisoprolol, Apixaban, Tiotropium Bromide, Lansoprazole, Salbutamol PRN
**SH:** Retired musician, ex-smoker, drinks 10 units of alcohol per week

What has brought you in to see us today?

I'm having difficulty swallowing.

Can you tell me more about what has happened?

It's been going on for 4 weeks. It started with just the sensation of solids getting stuck but I'm struggling with liquids now. I have lost about 8 kg since it started because eating is difficult.

I'm going to ask a few more specific questions.

I had a camera test 4 years ago which found a hiatus hernia, so it could be because of that. I'm concerned because of how much weight I've lost.

**Intraluminal**
Food Bolus

**Intramural**
Oesophageal Cancer
Oesophagitis
Pharyngeal Pouch
Achalasia

**Extramural**
Hiatus Hernia
Lung Cancer

**Neurological**
Stroke
Parkinson's Disease
Multiple Sclerosis

Weight Loss

Progressive Symptoms

Malignancy

Is there anything you've had to see a doctor about in the past?

Are there any medical conditions that affect your close family?

I'm going to ask a few questions about your lifestyle.

I have some heart problems and COPD.

Not that I'm aware of.

I used to smoke 40 per day but I have since quit. I drink occasionally.

ICE

Examination

**NEWS: 0**
HR 88
BP 152/102
RR 16
SaO$_2$ 99% on A
Temp 37.0

Patient is wearing loose fitting clothing
Abdomen is soft and non-tender with no palpable masses
Neck examination is normal

Based on what you have told me, I am concerned about a possible diagnosis of **oesophageal cancer**.

Definition

Oesophageal Cancer

Management

**Adenocarcinoma**
*Associated with GORD and tends to affect the lower third of the oesophagus.*

**Squamous Cell Carcinoma**
*Associated with smoking and alcohol and tends to the affect the upper and middle third of the oesophagus.*

Investigations

Bloods

FBC
U&E

Imaging/ Other

OGD & Biopsy
CT TAP

Superficial/ Locally Advanced Tumours

Often Unresectable

Curative treatment with surgical resection +/- chemotherapy

# Patient Background

> **Patient Background**
> 77-year-old male
>
> **PMH:** Hypertension, AF, Hypercholesterolaemia, TIA, COPD, Hiatus Hernia
> **DH:** Amlodipine, Atorvastatin, Bisoprolol, Apixaban, Tiotropium Bromide, Lansoprazole, Salbutamol PRN
> **SH:** Retired musician, ex-smoker, drinks 10 units of alcohol per week

Oesophageal cancer typically develops in people **over the age of 40 years** and is most common in those over the age of 80 years. It is much more common in **men**. Patients who **smoke heavily** or have a background of **alcohol excess** are at increased risk of developing oesophageal cancer (especially squamous cell carcinoma). The patient's background may also note a previous history of **gastro-oesophageal reflux disease** which is associated with an increased risk of developing oesophageal adenocarcinoma.

Furthermore, the presence of comorbid neurological conditions (e.g. stroke and Parkinson's disease) may allude to dysphagia arising as a consequence of these diseases.

# Differential Diagnosis

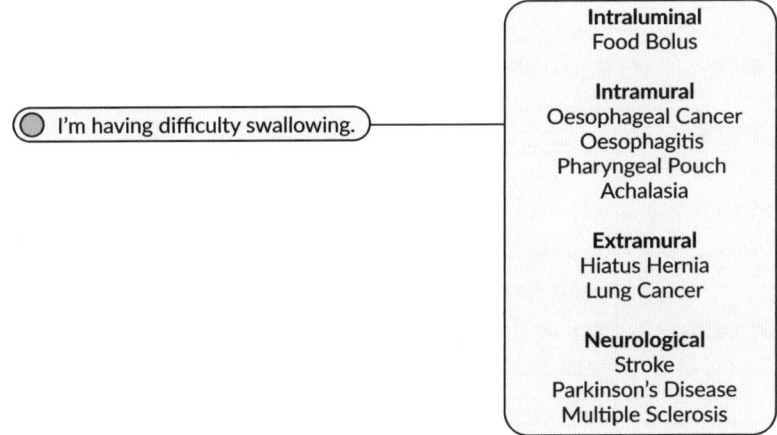

I'm having difficulty swallowing.

**Intraluminal**
Food Bolus

**Intramural**
Oesophageal Cancer
Oesophagitis
Pharyngeal Pouch
Achalasia

**Extramural**
Hiatus Hernia
Lung Cancer

**Neurological**
Stroke
Parkinson's Disease
Multiple Sclerosis

The differentials for dysphagia can be divided based on the location of the pathological process. A foreign body, such as a food bolus, can obstruct the lumen of the oesophagus causing dysphagia. This is an example of an **intraluminal** obstruction.

Defects of the tissues that make up the oesophagus can cause an **intramural** obstruction resulting in dysphagia. Examples of such diseases include oesophageal malignancy, pharyngeal pouch and achalasia (failure of relaxation of the lower oesophageal sphincter due to absence of the myenteric plexus ganglion cells).

Masses that lie within the chest cavity but outside the oesophagus can also externally compress the oesophagus leading to fixed dysphagia. Causes of **extramural** compression include enlarged lymph nodes, hiatus hernia and bronchial tumours.

The swallow mechanism involves the coordinated action of cranial nerves V, VII, IX, X and XII. Therefore, **neurological conditions** such as stroke, Parkinson's disease and multiple sclerosis can affect the function of these nerves, thereby impairing the patient's swallow. The dysphagia described may be fixed in some of these cases (e.g. stroke) or fluctuant (e.g. Parkinson's disease).

Read through the classical presentations table in the following section to develop an understanding of how the main differentials are classically present.

## Classical Presentations

| Differential | Classical Presentation |
|---|---|
| **Food Bolus** | Sudden onset coughing and difficulty swallowing after ingesting a large food bolus. If severe, it can cause airway obstruction. |
| **Oesophageal Cancer** | Subacute history of progressive dysphagia to solids followed by liquids. May be associated with haematemesis and melaena. Patients have often lost a considerable amount of weight. |
| **Oesophagitis** | Chronic history of discomfort when swallowing associated with burning retrosternal chest pain. Can be precipitated by certain drugs (e.g. NSAIDs and doxycycline). |

| Pharyngeal Pouch | Persistent dysphagia associated with regurgitation of undigested food, aspiration and halitosis. Typically occurs in elderly patients. |
|---|---|
| Achalasia | Intermittent dysphagia to both solids and liquids. |
| Hiatus Hernia | A common incidental finding on chest X-rays. If symptomatic, it tends to present with persistent dyspepsia that does not respond well to antacid treatment. |
| Lung Cancer | Several months of history of a persistent cough and, sometimes, haemoptysis. It is much more common in smokers and may be associated with unintentional weight loss. If compressing the oesophagus, it can cause fixed dysphagia. |
| Stroke | Sudden onset neurological impairment (e.g. sensory or motor defect). |
| Parkinson's Disease | Gradual onset history of worsening mobility. Classically presenting with bradykinesia, rigidity, postural instability and a stooped, shuffling gait. Subsequent autonomic dysfunction can lead to constipation and urinary incontinence. |
| Multiple Sclerosis | Classically presents with two or more episodes of acute neurological defects (e.g. optic neuritis) and can follow a relapsing–remitting, primary progressive or secondary progressive pattern. Dysphagia is often a late feature. |

# Red Flags

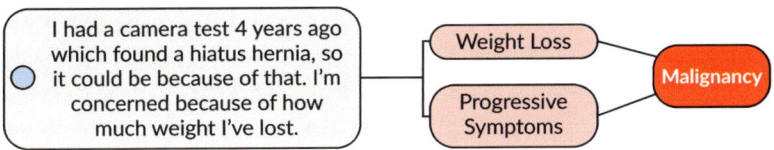

When taking a history from a patient presenting with dysphagia, it should be clarified whether the dysphagia has been intermittent or

**progressive**. Progressive dysphagia is suggestive of a gradually enlarging mass that initially makes it difficult to swallow solids and then liquids. Patients with dysphagia due to oesophageal cancer also tend to present with a **subacute history** usually spanning several weeks or months.

**Weight loss** can be a difficult associated symptom to interpret in the context of a patient with dysphagia. Benign causes of dysphagia, such as a pharyngeal pouch or achalasia, can cause a degree of weight loss because patients will tend to eat less if they are finding it difficult to swallow. The weight loss in oesophageal cancer is likely to be more rapid and pronounced as patients will be losing weight due to a combination of dysphagia causing reduced oral intake and the catabolic nature of the disease process.

# Assessment

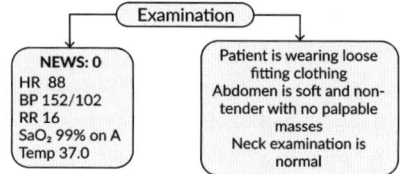

## Observations

Generally speaking, patients presenting with dysphagia will have normal observations.

## Examination

Most causes of dysphagia are likely to cause a degree of weight loss, with malignancy causing particularly pronounced weight loss. The abdomen is likely to be soft and non-tender. In some cases of oesophageal cancer, **Virchow's node** (left-sided supraclavicular lymph node) may be enlarged.

# Oesophageal Cancer

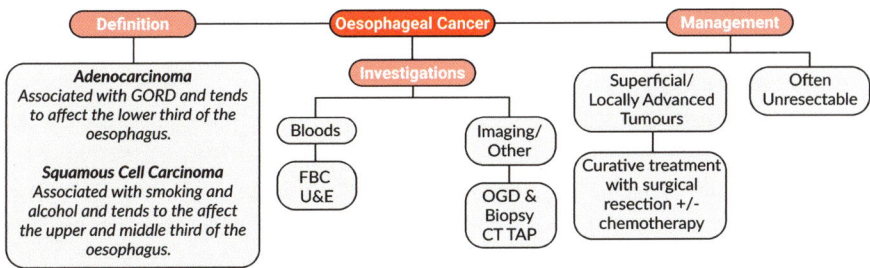

## Definition

There are two main forms of oesophageal cancer that differ in terms of their usual locations and key risk factors. **Adenocarcinoma** is the most common form of oesophageal cancer in the UK and is usually found in the lower third of the oesophagus. It arises from glandular epithelium and is strongly associated with gastro-oesophageal reflux disease. **Squamous cell carcinoma** is the most common type of oesophageal cancer worldwide and usually arises in the middle third of the oesophagus. It is strongly associated with smoking and alcohol.

## Investigations

A full blood count (**FBC**) will likely be sent as part of the initial blood tests in a patient presenting with dysphagia. Chronic bleeding from the friable oesophageal mucosa of a patient with oesophageal cancer can cause microcytic anaemia. It is worth noting, however, that undernourishment associated with dysphagia, even due to benign causes, can lead to anaemia due to nutrient deficiencies (e.g. folate).

The gold standard for investigating suspected oesophageal malignancy is an **oesophagogastroduodenoscopy (OGD)** with a **biopsy** taken of any masses that are identified. Alongside a histological diagnosis, a **CT thorax, abdomen and pelvis (CT TAP)** will likely be arranged to assess the degree of spread and, hence, stage the malignancy and plan surgical interventions.

## Management

Oesophageal cancer carries a poor prognosis as it is often quite advanced by the time it presents itself. In cases of superficial or locally advanced tumours without distant metastases, curative treatment could be achieved with a combination of complex upper gastrointestinal surgery (e.g. Ivor Lewis oesophagectomy) and chemotherapy. In many cases, however, the tumour will be unresectable by the time of diagnosis and treatment will be largely symptomatic with the involvement of the palliative care team.

# Bridge Box

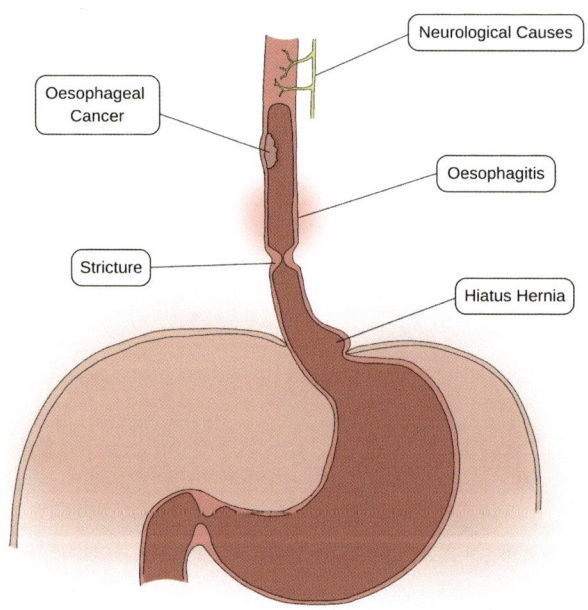

Differentials for dysphagia.

# Chapter 5

# Nausea and Vomiting

Nausea has a very broad differential. Surgical causes should always be considered, particularly in patients with a previous surgical history.

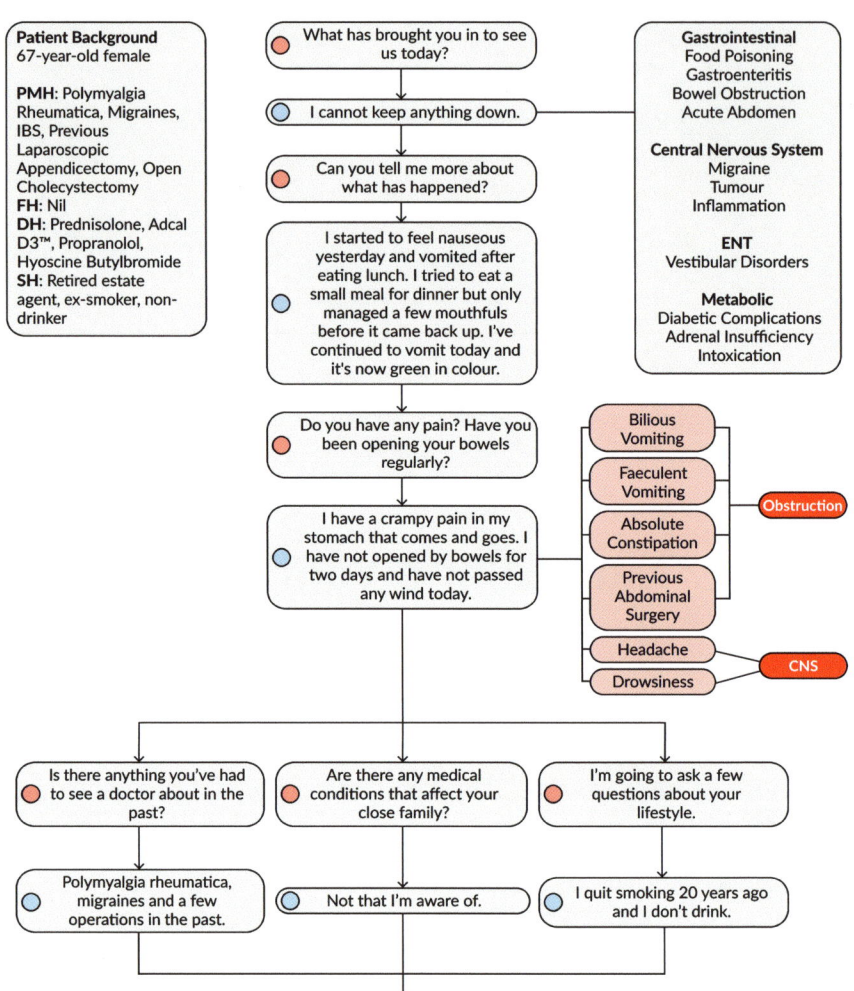

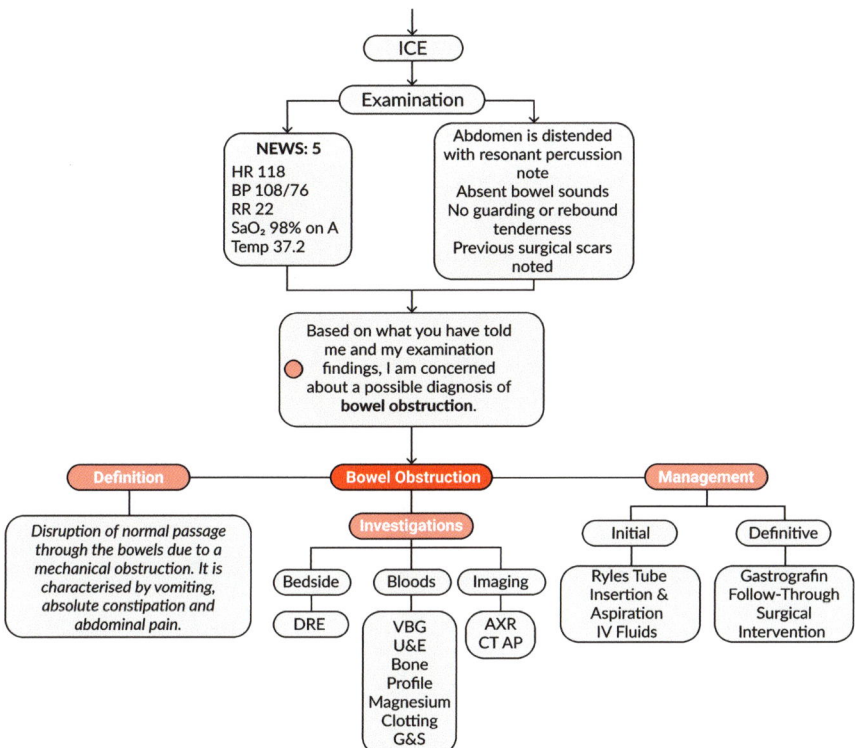

# Patient Background

**Patient Background**
67-year-old female

**PMH**: Polymyalgia Rheumatica, Migraines, IBS, Previous Laparoscopic Appendicectomy, Open Cholecystectomy
**FH**: Nil
**DH**: Prednisolone, Adcal D3™, Propranolol, Hyoscine Butylbromide
**SH**: Retired estate agent, ex-smoker, non-drinker

The patient's medical background can provide some clues about the possible cause of their nausea and vomiting. Patients should be asked about any **previous surgical interventions** involving the abdomen as this could result in the formation of adhesions which, in turn, can cause bowel obstruction. Older patients are also often on a concoction of several medications to manage various comorbidities — enquiring about **recent changes to their medications** may point you towards an adverse drug reaction that is causing the nausea and vomiting. Particularly in younger patients, you should sensitively probe about **recreational drug use** as both intoxication and regular use can lead to vomiting (e.g. cyclical vomiting syndrome in long-term cannabis users).

# Differential Diagnosis

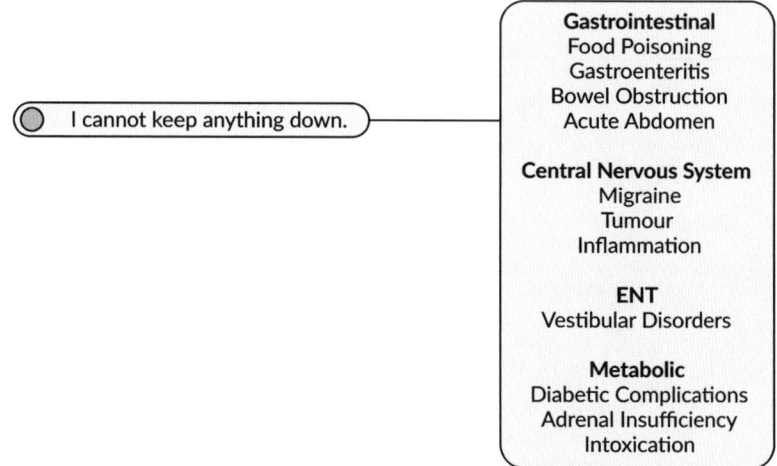

I cannot keep anything down.

**Gastrointestinal**
Food Poisoning
Gastroenteritis
Bowel Obstruction
Acute Abdomen

**Central Nervous System**
Migraine
Tumour
Inflammation

**ENT**
Vestibular Disorders

**Metabolic**
Diabetic Complications
Adrenal Insufficiency
Intoxication

Broadly speaking, the differentials for nausea and vomiting can be divided into gastrointestinal, central nervous system-related, ENT-related and metabolic causes.

## *Gastrointestinal*

Asking about **abdominal pain** can point you towards gastrointestinal causes of nausea and vomiting. **Changes in bowel habit** can help refine the differential diagnosis — bowel obstruction will cause absolute constipation whereas gastroenteritis and inflammatory bowel conditions will more likely cause diarrhoea.

## *Central Nervous System*

Many patients who are unwell may complain of a **headache**, but, in the absence of abdominal pain, a headache associated with nausea and vomiting should alert you to the possibility of a central cause such as intracranial infection, tumours and migraines.

### *ENT-Related*

Patients presenting with **hearing changes** and **vertiginous symptoms** will likely have developed a vestibular disorder (e.g. Meniere's disease and viral labyrinthitis). A relatively rare but important consideration is that posterior circulation strokes can also cause persistent vertigo — the risk can be assessed based on examination findings (e.g. **HINTS Exam**) and the patient's risk factor profile.

### *Metabolic*

Finally, complications of diabetes such as **diabetic ketoacidosis** and **hyperosmolar hyperglycaemic state** can lead to nausea and vomiting, so checking the patient's capillary glucose is a useful bedside investigation to perform. Adrenal insufficiency is a rare cause of nausea and vomiting that presents with relatively subtle features, but it should be considered in those presenting with a subacute history of **fatigue** who may also have other classical features such as **postural hypotension** and **skin pigmentation**. The initial panel of blood tests will also likely reveal an **electrolyte derangement** (hyperkalaemia and hyponatraemia) that is in keeping with a diagnosis of adrenal insufficiency.

Read through the classical presentations table in the following section to develop an understanding of how the main differentials are classically present.

## Classical Presentations

| Differential | Classical Presentation |
|---|---|
| **Gastroenteritis** | Acute onset diarrhoea, vomiting and abdominal pain that are usually associated with recently eating an unusual meal. Patients often have close contact with similar symptoms. |

| Bowel Obstruction | Acute onset generalised abdominal pain and distension associated with severe nausea and vomiting. Patients will not have opened their bowels and may not have passed flatus (absolute constipation). |
|---|---|
| Acute Abdomen | **Cholecystitis**: Acute onset persistent right upper quadrant pain associated with nausea and vomiting. This may occur on a background of intermittent, less intense right upper quadrant pain after meals (biliary colic). **Appendicitis**: Acute onset periumbilical pain associated with anorexia, nausea and vomiting that migrates to the right iliac fossa over time. **Pancreatitis**: Acute onset severe epigastric pain associated with nausea and vomiting. **Diverticulitis**: Acute onset left iliac fossa pain that may be associated with diarrhoea and fresh rectal bleeding. More common in older patients. **Perforated Peptic Ulcer**: Acute onset generalised abdominal pain in a patient with a rigid and tender abdomen. May have a preceding history of intermittent epigastric pain and regular use of erosive medications (e.g. NSAIDs). |
| Migraine | Acute onset unilateral throbbing headache associated with photophobia and phonophobia. Patients may feel nauseous, and some may experience an aura before the onset of the headache. |
| Brain Tumour | Persistent headaches that are worse when lying down and in the mornings. May be associated with nausea and vomiting. |

| | |
|---|---|
| **CNS Inflammation** | Generally unwell with a fever, generalised headache, photophobia and neck stiffness. Some patients may have a rash. Patients with *encephalitis* may develop seizures and reduced GCS. |
| **Vestibular Disorders** | Sensation of the room spinning and being unable to balance. Depending on the cause, the episodes may be triggered by certain head movements (BPPV), be associated with hearing impairment and aural fullness (Meniere's disease) or recent viral infection (viral labyrinthitis). |
| **Diabetic Complications** | **Diabetic Ketoacidosis**: Classically occurs in patients with type 1 diabetes mellitus and presents with polyuria, polydipsia, drowsiness, nausea and abdominal pain. It may be triggered by an underlying infection. **Hyperosmolar Hyperglycaemic State**: Classically occurs in patients with type 2 diabetes mellitus and presents with polyuria and polydipsia. Patients may appear confused and will be profoundly dehydrated. |
| **Adrenal Insufficiency** | Subtle and insidious presentation involving complaints of fatigue associated with orthostatic hypotension and skin pigmentation. Initial blood may reveal hyponatraemia and hyperkalaemia. |
| **Intoxication** | Depends largely on the drug that is consumed. May be associated with nausea and vomiting. |

## Red Flags

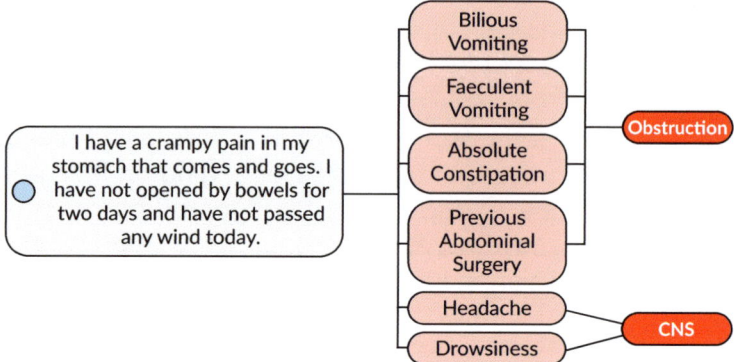

The main features suggestive of bowel obstruction include **absolute constipation**, **abdominal distension** and a background of **previous abdominal surgery**. It is worth noting that excessive vomiting may not always be a feature of bowel obstruction, especially if the obstruction is at the distal end of the gastrointestinal tract.

Central causes of nausea and vomiting, such as intracranial bleeds, tumours and infections, can cause a rapid deterioration in the patient's clinical state so it requires prompt identification and management. **Headache**, **drowsiness**, **seizures** and **confusion** are associated symptoms that may raise suspicion of a potential central cause and be used to justify cross-sectional brain imaging.

## Assessment

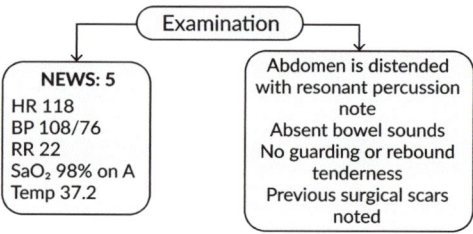

## *Observations*

If patients have been vomiting profusely, they are likely to have become dehydrated. This may make the patient **tachycardic** and **hypotensive** though younger patients with a greater physiological reserve may be able to compensate well. The presence of a **fever** will alert you of the possibility of an infection driving nausea (e.g. intra-abdominal infection). In frail patients who have been vomiting, the possibility of them having aspirated should be considered. This may lead to **tachypnoea** and **desaturation**.

## *Examination*

**Abdominal tenderness**, in general, is suggestive of a visceral cause of nausea and vomiting and the specific region that is tender will provide more useful information about the possible underlying diagnosis (e.g. right iliac fossa pain in appendicitis and right upper quadrant pain in biliary diseases). **Abdominal distension** in the context of significant vomiting is highly suggestive of bowel obstruction. You may also be able to elicit a **resonant percussion note** and **tinkling or absent bowel sounds**.

If the cause of nausea and vomiting is not thought to be intra-abdominal, attention should be paid to any neurological features that the patient is demonstrating. A **reduced GCS** may be seen in intracranial pathology (e.g. infection) and in metabolic disorders (e.g. hypoglycaemia, intoxication and adrenal crises). The presence of **nystagmus** indicates that there may be a vertiginous cause. A **HINTS Exam** can be performed to clinically distinguish between central and peripheral causes of vertigo.

# Bowel Obstruction

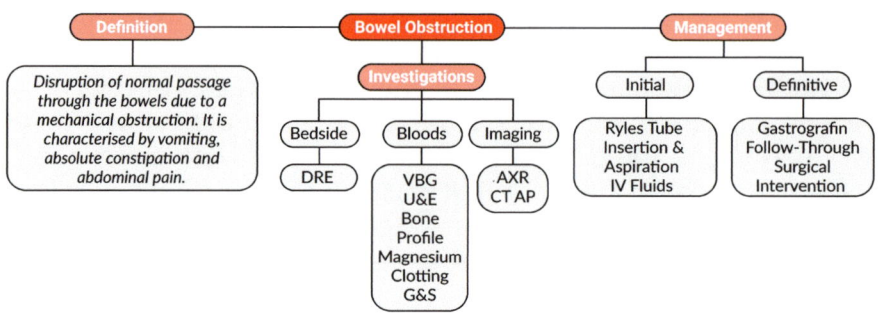

## *Definition*

Bowel obstruction classically presents with absolute constipation and severe vomiting. It may be caused by adhesions secondary to previous abdominal surgery, tumours, volvulus and hernias.

## *Investigations*

A **digital rectal examination** may be performed to confirm that the rectum is empty and that the abdominal distension and vomiting are not caused by severe constipation.

A **venous blood gas** provides several useful pieces of information. First and foremost, it will reveal whether the patient has **lactic acidosis**. This may occur secondary to dehydration from vomiting or tissue hypoxia in bowel obstruction. It will also provide an early indication of **electrolyte derangements** that can arise because of the vomiting or be a potential cause of pseudo-obstruction of the bowel. The electrolytes should be formally assessed by requesting a **U&E**, **bone profile** and **magnesium level**.

An **abdominal X-ray** is often performed as the initial investigation in suspected bowel obstruction, but this will often be followed by a **CT abdomen and pelvis with contrast** to help identify the likely underlying cause (e.g. tumour).

## *Management*

The initial management of bowel obstruction is by taking a **'drip and suck'** approach. This involves inserting a **Ryles tube** to aspirate stomach contents and decompress the system and providing **IV fluids** as the patient is likely to be significantly dehydrated after several bouts of vomiting, and they should be kept nil-by-mouth while awaiting surgical review.

In many cases of small bowel obstruction, **gastrografin follow-through** can be used as a diagnostic and therapeutic intervention as it can reduce small bowel oedema and relieve the obstruction. If there are any concerns about bowel ischaemia, a patient will likely undergo an **emergency laparotomy** to relieve the obstruction or resect bowel that is no longer viable. If patients have extensive adhesions, **adhesiolysis** may be performed, and if a hernia was responsible for the bowel obstruction, **hernia repair** may be considered. In cases of large bowel obstruction caused by a sigmoid volvulus, a **flatus tube** can be inserted to decompress the loop of the bowel. If the obstruction is caused by a tumour, the patient is likely to require a laparotomy to resect the affected section of the bowel.

# Bridge Box

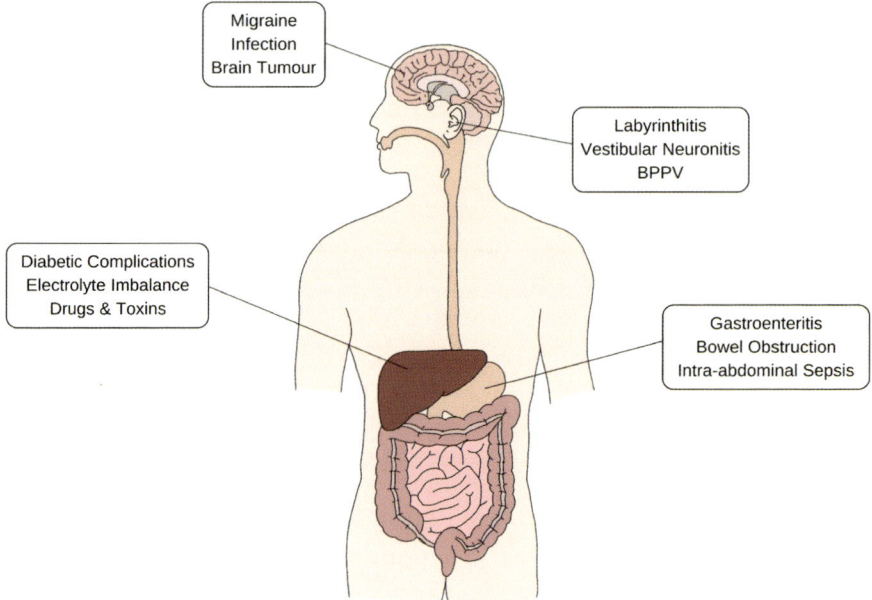

Differentials for nausea and vomiting.

# Chapter 6

# Haematemesis

Haematemesis is a startling symptom for any patient to experience. Large-volume haematemesis is likely to present as a major haemorrhage call and require urgent resuscitation. Even smaller volume haematemesis may be suggestive of a dangerous underlying cause that will require further investigation.

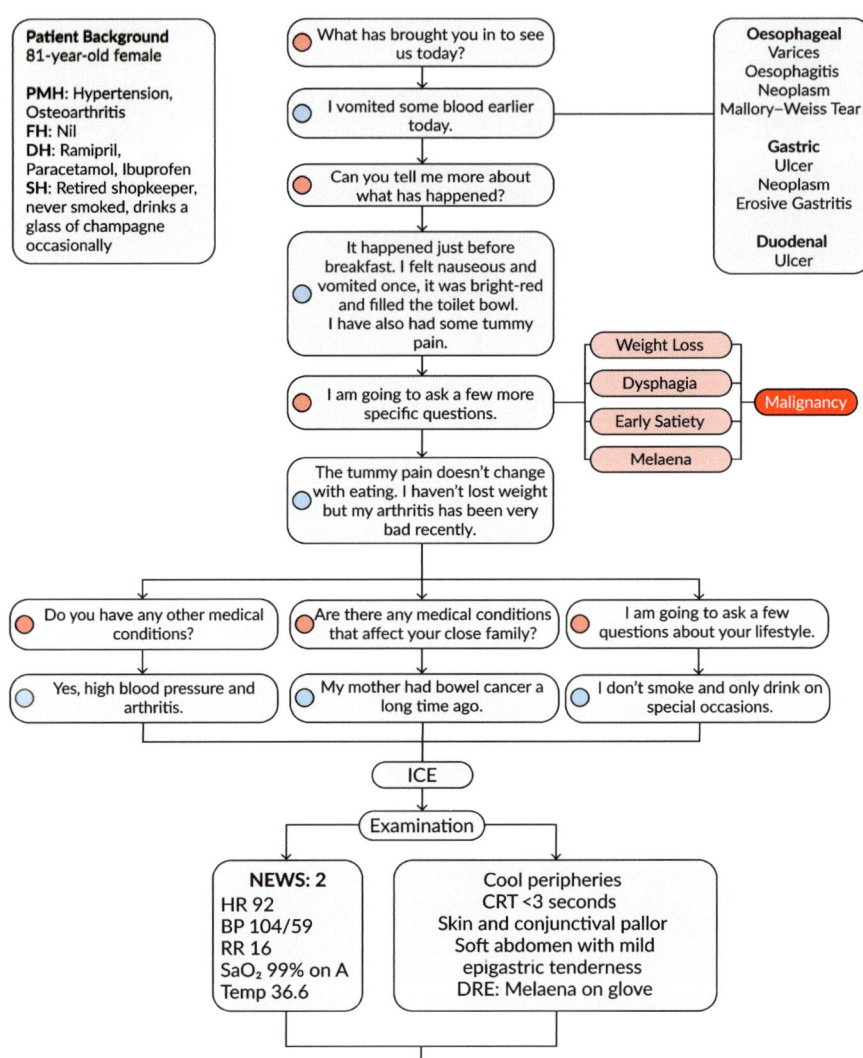

**Patient Background**
81-year-old female

**PMH:** Hypertension, Osteoarthritis
**FH:** Nil
**DH:** Ramipril, Paracetamol, Ibuprofen
**SH:** Retired shopkeeper, never smoked, drinks a glass of champagne occasionally

What has brought you in to see us today?

I vomited some blood earlier today.

Can you tell me more about what has happened?

It happened just before breakfast. I felt nauseous and vomited once, it was bright-red and filled the toilet bowl. I have also had some tummy pain.

I am going to ask a few more specific questions.

The tummy pain doesn't change with eating. I haven't lost weight but my arthritis has been very bad recently.

**Oesophageal**
Varices
Oesophagitis
Neoplasm
Mallory–Weiss Tear

**Gastric**
Ulcer
Neoplasm
Erosive Gastritis

**Duodenal**
Ulcer

Weight Loss
Dysphagia
Early Satiety
Melaena

Malignancy

Do you have any other medical conditions?

Yes, high blood pressure and arthritis.

Are there any medical conditions that affect your close family?

My mother had bowel cancer a long time ago.

I am going to ask a few questions about your lifestyle.

I don't smoke and only drink on special occasions.

ICE

Examination

**NEWS: 2**
HR 92
BP 104/59
RR 16
SaO₂ 99% on A
Temp 36.6

Cool peripheries
CRT <3 seconds
Skin and conjunctival pallor
Soft abdomen with mild epigastric tenderness
DRE: Melaena on glove

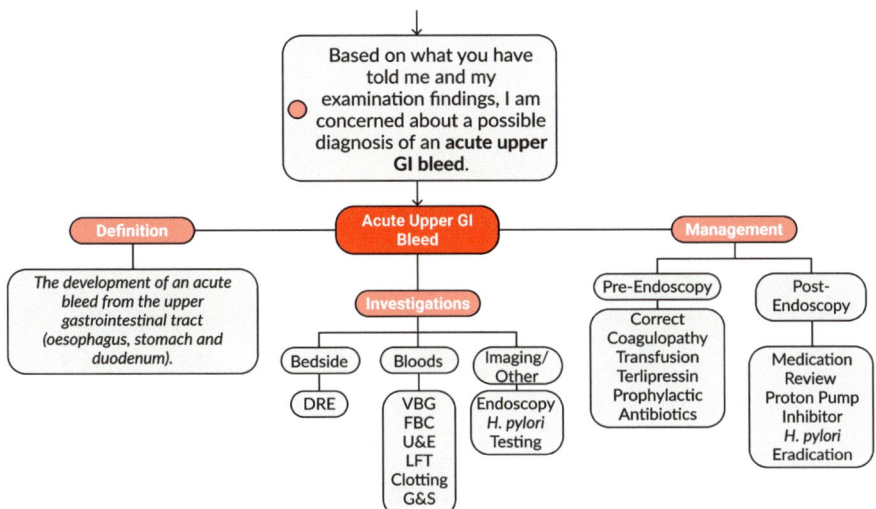

# Patient Background

**Patient Background**
81-year-old female

**PMH:** Hypertension, Osteoarthritis
**FH:** Nil
**DH:** Ramipril, Paracetamol and Ibuprofen
**SH:** Retired shopkeeper, never smoked, drinks a glass of champagne occasionally

Haematemesis is a distressing symptom to witness or experience and, unlike many other presentations, the age and sex of the patient are unlikely to provide much of an inkling about the potential underlying cause. The social and drug history, on the other hand, can provide some important clues. Common drugs that can increase the risk of peptic ulcer disease include **NSAIDs**, **steroids and bisphosphonates**. Furthermore, patients on **antiplatelets** and **anticoagulants** are at increased risk of significant bleeds. The most important social factor to note in a patient presenting with haematemesis is a background of **alcohol excess**. This may indicate that the patient is at risk of having oesophageal varices which can give rise to massive upper gastrointestinal bleeds. Similarly, a background of **liver disease** due to other causes (e.g. viral hepatitis) should also be noted in the patient's past medical history.

## Differential Diagnosis

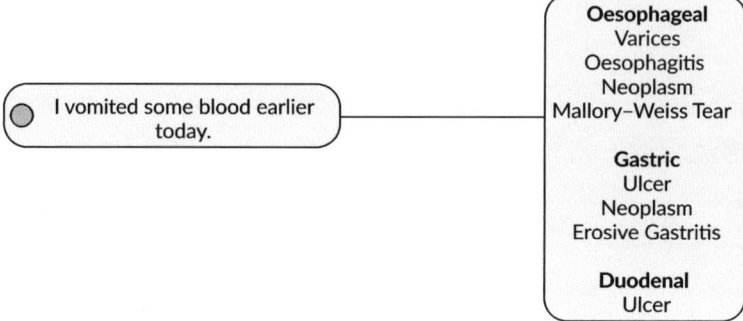

The causes of haematemesis can be divided anatomically into **oesophageal**, **gastric** and **duodenal**.

**Oesophageal varices** are a common cause of significant upper gastrointestinal bleeds in patients with a background of liver disease. It is worth checking previous hospital records to see whether the patient had previous cross-sectional imaging or endoscopies that may have identified varices. **Oesophagitis** and **oesophageal cancer** can also present with haematemesis though they are more commonly present with a subacute history of dysphagia. **Mallory–Weiss tears** are superficial tears of the mucous lining of the oesophagus that typically occur after a bout of vomiting. They may cause mild haematemesis and usually resolve without intervention.

In the stomach, **peptic ulcers**, **gastric cancer** and **gastritis** can all result in haematemesis. Peptic ulcers can also arise in the duodenum.

Read through the classical presentations table in the following section to develop an understanding of how the main differentials are classically present.

## Classical Presentations

| Differential | Classical Presentation |
|---|---|
| Oesophageal Varices | Profuse haematemesis in a patient with a background of chronic liver disease. |

| Oesophagitis | Chronic history of discomfort when swallowing associated with burning retrosternal chest pain. Can be precipitated by certain drugs (e.g. NSAIDs and doxycycline). |
| --- | --- |
| Oesophageal Cancer | Subacute history of progressive dysphagia to solids followed by liquids. May be associated with haematemesis and melaena. Patients have often lost a considerable amount of weight. |
| Mallory–Weiss Tear | A small amount of fresh blood appearing in the vomitus of a patient who has been vomiting or retching frequently. |
| Gastric Cancer | Patients may describe a preceding history of early satiety and abdominal fullness. They may also have lost weight. |
| Peptic Ulcer Disease | Chronic history of burning epigastric pain that may occur at the time of a meal (gastric ulcer) or a few hours afterwards (duodenal ulcer). If the ulcer is bleeding, the patient may also describe melaena. |

# Red Flags

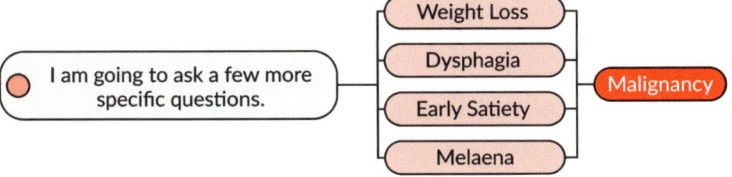

In patients presenting with haematemesis or melaena who do not have a background of liver disease or long-term use of drugs that can damage the lining of the stomach, oesophageal or gastric malignancy should be considered. Both types of malignancy can cause **weight loss**, **dyspepsia** and **melaena**. Patients with gastric cancer may also note that they experience a sensation of **early satiety** and have, therefore, reduced their oral intake leading to weight loss. Oesophageal cancer also classically causes **dysphagia** initially to solids and then to liquids.

# Assessment

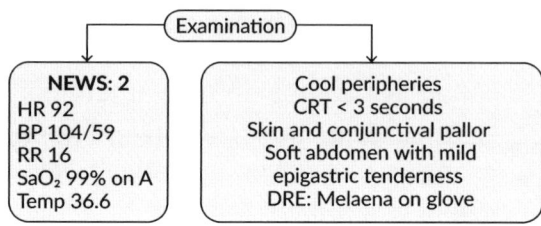

Examination

| NEWS: 2 | Cool peripheries |
| HR 92 | CRT < 3 seconds |
| BP 104/59 | Skin and conjunctival pallor |
| RR 16 | Soft abdomen with mild |
| SaO₂ 99% on A | epigastric tenderness |
| Temp 36.6 | DRE: Melaena on glove |

## *Observations*

Patients presenting with large-volume haematemesis may show evidence of **haemodynamic compromise** (hypotension and tachycardia). Any patient who is vomiting is also at risk of aspiration, which can lead to **hypoxia** and **tachypnoea**.

## *Examination*

The patient should be assessed for signs of **hypovolaemic shock** (e.g. cool peripheries with delayed capillary refill time). Abdominal examination may reveal a **palpable mass** (in the case of malignancy) or may reveal evidence of **peritonism** (in the case of a perforated peptic ulcer). A digital rectal examination may be performed to demonstrate the presence of **melaena**.

# Acute Upper Gastrointestinal Bleed

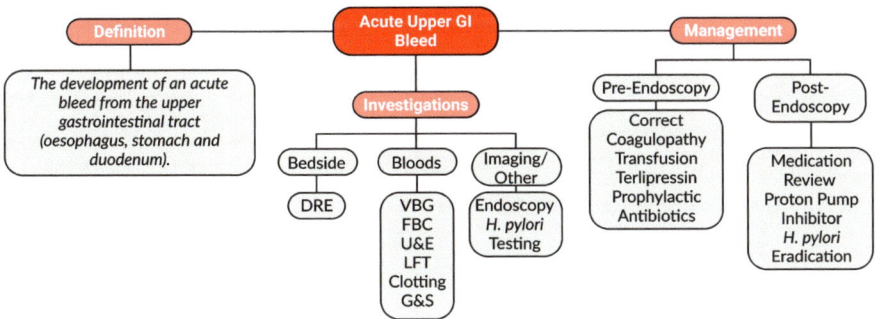

## *Definition*

An acute upper gastrointestinal (GI) bleed is a medical emergency. It refers to any circumstance in which a patient is thought to have lost a significant amount of blood from the upper part of the gastrointestinal tract (oesophagus, stomach and duodenum).

## *Investigations*

A venous blood gas (**VBG**) should be run as it will provide an early indication of the patient's haemoglobin as well as the lactate concentration which would be raised in the case of hypovolaemic shock. If patients are being assessed immediately after having a bleed, their haemoglobin may initially appear normal as they have lost red cells and plasma in equal measure and have not had enough time to expand their plasma volume in response to the bleed.

The haemoglobin can be confirmed on an **FBC** which will also reveal the platelet concentration. **U&E** is particularly useful in cases where there is no physical evidence of haematemesis or melaena as the urea is likely to be raised (it is a product of the digestion of red cells within the stomach). In any presentation that involves significant bleeding, a **clotting screen** should be sent in case there are any clotting derangements that have precipitated or worsened the bleed. As some of these patients will require blood transfusions, it is also important to send a **G&S**.

A patient with haematemesis will require an **endoscopy** to visualise the oesophagus and stomach to identify the source of the bleed. How urgently the patient needs an endoscopy depends on the nature of the presentation (e.g. severe haematemesis brought in by ambulance to A&E vs isolated episode presenting to primary care) and there are scoring tools to help assess the urgency (e.g. Glasgow–Blatchford score). In patients with presumed gastritis or peptic ulcer disease who do not respond to initial treatment with proton pump inhibitors, *Helicobacter pylori* testing should be considered.

## Management

In patients presenting with acute upper gastrointestinal bleeds, it may not be known whether the cause is likely to be variceal, arising from a peptic ulcer or from a malignancy, therefore, treatment is often initiated to cover multiple possible causes. Nonetheless, management hinges upon a comprehensive **A to E assessment** with a likely focus on circulation. **Coagulopathy should be corrected** where appropriate and **transfusions** should be arranged aiming for a haemoglobin of over 70 g/l (over 80 g/l in patients with a background of acute coronary syndrome). **Terlipressin** (vasopressin analogue) is usually given as it causes splanchnic vasoconstriction and reduces blood flow to bleeding oesophageal varices. **Prophylactic antibiotics** have also been shown to improve outcomes in patients presenting with upper gastrointestinal bleeds. **Proton pump inhibitors** are generally avoided prior to endoscopy as they can make some of the endoscopy findings difficult to interpret. They are, however, often given after an endoscopy has been performed and biopsies have been taken. **Medications should be reviewed** and rationalised if they are thought to be contributing to the development of peptic ulcers. If *H. pylori* infection is identified, it should be treated using **triple therapy** (PPI and two antibiotics).

# Bridge Box

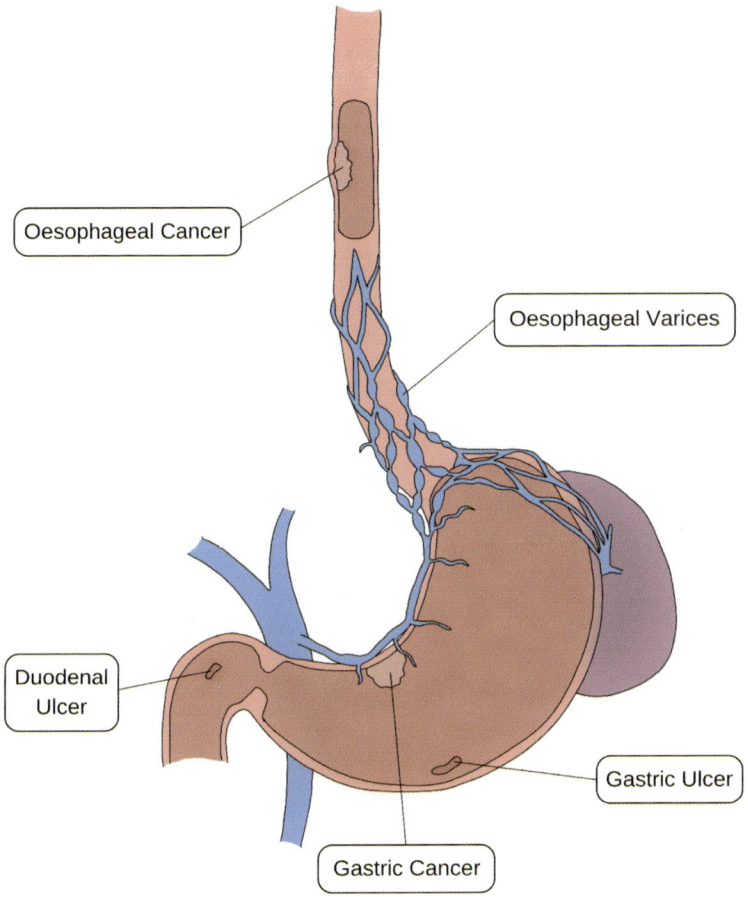

Differentials for haematemesis.

# Chapter 7

# Chest Pain

Chest pain is a very common presenting complaint seen in A&E. Much of the time, it can be attributed to benign causes, however, it is important to take a systematic approach to avoid missing life-threatening underlying conditions.

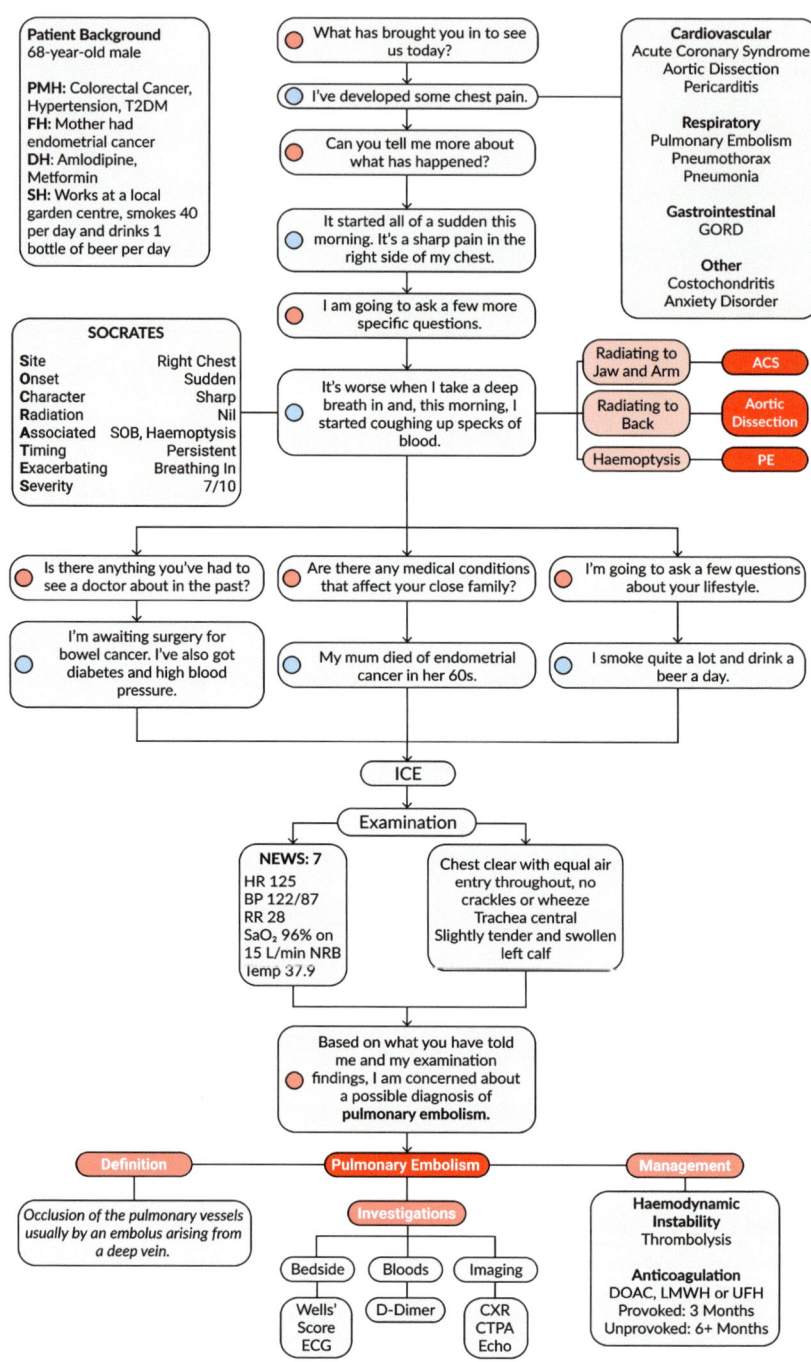

**Patient Background**
68-year-old male

**PMH:** Colorectal Cancer, Hypertension, T2DM
**FH:** Mother had endometrial cancer
**DH:** Amlodipine, Metformin
**SH:** Works at a local garden centre, smokes 40 per day and drinks 1 bottle of beer per day

What has brought you in to see us today?

I've developed some chest pain.

Can you tell me more about what has happened?

It started all of a sudden this morning. It's a sharp pain in the right side of my chest.

I am going to ask a few more specific questions.

**Cardiovascular**
Acute Coronary Syndrome
Aortic Dissection
Pericarditis

**Respiratory**
Pulmonary Embolism
Pneumothorax
Pneumonia

**Gastrointestinal**
GORD

**Other**
Costochondritis
Anxiety Disorder

**SOCRATES**

| | |
|---|---|
| Site | Right Chest |
| Onset | Sudden |
| Character | Sharp |
| Radiation | Nil |
| Associated | SOB, Haemoptysis |
| Timing | Persistent |
| Exacerbating | Breathing In |
| Severity | 7/10 |

It's worse when I take a deep breath in and, this morning, I started coughing up specks of blood.

Radiating to Jaw and Arm → **ACS**
Radiating to Back → **Aortic Dissection**
Haemoptysis → **PE**

Is there anything you've had to see a doctor about in the past?

I'm awaiting surgery for bowel cancer. I've also got diabetes and high blood pressure.

Are there any medical conditions that affect your close family?

My mum died of endometrial cancer in her 60s.

I'm going to ask a few questions about your lifestyle.

I smoke quite a lot and drink a beer a day.

ICE

Examination

**NEWS: 7**
HR 125
BP 122/87
RR 28
SaO$_2$ 96% on 15 L/min NRB
Temp 37.9

Chest clear with equal air entry throughout, no crackles or wheeze
Trachea central
Slightly tender and swollen left calf

Based on what you have told me and my examination findings, I am concerned about a possible diagnosis of **pulmonary embolism**.

**Definition**

*Occlusion of the pulmonary vessels usually by an embolus arising from a deep vein.*

**Pulmonary Embolism**

**Investigations**

| Bedside | Bloods | Imaging |
|---|---|---|
| Wells' Score ECG | D-Dimer | CXR CTPA Echo |

**Management**

**Haemodynamic Instability**
Thrombolysis

**Anticoagulation**
DOAC, LMWH or UFH
Provoked: 3 Months
Unprovoked: 6+ Months

# Patient Background

Patient Background
68-year-old male

**PMH:** Colorectal Cancer, Hypertension, T2DM
**FH:** Mother had endometrial cancer
**DH:** Amlodipine, Metformin
**SH:** Works at a local garden centre, smokes 40 per day and drinks 1 bottle of beer per day

There should be a low threshold for considering serious cardiovascular causes of chest pain (e.g. acute coronary syndrome (ACS) and aortic dissection) in **older patients**, especially those with a known background of ischaemic heart disease or risk factors for cardiovascular disease (e.g. diabetes mellitus, hypertension and heavy smoking). As pulmonary embolism is another worrying cause of chest pain, **risk factors for venous thromboembolism** in the patient's history should also be noted (e.g. active cancer and immobility).

# Differential Diagnosis

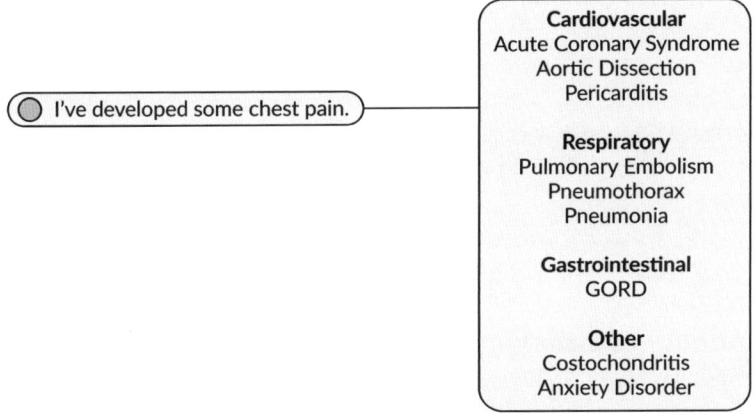

I've developed some chest pain.

**Cardiovascular**
Acute Coronary Syndrome
Aortic Dissection
Pericarditis

**Respiratory**
Pulmonary Embolism
Pneumothorax
Pneumonia

**Gastrointestinal**
GORD

**Other**
Costochondritis
Anxiety Disorder

The causes of chest pain can be broadly categorised based on the organ systems affected. The main cardiovascular causes include **ACS**, **aortic dissection** and **pericarditis**. As ACS, in particular, is relatively common and can be dangerous, the diagnostic work-up of a patient with chest pain often involves requesting investigations that can help exclude ACS (e.g. ECG and troponin).

Respiratory causes of acute chest pain include **pulmonary embolism** and **pneumothorax**. **Pneumonia** can cause some pleural irritation resulting in sharp chest pain, but this is more likely to have a subacute onset. Benign causes of chest pain include **GORD, costochondritis** and **anxiety disorder**.

# SOCRATES

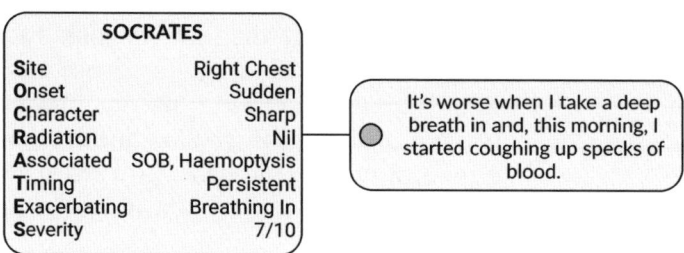

There are a few patterns of symptoms that are worth keeping at the back of your mind while you explore SOCRATES in a patient presenting with chest pain.

- **Site**
  - o **Central**: ACS, aortic dissection, pericarditis, GORD, costochondritis and anxiety disorder
  - o **Lateralising**: PE, pneumothorax and pneumonia
- **Onset**
  - o **Sudden**: ACS, aortic dissection, PE and pneumothorax
  - o **Gradual**: Pericarditis, GORD, costochondritis and pneumonia
- **Character**
  - o **Aching or Crushing**: ACS and anxiety
  - o **Sharp**: Pericarditis, PE and pneumothorax
  - o **Tearing**: Aortic dissection
- **Radiation**
  - o **To Shoulder, Arm or Jaw**: ACS
  - o **To Back (Between the Scapulae)**: Aortic dissection
- **Associated Symptoms**
  - o **Shortness of Breath**: PE, pneumothorax, pneumonia and anxiety
  - o **Cough**: PE and pneumonia
  - o **Sweating**: ACS
  - o **Fever and Fatigue**: Pericarditis and pneumonia

- **Timing**
  - **Persistent**: ACS, PE, pneumothorax, pneumonia and pericarditis
  - **Intermittent**: GORD and anxiety
- **Exacerbating**
  - **Breathing In**: PE, pneumothorax, pneumonia, pericarditis and costochondritis
  - **Lying Down**: GORD
- **Severity**: Varies considerably for each diagnosis.

Read through the classical presentations table in the following section to develop an understanding of how the main differentials are classically present.

## Classical Presentations

| Differential | Classical Presentation |
|---|---|
| **Acute Coronary Syndrome** | Classically presents with central crushing chest pain that radiates to the jaw. Associated with sweating, anxiety and nausea. Patients may describe a prior history of experiencing chest pain on exertion that is relieved by rest (stable angina). |
| **Aortic Dissection** | Sudden onset tearing central chest pain that radiates to the back, in between the scapulae. It may result in syncope and arm pain. Associated risk factors include hypertension and connective tissue disorders (e.g. Marfan syndrome). |
| **Pericarditis** | Gradual onset sharp central chest pain that is worsened by breathing in and lessened by leaning forward. Patients with viral pericarditis may have preceding viral symptoms (e.g. fever and lethargy). |

| | |
|---|---|
| **Pulmonary Embolism** | Sudden onset sharp chest pain associated with shortness of breath. The pain is worsened by taking a deep breath in. Patients may have concomitant unilateral leg swelling (suggestive of a deep vein thrombosis (DVT)) and may have risk factors for venous thromboembolism (e.g. immobility, active cancer and recent surgery). |
| **Pneumothorax** | Sudden onset chest pain and shortness of breath in a tall, thin patient (spontaneous) or in a patient with underlying lung disease (secondary). It can also occur following trauma to the chest (e.g. rib fracture). |
| **Pneumonia** | Gradual onset chest discomfort, shortness of breath and cough productive of yellow-green sputum. May be accompanied by a fever and lethargy. |
| **GORD** | Chronic history of epigastric discomfort that is worsened by spicy meals. Patients may also complain of an unpleasant taste at the back of their mouth that is worse when lying flat. |
| **Costochondritis** | Gradual onset anterior chest wall pain and reproducible tenderness that may make it difficult to take a deep breath in. |
| **Anxiety Disorder** | Episodic chest discomfort that may be associated with times of increased stress. May also be accompanied by shortness of breath, palpitations and difficulty swallowing (globus). |

# Red Flags

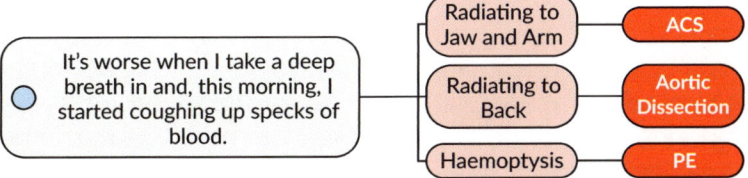

Aching central chest pain that **radiates to the left jaw and/or arm** in the context of a patient with cardiovascular risk factors is highly suggestive of ACS. Other associated symptoms include sweating and nausea. Tearing central chest pain that **radiates to the back** is classical of aortic dissection. Sudden onset sharp chest pain associated with shortness of breath and **haemoptysis** is highly suggestive of PE.

# Assessment

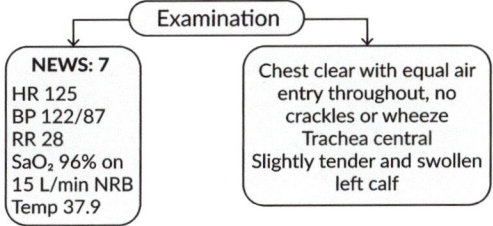

## *Observations*

In respiratory causes of chest pain, you are likely to notice **tachypnoea** or **desaturation**. Furthermore, in infectious or inflammatory causes, such as pneumonia and pericarditis, patients may have a **fever**. **Elevated blood pressure** may be seen in patients presenting with an aortic dissection as it is a major risk factor. Anxious patients may be **tachycardic** and **tachypnoeic,** but the blood pressure and oxygen saturation are likely to be maintained.

## Examination

Upon auscultation of the precordium, a **pericardial friction rub** may be heard in some cases of pericarditis. On the other hand, if there is a pericardial effusion, the heart sounds may be muffled. In a pneumothorax, there will likely be **reduced air entry** on the affected side with **asymmetrical chest expansion** and, possibly, **tracheal deviation**. In patients with pneumonia, **coarse crackles** or **bronchial breath sounds** may be heard over the affected area. Examination of the chest in patients with a pulmonary embolism will likely be normal. It is important to assess the patient's legs for **evidence of a DVT**. Costochondritis usually causes **reproducible chest wall tenderness** and GORD may be associated with some mild **epigastric tenderness**.

# Pulmonary Embolism

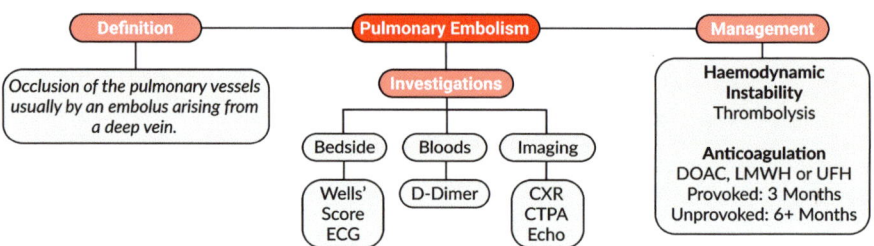

## Definition

Pulmonary embolism refers to the occlusion of a pulmonary artery due to a clot arising from a deep vein. It typically causes chest pain and shortness of breath.

## Investigations

At the bedside, the **Wells' score** can be calculated using aspects of the patient's history and their observations. This provides an early indication of the risk of pulmonary embolism as a diagnosis. An **ECG** is also an essential investigation — it is most likely to show sinus tachycardia, however, it may also demonstrate features of right heart strain (e.g. right bundle branch block and T wave inversion in V1 to V4). This, along with troponin and BNP, can help gauge the severity of the pulmonary embolism and its impact on cardiac function. In patients deemed low risk by the Wells' score, a **D-Dimer** should be sent. It has a high sensitivity as a test for venous thromboembolism.

A **chest X-ray** is often the initial investigation that is requested in a patient with chest pain and shortness of breath, primarily to rule out other causes (e.g. pneumothorax). A **CT pulmonary angiogram** is the gold standard investigation for diagnosing PE. A point-of-care **echocardiogram** may be performed by trained personnel to assess for features of right heart strain.

## *Management*

Haemodynamically unstable patients with PE should be considered for thrombolysis. If patients are stable, they require anticoagulation. If the PE is provoked (e.g. recent surgery), the anticoagulation can be discontinued after 3 months, whereas, if it is unprovoked, it should be continued for at least 6 months while the patient undergoes investigations for underlying causes (e.g. anti-thrombin III deficiency).

# Bridge Box

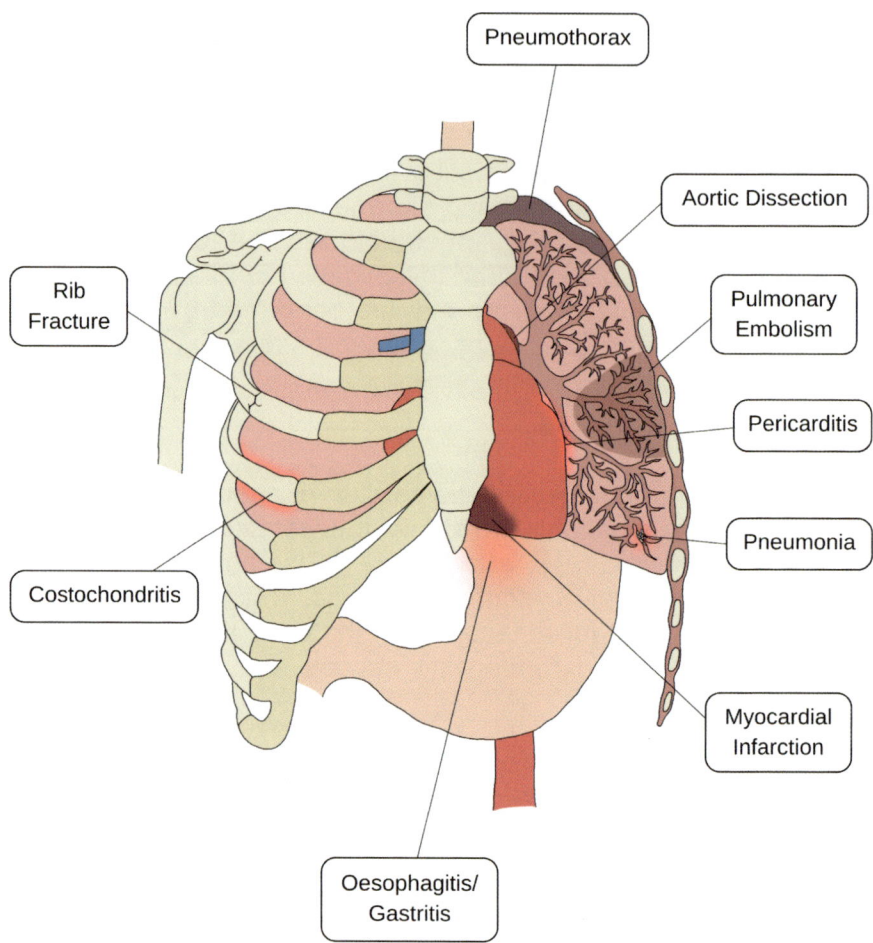

Differentials for chest pain.

# Chapter 8

# Cough

Most people will experience a cough at some point in their lives and most cases will be attributed to simple, self-limiting viral infections. A more persistent cough or an abnormal cough, however, may be suggestive of an underlying condition that requires active investigation and treatment.

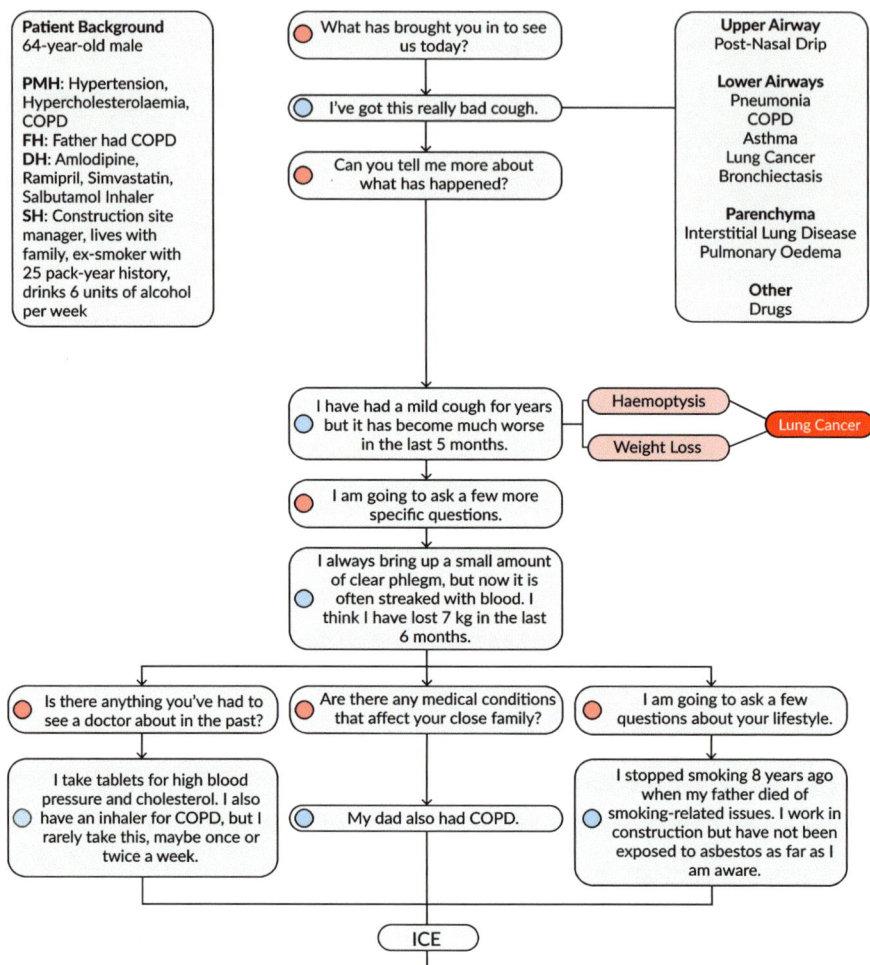

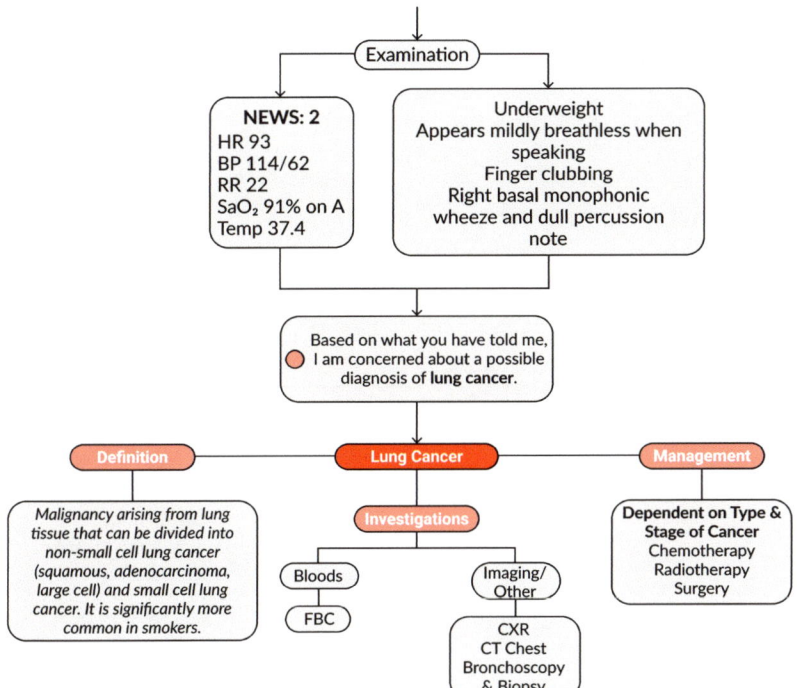

# Patient Background

**Patient Background**
64-year-old male

**PMH:** Hypertension, Hypercholesterolaemia, COPD
**FH:** Father had COPD
**DH:** Amlodipine, Ramipril, Simvastatin, Salbutamol Inhaler
**SH:** Construction site manager, lives with family, ex-smoker with 25 pack-year history, drinks 6 units of alcohol per week

Most causes of a cough can happen at any age; however, **older patients** are more likely to develop conditions, such as lung cancer, COPD and interstitial lung disease. A chronic cough in a young person is more likely to be due to postnasal drip or asthma. The drug history should also be screened for common **drugs** that can cause a cough (e.g. ACE inhibitors) and for drugs that can cause interstitial lung disease (e.g. methotrexate). Patients with known **underlying lung disease** presenting with a new cough or a change in their chronic cough may be suggestive of a superadded infection. Social history is of profound importance in a patient presenting with a chronic cough. A history of **heavy smoking** increases the risk of developing COPD and lung cancer. Furthermore, occupational exposure to certain organic or inorganic allergens can increase the risk of developing interstitial lung disease (extrinsic allergic alveolitis and pneumoconiosis).

## Differential Diagnosis

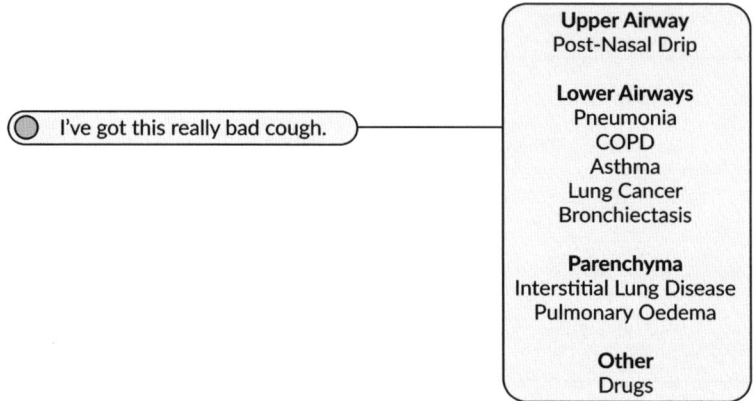

The causes of a cough can be divided into categories based on the likely location of the pathology. **Postnasal drip** is a very common cause of a chronic cough — it is a condition in which mucus from the nasal mucosa slides drips along the nasopharynx and into the larynx, triggering a cough.

Causes of chronic cough affecting the lower airways and lung parenchyma include **COPD**, **asthma**, **lung cancer**, **bronchiectasis** and **interstitial lung disease**. Patients with heart failure may develop a chronic cough due to **pulmonary oedema**. There are a variety of common **drugs** that can also cause a chronic cough, the best recognised of which are ACE inhibitors.

# Classical Presentations

| Differential | Classical Presentation |
|---|---|
| **Postnasal Drip** | Chronic nocturnal cough with no red flags. |
| **Pneumonia** | Gradual onset chest discomfort, shortness of breath and cough productive of yellow-green sputum. May be accompanied by a fever and lethargy. |
| **COPD** | Chronic history of worsening shortness of breath, reduced exercise tolerance and a persistent cough. Usually happens in patients with a significant smoking history. An exacerbation manifests with an acute worsening in their breathing which may be accompanied by features of infection (e.g. productive cough and fever). |
| **Asthma** | Chronic history of a dry nocturnal cough. Patients may also describe becoming breathless with a wheeze and noisy breathing at certain times. There may be clear precipitants, such as animal fur and exercise. |
| **Lung Cancer** | Several months' history of a persistent cough and, sometimes, haemoptysis. It is much more common in smokers and may be associated with unintentional weight loss. |
| **Bronchiectasis** | Chronic cough productive of copious volumes of sputum and sometimes haemoptysis. Patients also tend to get recurrent chest infections. |
| **Interstitial Lung Disease** | Chronic history of worsening shortness of breath associated with a dry cough. Some patients may have a background of occupational exposure to asbestos or coal dust. |

| | |
|---|---|
| **Pulmonary Oedema** | Gradual or rapid onset shortness of breath classically associated with a cough productive of pink, frothy sputum. Patients may also complain of ankle swelling, orthopnoea and paroxysmal nocturnal dyspnoea. If the episode was precipitated by an ischaemic event, they may complain of chest pain. |
| **Drug Side-Effect** | Persistent dry cough that arises soon after starting a new medication. ACE inhibitors are a cause that features commonly in exams. |

## Red Flags

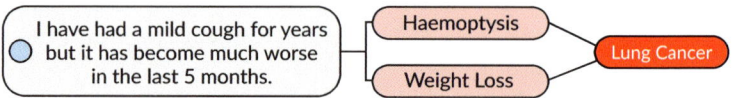

In most cases, patients presenting to primary care with a cough will have a lower respiratory tract infection which will resolve either spontaneously or with antibiotics. In some cases, however, a persistent dry cough may be the presenting symptom of underlying lung cancer. Such cases can be incredibly difficult to distinguish from more benign causes like lower respiratory tract infections and postnasal drip, but red flag features include **haemoptysis** and **weight loss**.

## Assessment

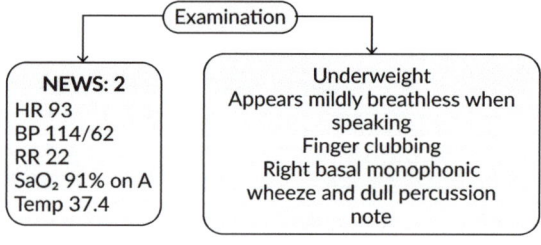

## *Observations*

In acute causes of cough (e.g. pneumonia and exacerbation of underlying lung disease), the patient may be **tachypnoeic** and may have **desaturated**. In chronic causes, on the other hand, the patient's observations may be normal. It is worth noting that if a patient has known underlying lung disease (e.g. COPD or interstitial lung disease), they may be a chronic carbon dioxide retainer, in which case their target oxygen saturations should remain around 88–92%. A **fever** would likely be suggestive of pneumonia or an infective exacerbation of pre-existing lung disease.

## *Examination*

Patients with lung cancer may appear cachectic and a **monophonic wheeze** may be heard in a discrete lung area (though this is a subtle sign). Patients with COPD, asthma and bronchiectasis may demonstrate a **polyphonic wheeze**. This may not be particularly apparent in patients with well-controlled disease. Patients with interstitial lung disease usually have **fine end-inspiratory crepitations**. **Finger clubbing** may be noted in patients with lung cancer, bronchiectasis and interstitial lung disease. Patients with pneumonia are likely to demonstrate **coarse crackles** and **bronchial breath sounds**.

# Lung Cancer

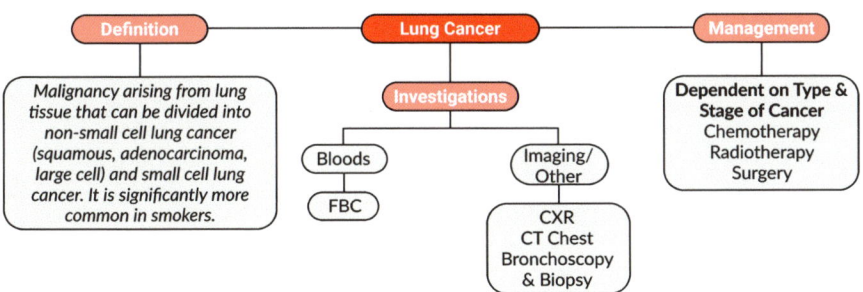

## Definition

Lung cancer is broadly divided into small cell lung cancer and non-small cell lung cancer (e.g. squamous cell, adenocarcinoma and large cell). It also encompasses neuroendocrine tumours and mesothelioma.

## Investigations

An **FBC** is a useful investigation, especially in patients with haemoptysis, as it may demonstrate a drop in haemoglobin. A **chest X-ray** is usually the first imaging modality that patients with suspected lung cancer will be exposed to. If large enough, it may reveal suspicious lung nodules. These can be further evaluated with a **CT scan**. Once the location has been identified, a **biopsy** may be taken for analysis either using **bronchoscopy** or **imaging-guided** techniques depending on the location of the mass.

## Management

The management of lung cancer depends largely on the type and stage of the tumour but will likely involve a combination of chemotherapy, radiotherapy and surgery (e.g. lobectomy).

# Bridge Box

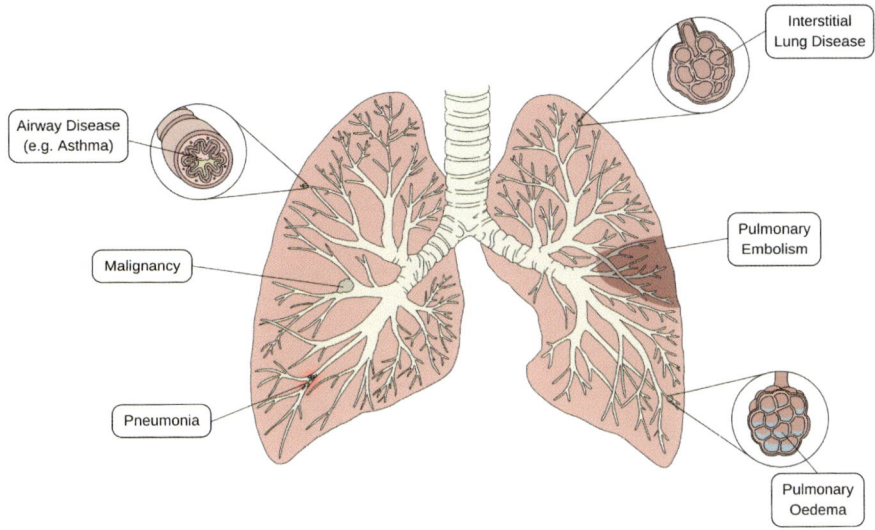

Differentials for cough.

# Chapter 9

# Shortness of Breath

Whether presenting acutely or with a prolonged history, shortness of breath is a concerning symptom for patients. Breathing issues must be taken seriously as patients can deteriorate rapidly.

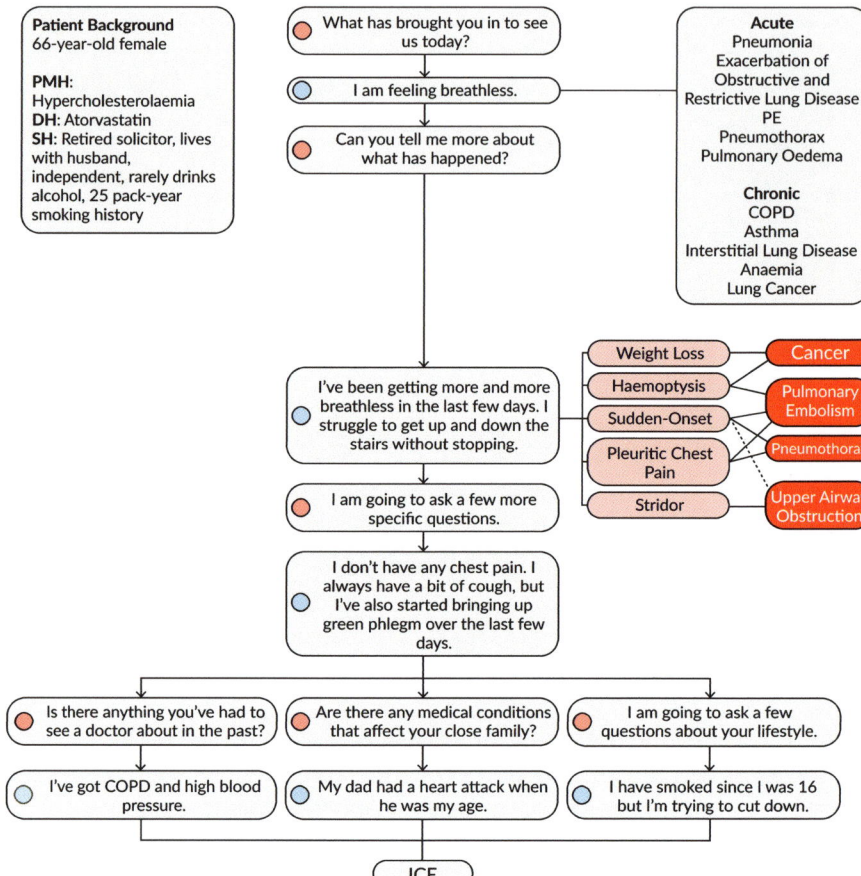

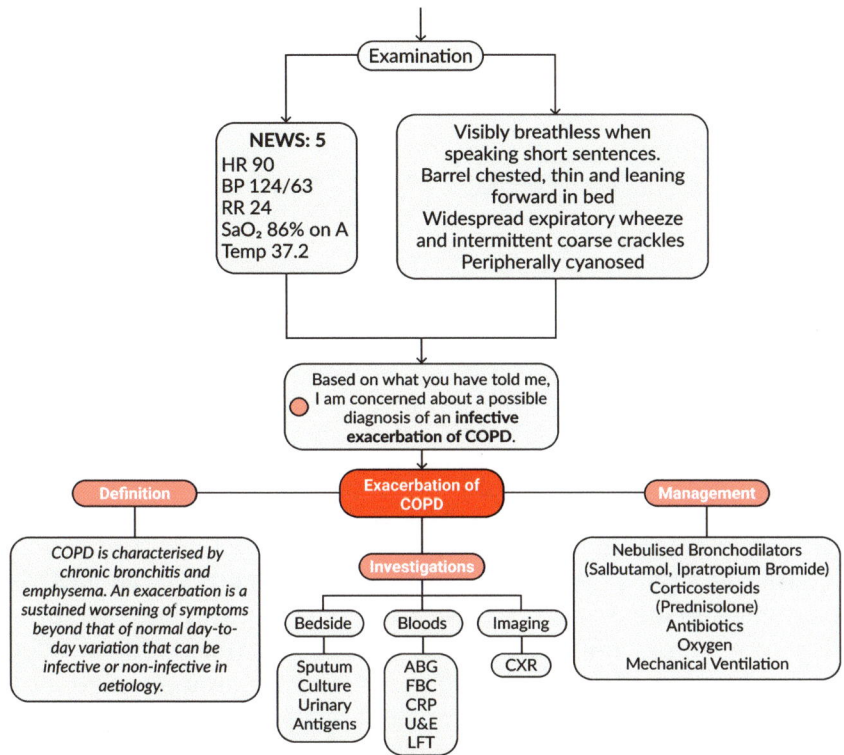

**Examination**

**NEWS: 5**
HR 90
BP 124/63
RR 24
$SaO_2$ 86% on A
Temp 37.2

Visibly breathless when
speaking short sentences.
Barrel chested, thin and leaning
forward in bed
Widespread expiratory wheeze
and intermittent coarse crackles
Peripherally cyanosed

Based on what you have told me,
I am concerned about a possible
diagnosis of an **infective
exacerbation of COPD.**

**Definition**

**Exacerbation of
COPD**

**Management**

COPD is characterised by
chronic bronchitis and
emphysema. An exacerbation is a
sustained worsening of symptoms
beyond that of normal day-to-
day variation that can be
infective or non-infective in
aetiology.

**Investigations**

| Bedside | Bloods | Imaging |
|---|---|---|
| Sputum Culture Urinary Antigens | ABG FBC CRP U&E LFT | CXR |

Nebulised Bronchodilators
(Salbutamol, Ipratropium Bromide)
Corticosteroids
(Prednisolone)
Antibiotics
Oxygen
Mechanical Ventilation

# Patient Background

**Patient Background**
66-year-old female

**PMH:**
Hypercholesterolaemia
**DH:** Atorvastatin
**SH:** Retired solicitor, lives
with husband,
independent, rarely drinks
alcohol, 25 pack-year
smoking history

Most causes of shortness of breath are more common in **older patients** (e.g. COPD, interstitial lung disease, pneumonia and heart failure). Causes that are more classically associated with **younger patients** include asthma and pneumothorax. The patient's **past medical history** can provide rather obvious clues about the likely cause of shortness of breath (e.g. a known background of COPD or heart disease). In patients presenting for the first time with shortness of breath, taking note of their **smoking status** can help determine their risk of developing certain diseases, such as COPD and heart failure.

# Differential Diagnosis

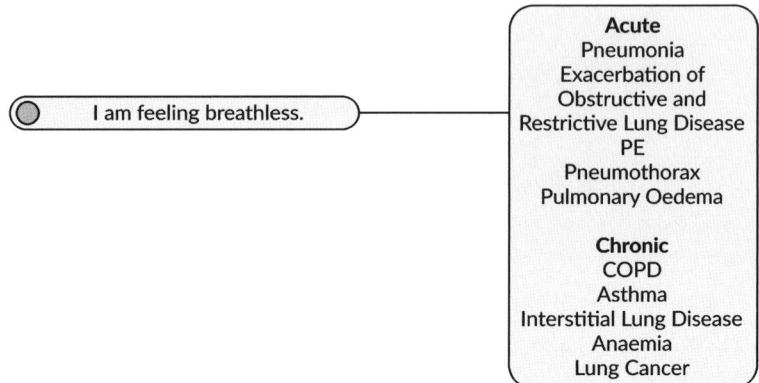

The causes of shortness of breath can be divided into **acute** and **chronic**, though there is a degree of overlap. Common acute causes include pneumonia and exacerbations of underlying obstructive disease (e.g. COPD and asthma) and restrictive disease (e.g. interstitial lung disease). Other acute causes include pulmonary embolism, pneumothorax and decompensated heart failure. Chronic causes of shortness of breath include COPD, interstitial lung disease, anaemia and lung cancer.

Though most causes of breathlessness are primary lung conditions, it is important to consider systemic conditions that could make patients breathless. For example, a patient with **metabolic acidosis** (e.g. due to diabetic ketoacidosis) will increase their minute ventilation in an attempt to blow off more carbon dioxide and compensate for the increase in metabolic acids within the blood. Similarly, if a patient is **anaemic**, the oxygen-carrying capacity of their blood and, hence, the oxygen delivery to tissues are compromised. At times of increased demand, this can lead to tissue hypoxia and lactic acidosis.

Read through the classical presentations table in the following section to develop an understanding of how the main differentials are classically present.

# Classical Presentations

| Differential | Classical Presentation |
|---|---|
| **Pneumonia** | Gradual onset chest discomfort, shortness of breath and cough productive of yellow-green sputum. May be accompanied by a fever and lethargy. |
| **Pulmonary Embolism** | Sudden onset sharp chest pain associated with shortness of breath. The pain is worsened by taking a deep breath in. Patients may have concomitant unilateral leg swelling (suggestive of a DVT) and may have certain risk factors (e.g. immobility, active cancer and recent surgery). |
| **Pneumothorax** | Sudden onset chest pain and shortness of breath in a tall, thin patient (spontaneous) or in a patient with underlying lung disease (secondary). It can also occur following trauma to the chest (e.g. rib fracture). |
| **Pulmonary Oedema** | Gradual or rapid onset shortness of breath classically associated with a cough productive of pink, frothy sputum. Patients may also complain of ankle swelling, orthopnoea and paroxysmal nocturnal dyspnoea. If the episode was precipitated by an ischaemic event, they may complain of chest pain. |
| **COPD** | Chronic history of worsening shortness of breath, reduced exercise tolerance and a persistent cough. Usually happens in patients with a significant smoking history. An exacerbation manifests with an acute worsening in their breathing which may be accompanied by features of infection (e.g. productive cough and fever). |

| Asthma | Chronic history of a dry nocturnal cough. Patients may also describe becoming breathless with a wheeze and noisy breathing at certain times. There may be clear precipitants, such as animal fur and exercise. |
|---|---|
| Interstitial Lung Disease | Chronic history of worsening shortness of breath associated with a dry cough. Some patients may have a background of occupational exposure to asbestos or coal dust. |
| Anaemia | Chronic history of shortness of breath, reduced exercise tolerance and fatigue. Patients may have an obvious source of excess bleeding (e.g. heavy menstrual bleeding) or it may be occult (e.g. colorectal malignancy). |
| Lung Cancer | Several months' history of a persistent cough and, sometimes, haemoptysis. It is much more common in smokers and may be associated with unintentional weight loss. |

## Red Flags

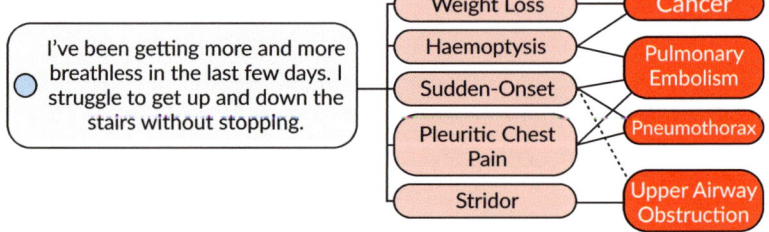

First, a patient with acute difficulty breathing and stridor requires emergency attention as it suggests that the airway is compromised. In such circumstances, an on-call anaesthetist should be bleeped (either directly or as part of a peri-arrest call) as the patient may require advanced airway management. Common causes of **stridor** that could be rapidly reversed include anaphylaxis and foreign-body inhalation.

Other causes of **acute shortness of breath** include pulmonary embolism and pneumothorax, both of which are associated with **pleuritic chest pain** (sharp pain that is worse when breathing in). Patients should also be screened for **risk factors for venous thromboembolism** (e.g. immobility, recent surgery and active cancer). Pulmonary oedema can also develop rapidly in patients who usually have a background of heart, liver or renal failure but may also present insidiously with worsening exercise tolerance and orthopnoea.

In patients presenting with a chronic history of shortness of breath, the presence of **haemoptysis** and **weight loss** may be suggestive of an underlying diagnosis of lung cancer. This is of particular concern if the patient has a significant smoking history.

## Assessment

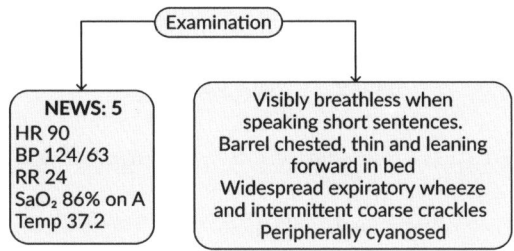

### *Observations*

Patients who are short of breath are likely to be **tachypnoeic** and may be **desaturating**. These parameters, along with the NEWS score, will help assess the severity of the patient's condition. Caution should be taken when interpreting the oxygen saturations at first glance in a patient with established lung disease, as they may be a chronic carbon dioxide retainer whose target saturations should be 88–92%. Nonetheless, in acutely breathless and desaturating patients, high-flow oxygen should be applied while their retainer status is established. **Tachycardia** is also associated with many causes of shortness of breath (e.g. exacerbations of COPD, pneumonia and PE). It is worth noting that, sometimes, PEs can present with subtle features such as tachycardia and chest pain without obvious tachypnoea or desaturation — these patients should be further evaluated based on their Wells' score. Patients with an infective exacerbation of underlying lung disease and patients presenting with pneumonia may have a **fever**.

## Examination

On inspection, the patient may be noted to have a **barrel chest** due to hyperinflation of the lungs (most commonly seen in COPD). On the other hand, patients with severe **chest wall and spinal abnormalities** such as pectus excavatum and kyphoscoliosis may have a lower threshold for developing breathlessness because their lung capacity is reduced at baseline. Visible **cyanosis** is a marker of significant hypoxia. Patients with COPD may also be seen performing **pursed lip breathing**.

The findings on auscultation can provide useful information about the likely underlying cause of the shortness of breath. Some common features are listed in the following:

- **Focal Bronchial Breath Sounds and Coarse Crackles**: Pneumonia
- **Widespread Polyphonic Wheeze**: Obstructive lung disease (COPD and asthma)
- **Focal Monophonic Wheeze**: Bronchial mass (e.g. cancer)
  - A monophonic wheeze is a single high-pitched whistling sound whereas a polyphonic wheeze consists of multiple sounds of different pitches. This is because, in COPD and Asthma, the airways are narrowed at multiple locations, whereas in lung cancer, there will only likely be a single, discrete narrowing.
- **Widespread Fine End-Inspiratory Crackles**: Interstitial lung disease
- **Bibasal Soft Inspiratory Crepitations**: Pulmonary oedema
- **Reduced Air Entry**: Pneumothorax, life-threatening asthma, pleural effusion

# Exacerbation of COPD

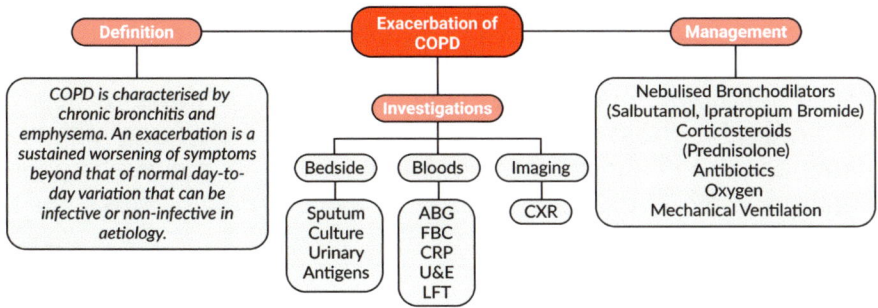

## Definition

An exacerbation of COPD is a very common presentation in A&E. Patients may be brought in by ambulance having desaturated significantly and can deteriorate rapidly. It refers to an acute worsening in the symptoms of a patient with COPD and can be described as *infective* (evidence of lung infection) or *non-infective*. This can be determined based on the history and the investigation findings.

## Investigations

At the bedside, if the patient has a productive cough, a **sputum sample** should be taken and sent for microscopy and culture. It may help guide antibiotic treatment at a later stage. A **urine sample** may also be sent to check for Legionella and Streptococcal antigens. Much of the time, exacerbations of COPD are caused by viruses, such as influenza and COVID, so a **respiratory viral screen** should also be sent.

In acutely desaturating patients, an **ABG** will allow you to assess their gas exchange and determine if they have developed respiratory failure and, hence, assess the need for higher-level care (e.g., non-invasive ventilation (NIV) and ICU). By looking at the bicarbonate concentration, the retainer status of the patient can also be established. An **FBC** and a **CRP** may reveal raised inflammatory markers in keeping with an infectious process. It is worth noting that many COPD patients will have a rescue pack at home containing antibiotics and steroids at home — if they have taken some steroids before arriving at the hospital, they will likely have a neutrophilia secondary to steroid-induced demargination of neutrophils. **U&E** and **LFT** are useful tests to request as atypical infections can cause derangements, such as hyponatraemia and transaminitis.

An urgent **chest X-ray** should be requested as it may demonstrate an area of consolidation in keeping with an infective exacerbation or may reveal other causes of acute breathlessness, such as a secondary pneumothorax.

## Management

The initial management of any acutely desaturating patient involves applying **high-flow oxygen**. This step should be taken even if the patient is a known carbon dioxide retainer as acute hypoxia is likely to kill a patient faster than carbon dioxide retention secondary to over-oxygenation. The oxygen can be titrated down once the patient has stabilised. **Nebulised bronchodilators** (salbutamol and ipratropium) are often effective at opening the airways and allowing the patient to breathe more comfortably. Patients should also be promptly started on **steroids** (e.g. oral prednisolone) to settle their airway inflammation and **antibiotics** (based on trust guidelines) if there is convincing evidence of concurrent bacterial infection (e.g. productive cough and consolidation on X-ray). If patients fail to improve sufficiently with these measures, they should be considered for **NIV** and **ITU input**.

# Bridge Box

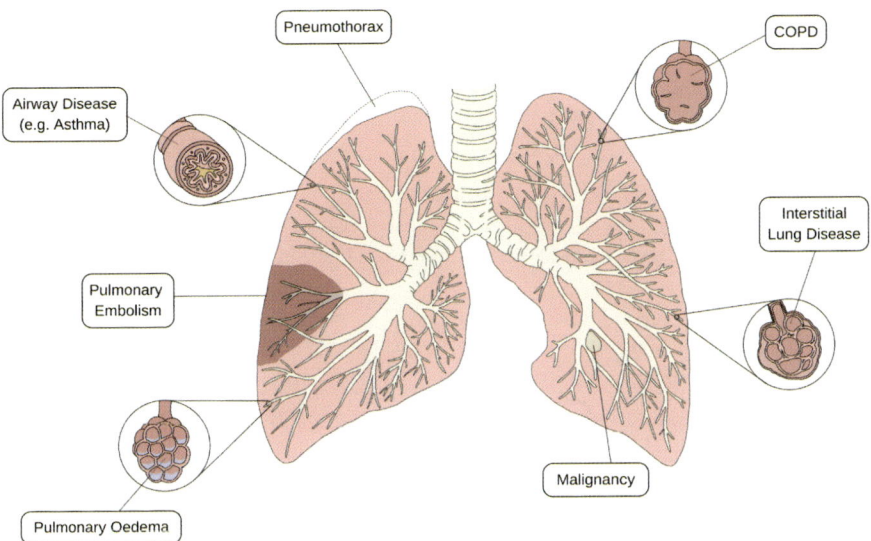

Pneumothorax

COPD

Airway Disease
(e.g. Asthma)

Interstitial
Lung Disease

Pulmonary
Embolism

Pulmonary Oedema

Malignancy

Differentials for shortness of breath.

# Chapter 10

# Epigastric Pain

As it relates to the junction between the chest and the abdomen, epigastric pain can be suggestive of underlying abdominal or chest pathology. A careful review of the associated symptoms is required to identify the relevant organ system involved and, hence, the underlying cause.

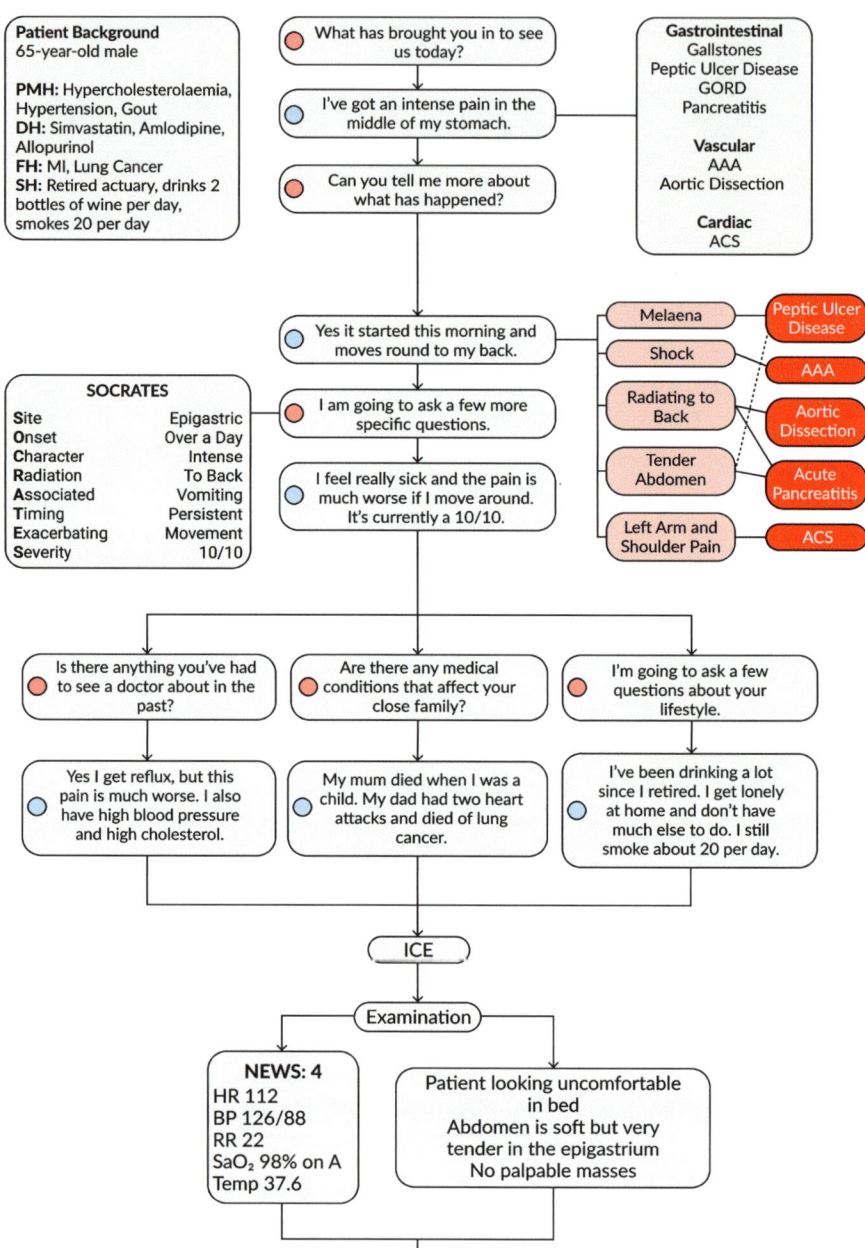

**Patient Background**
65-year-old male

**PMH:** Hypercholesterolaemia, Hypertension, Gout
**DH:** Simvastatin, Amlodipine, Allopurinol
**FH:** MI, Lung Cancer
**SH:** Retired actuary, drinks 2 bottles of wine per day, smokes 20 per day

What has brought you in to see us today?

I've got an intense pain in the middle of my stomach.

Can you tell me more about what has happened?

**Gastrointestinal**
Gallstones
Peptic Ulcer Disease
GORD
Pancreatitis

**Vascular**
AAA
Aortic Dissection

**Cardiac**
ACS

Yes it started this morning and moves round to my back.

I am going to ask a few more specific questions.

I feel really sick and the pain is much worse if I move around. It's currently a 10/10.

**SOCRATES**

| | |
|---|---|
| Site | Epigastric |
| Onset | Over a Day |
| Character | Intense |
| Radiation | To Back |
| Associated | Vomiting |
| Timing | Persistent |
| Exacerbating | Movement |
| Severity | 10/10 |

Melaena — Peptic Ulcer Disease

Shock — AAA

Radiating to Back — Aortic Dissection

Tender Abdomen — Acute Pancreatitis

Left Arm and Shoulder Pain — ACS

Is there anything you've had to see a doctor about in the past?

Are there any medical conditions that affect your close family?

I'm going to ask a few questions about your lifestyle.

Yes I get reflux, but this pain is much worse. I also have high blood pressure and high cholesterol.

My mum died when I was a child. My dad had two heart attacks and died of lung cancer.

I've been drinking a lot since I retired. I get lonely at home and don't have much else to do. I still smoke about 20 per day.

ICE

Examination

**NEWS: 4**
HR 112
BP 126/88
RR 22
SaO₂ 98% on A
Temp 37.6

Patient looking uncomfortable in bed
Abdomen is soft but very tender in the epigastrium
No palpable masses

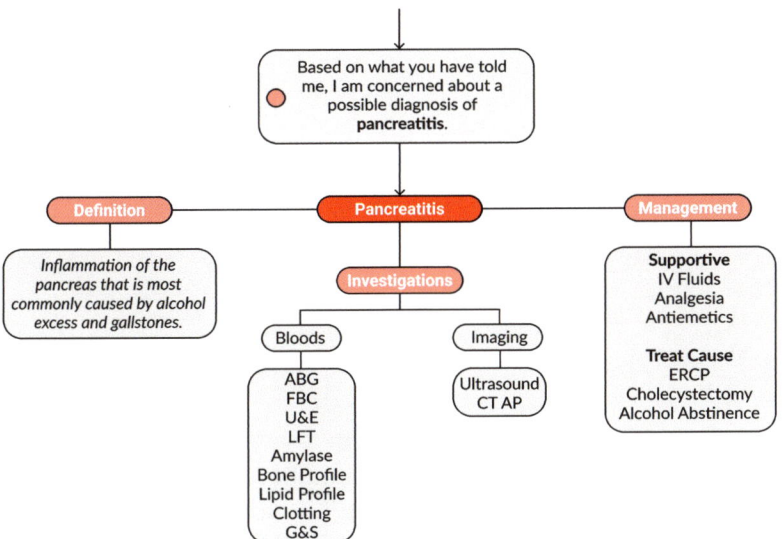

## Patient Background

**Patient Background**
65-year-old male

**PMH:** Hypercholesterolaemia, Hypertension, Gout
**DH:** Simvastatin, Amlodipine, Allopurinol
**FH:** MI, Lung Cancer
**SH:** Retired actuary, drinks 2 bottles of wine per day, smokes 20 per day

Most causes of epigastric pain can occur at a broad range of ages and in both men and women. **Alcohol excess** is a very common cause of acute pancreatitis which should be screened for when enquiring about their lifestyle. In addition, **overweight female** patients **over the age of 40 years** are at an increased risk of developing gallstone-related diseases (e.g. biliary colic and gallstone pancreatitis). In **middle-aged and elderly men** presenting with epigastric pain, serious cardiac and vascular pathology should be considered (e.g. ACS, aortic dissection and abdominal aortic aneurysm (AAA)). GORD is a very common cause of epigastric discomfort and can be significantly worsened by certain common **medications** that irritate the lining of the stomach (e.g. NSAIDs and steroids).

## Differential Diagnosis

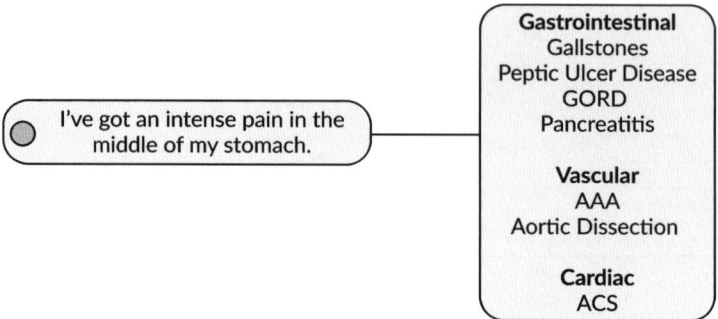

The causes of epigastric pain can be divided based on the organ systems affected. Most cases of epigastric pain will be caused by a disease that affects the gastrointestinal tract. In primary care, **gastro-oesophageal reflux disease** and **peptic ulcer disease** are very common causes that can usually be managed well in the community. Patients presenting more acutely to A&E with severe pain may have more serious conditions, such as **acute pancreatitis** or **gallstone diseases**.

It is important to consider the other important structures that lie within or in close proximity to the epigastrium — notably the heart and the aorta. Particularly in middle-aged and older men, it is important to consider **acute coronary syndrome** and **aortic dissection** as a cause of epigastric pain. Furthermore, if the patient is very unwell and showing signs of shock upon initial assessment, the possibility of a **leaking or ruptured AAA** should be considered.

# SOCRATES

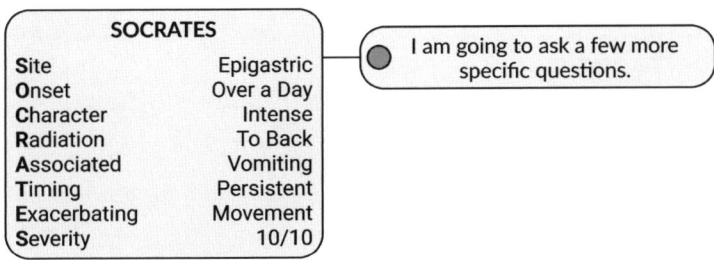

There are a few patterns of symptoms that are worth keeping at the back of your mind while you explore SOCRATES in a patient presenting with epigastric pain.

- **Site**
  - **Involving Chest**: ACS and aortic dissection
  - **Mainly Abdomen**: Gallstones, peptic ulcer disease, GORD, pancreatitis and AAA complication
- **Onset**
  - **Sudden**: Aortic dissection, AAA complication and ACS
  - **Over a Day**: Pancreatitis
  - **Over Several Days or Weeks**: GORD and peptic ulcer disease
    - It is important to note that peptic ulcers can present very acutely if it perforates or causes a large bleed.
- **Character**
  - **Crushing**: ACS
  - **Burning**: GORD and peptic ulcer disease
  - **Intense**: AAA complication, aortic dissection and pancreatitis
- **Radiation**
  - **To Shoulder and Jaw**: ACS
  - **To Between Shoulder Blades**: Aortic dissection
  - **To Back**: Pancreatitis
- **Associated Symptoms**
  - **Vomiting**: Gallstones and pancreatitis
  - **Sweating**: ACS and AAA complication
  - **Change in Bowel Habit**: Gallstones (steatorrhoea) and peptic ulcer disease (melaena)

- **Timing**
  - ○ **Persistent**: Most causes of epigastric pain
  - ○ **Intermittent**: GORD, peptic ulcer disease and biliary colic
- **Exacerbating**
  - ○ **Eating**: Peptic ulcer disease, GORD and gallstone disease
  - ○ **Lying Down**: GORD
- **Severity**
  - ○ **Generally Mild**: Peptic ulcer disease and GORD
  - ○ **Very Severe**: AAA complication, aortic dissection, ACS, gallstone disease and pancreatitis

Read through the classical presentations table in the following section to develop an understanding of how the main differentials are classically present.

## Classical Presentations

| Differential | Classical Presentation |
| --- | --- |
| Gallstone Disease | **Biliary Colic**: Intermittent epigastric and right upper quadrant pain that is worse after eating a fatty meal.<br>**Cholecystitis**: Persistent right upper quadrant pain associated with nausea, vomiting and a fever. Patients may have a preceding history of biliary colic.<br>**Acute Cholangitis**: Characterised by persistent right upper quadrant pain, jaundice and a fever (Charcot's triad). Patients are usually very unwell and require urgent intervention. |
| Peptic Ulcer Disease | Chronic history of burning epigastric pain that may occur at the time of a meal (gastric ulcer) or a few hours afterwards (duodenal ulcer). If the ulcer is bleeding, the patient may also describe melaena. |
| GORD | Chronic history of epigastric discomfort that is worsened by spicy meals. Patients may also complain of an unpleasant taste at the back of their mouth that is worse when lying flat. |

| Pancreatitis | Gradual onset severe epigastric pain associated with nausea and vomiting. Patients may have a history of alcohol excess or known gallstones. |
|---|---|
| Abdominal Aortic Aneurysm | May present with an insidious history of backache, classically in men over the age of 60 years. If the aneurysm is **leaking** or **ruptured**, patients may present with acute onset central abdominal pain with evidence of hypovolaemic shock (low blood pressure and tachycardia). |
| Aortic Dissection | Sudden onset tearing central chest pain that radiates to the back, in between the scapulae. It may result in syncope and arm pain. Associated risk factors include hypertension and connective tissue disorders (e.g. Marfan syndrome). |
| Acute Coronary Syndrome | Classically presents with central crushing chest pain that radiates to the jaw. Associated with sweating, anxiety and nausea. Patients may describe a prior history of experiencing chest pain on exertion that is relieved by rest (stable angina). |

# Red Flags

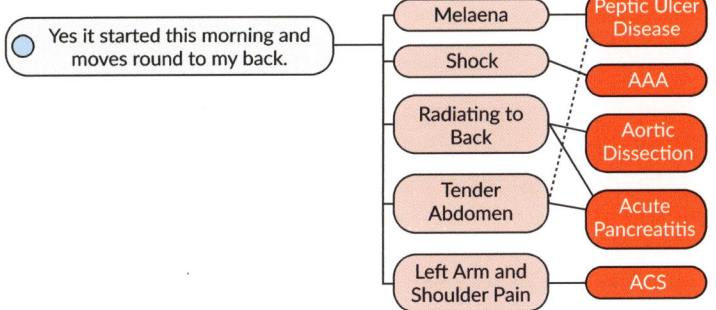

Some of the acute causes of epigastric pain have the potential to cause a rapid deterioration in the patient's clinical state so there are a few important questions and clinical features that should be explored to assess for these dangerous causes.

Patients with a bleeding peptic ulcer may mention a change in the colour of their stools (**melaena**). This may be associated with **haematemesis** and features of anaemia, such as shortness of breath and fatigue. AAA complications should be considered in any patient, especially older men, presenting to A&E in a **shocked** state with severe abdominal pain. They often require aggressive resuscitation and urgent investigations (point-of-care ultrasound and CT aortogram). Pain that **radiates to the back** may be suggestive of an aortic dissection (usually associated with chest pain radiating to a point between the shoulder blades) or pancreatitis. A very **tender abdomen** is a feature that is often associated with acute pancreatitis in the context of epigastric pain but will also be seen in patients with a perforated ulcer and gallstone diseases. In ACS, the pain classically **radiates towards the left arm, jaw and shoulder**.

# Examination

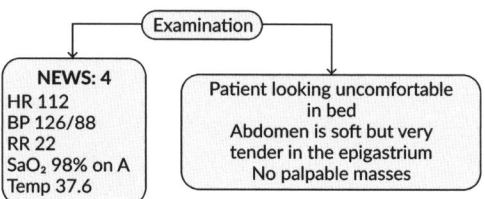

Observations section diagram:

**Examination**

| NEWS: 4 |
|---|
| HR 112 |
| BP 126/88 |
| RR 22 |
| SaO₂ 98% on A |
| Temp 37.6 |

Patient looking uncomfortable in bed
Abdomen is soft but very tender in the epigastrium
No palpable masses

## *Observations*

Patients who are in considerable pain, regardless of the cause, are likely to be **tachycardic**. The presence of **hypotension** should alert you to the possibility of a major vascular abnormality such as a leaking or ruptured AAA, though patients with inflammatory conditions (e.g. pancreatitis) or other significant bleeds (e.g. bleeding peptic ulcer) may also present in a state of shock. Patients who are **desaturating** in the context of severe epigastric pain may have developed acute respiratory distress syndrome (ARDS) secondary to pancreatitis (a marker of severity). A **fever** may be seen in both pancreatitis and infections of the biliary tree (e.g. cholangitis).

## *Examination*

Gastrointestinal causes of epigastric pain are likely to cause some discomfort upon palpation of the epigastrium. The epigastrium is likely to be **exquisitely tender** in patients with acute pancreatitis, biliary infections and perforated peptic ulcers due to the localised peritonism. In severe cases of pancreatitis, evidence of retroperitoneal haemorrhage may be noted (**Grey Turner** and **Cullen's signs**) and **widespread inspiratory crepitations** may be heard upon auscultation of the chest (ARDS). The patient should be assessed for **Murphy's sign** as this may be suggestive of cholecystitis presenting with epigastric pain. In cases of an AAA, a **centrally expansile and pulsatile mass** may be felt.

# Pancreatitis

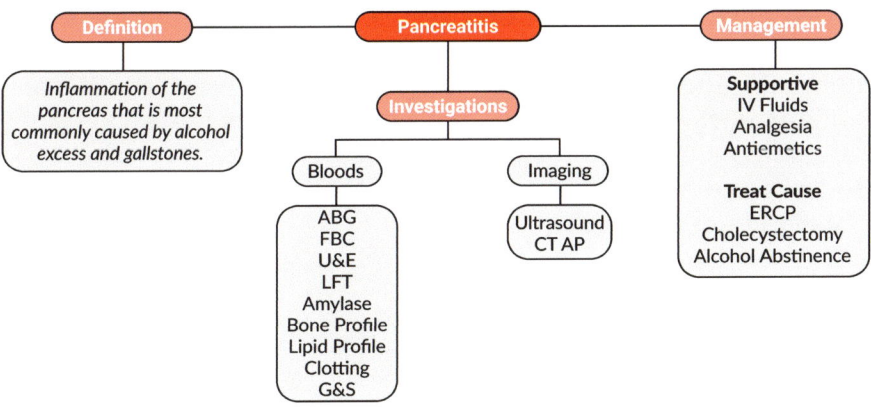

## *Definition*

Acute pancreatitis refers to inflammation of the pancreas resulting in epigastric pain and systemic upset. It is most commonly caused by alcohol excess and gallstones, though there are several other causes that are recalled using the mnemonic '**GET SMASHED**'.

## Investigations

The clinical presentation, examination findings and patient factors (e.g. background of alcohol excess or known gallstones) can provide useful evidence to make a clinical diagnosis of acute pancreatitis. An **FBC** will likely reveal a raised white cell count and an **amylase** level is likely to be significantly elevated in patients with acute pancreatitis (though it may not be raised in chronic pancreatitis). As acute pancreatitis can occur secondary to gallstones, an **LFT** should be requested — this may show an obstructive pattern (i.e. significantly raised ALP and GGT). Pancreatitis causes significant third spacing of fluid and, hence, intravascular depletion so it may lead to an AKI which would be noted on the **U&E**. Acute pancreatitis can be *caused* by hypercalcaemia and can *lead to* hypocalcaemia (due to saponification), so a **bone profile** is also a useful test to request. Similarly, hyperlipidaemia is a recognised cause of acute pancreatitis which can be identified on a **lipid profile**. If there is any evidence of respiratory compromise (suggestive of ARDS), an **ABG** should be performed — the $PaO_2$ is part of the Glasgow-Imrie criteria for severity of acute pancreatitis.

An **abdominal ultrasound** enables visualisation of the biliary tree to check for duct dilatation suggestive of an obstructing gallstone. **CT abdomen and pelvis with contrast** provides the most comprehensive radiographic assessment of pancreatitis and may reveal features, such as parenchymal enlargement, pancreatic oedema and retroperitoneal fat stranding. It will also allow the identification of pseudocysts.

## Management

Initial management involves resuscitation with **IV fluids** and controlling the symptoms with strong **analgesia** and **antiemetics**. It is important to note that patients may have a fever as pancreatitis causes a systemic inflammatory response, however, in the absence of any more compelling evidence of infection, antibiotics should *not* be routinely started in patients with acute pancreatitis.

If the episode of pancreatitis is caused by alcohol, the mainstay of treatment is managing symptoms, fluid resuscitation and enabling the patient to reduce or **eliminate their alcohol intake**. The management of gallstone pancreatitis involves either removing the obstructing gallstone (by **ERCP**), draining the obstructed system (via a **cholecystostomy** or **percutaneous transhepatic biliary drainage**) or removing the source of the gallstones (**cholecystectomy**) based on the context.

## Bridge Box

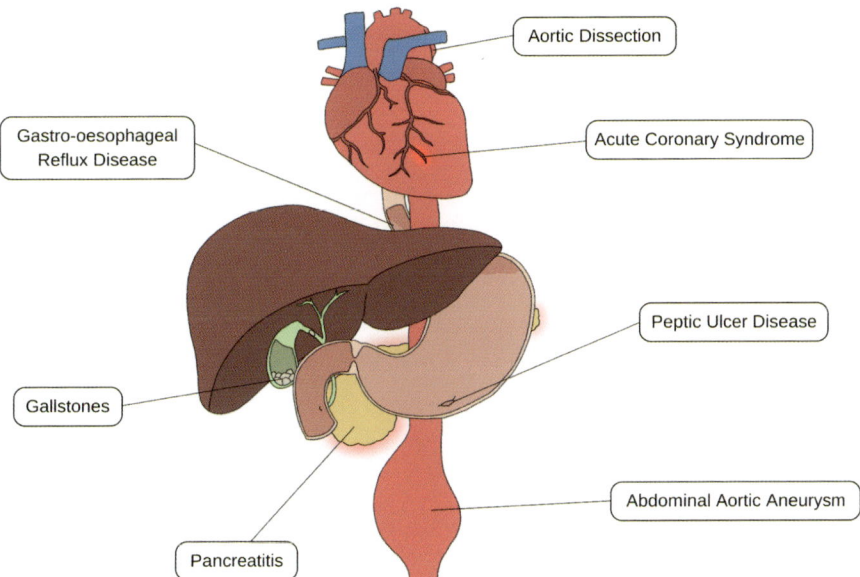

Differentials for epigastric pain.

# Chapter 11

# Jaundice

Jaundice is a serious symptom that may be suggestive of a sinister underlying cause. The causes of jaundice are manifold, and an understanding of bilirubin metabolism will aid your approach to distinguishing these causes.

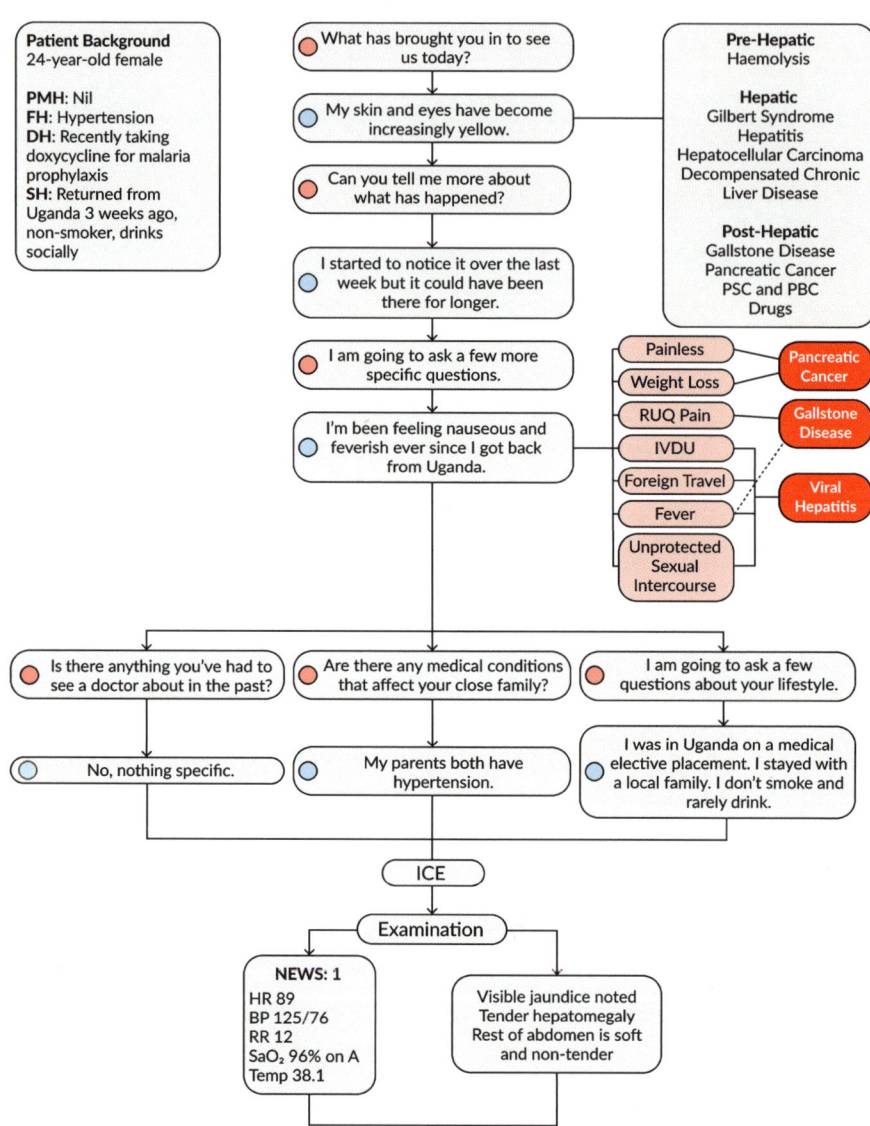

**Patient Background**
24-year-old female

**PMH:** Nil
**FH:** Hypertension
**DH:** Recently taking doxycycline for malaria prophylaxis
**SH:** Returned from Uganda 3 weeks ago, non-smoker, drinks socially

What has brought you in to see us today?

My skin and eyes have become increasingly yellow.

Can you tell me more about what has happened?

I started to notice it over the last week but it could have been there for longer.

I am going to ask a few more specific questions.

I'm been feeling nauseous and feverish ever since I got back from Uganda.

**Pre-Hepatic**
Haemolysis

**Hepatic**
Gilbert Syndrome
Hepatitis
Hepatocellular Carcinoma
Decompensated Chronic Liver Disease

**Post-Hepatic**
Gallstone Disease
Pancreatic Cancer
PSC and PBC
Drugs

Painless
Weight Loss
RUQ Pain
IVDU
Foreign Travel
Fever
Unprotected Sexual Intercourse

Pancreatic Cancer
Gallstone Disease
Viral Hepatitis

Is there anything you've had to see a doctor about in the past?

Are there any medical conditions that affect your close family?

I am going to ask a few questions about your lifestyle.

No, nothing specific.

My parents both have hypertension.

I was in Uganda on a medical elective placement. I stayed with a local family. I don't smoke and rarely drink.

ICE

Examination

**NEWS: 1**
HR 89
BP 125/76
RR 12
$SaO_2$ 96% on A
Temp 38.1

Visible jaundice noted
Tender hepatomegaly
Rest of abdomen is soft and non-tender

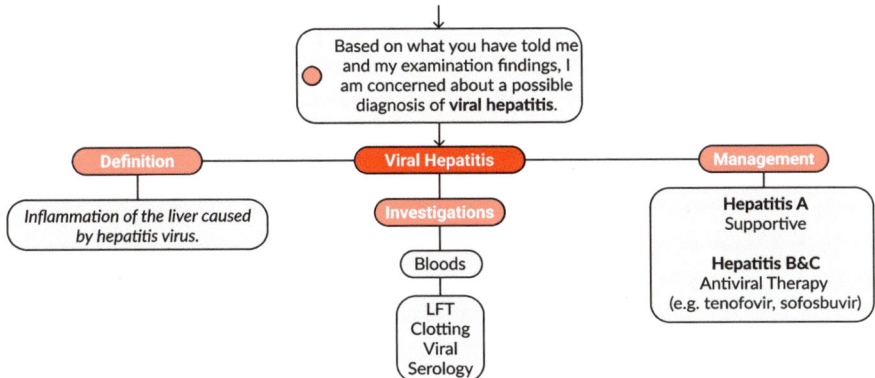

# Patient Background

**Patient Background**
24-year-old female

**PMH:** Nil
**FH:** Hypertension
**DH:** Recently taking doxycycline for malaria prophylaxis
**SH:** Returned from Uganda 3 weeks ago, non-smoker, drinks socially

There are several risk factors for viral hepatitis that can be gleaned from the patient's background. For example, having spent time in a **viral hepatitis endemic region**, **unsafe sex** and **intravenous drug** use all increase the risk of contracting viral hepatitis. The patient's **drug history** should also be screened to check for medications that are known to affect liver function — this may be acute (e.g. cholestasis secondary to co-amoxiclav) or chronic (e.g. methotrexate). Patients who drink **alcohol to excess** are, of course, at increased risk of developing alcoholic liver disease.

**Overweight patients** (especially women over the age of 40 years) are at increased risk of developing gallstone disease and non-alcoholic fatty liver disease. A background of **haemolytic conditions** (e.g. sickle cell disease and G6PD deficiency) should prompt you to consider pre-hepatic causes of jaundice. Furthermore, a history of **autoimmune conditions** (e.g. SLE) may suggest that autoimmune haemolytic anaemia and autoimmune hepatitis are possible causes of jaundice.

On the contrary, patients who are otherwise completely well with no past medical history or risk factors presenting with mild asymptomatic jaundice may have **Gilbert syndrome**.

## Differential Diagnosis

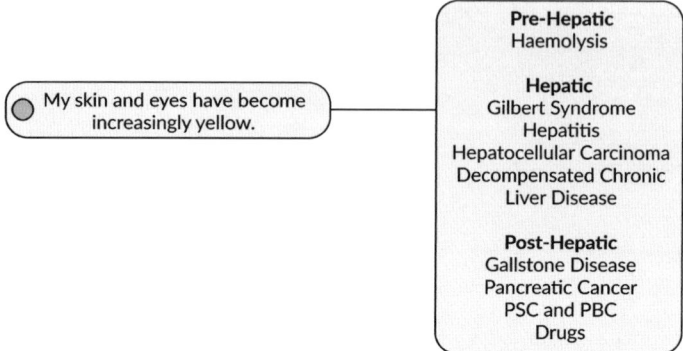

A rise in serum bilirubin can occur due to abnormalities at any of the three stages of bilirubin metabolism and excretion. These are detailed in the **Bridge Box** section.

**Haemolytic conditions** (characterised by reduced red cell survival) lead to an increased turnover of red cells thereby releasing more bilirubin within the circulation. Causes of haemolysis include sickle cell disease, G6PD deficiency and autoimmune haemolytic anaemia. Jaundice occurs when the rate of generation of bilirubin exceeds the capacity of the liver to metabolise it.

**Hepatic** causes of jaundice are related to defects in the liver's ability to conjugate bilirubin and excrete it into the biliary canaliculi. Gilbert syndrome is a common, benign condition that is characterised by decreased activity of UDP glucuronyltransferase. It usually manifests with mild jaundice in the context of a recent illness. All the causes of hepatitis (alcoholic, viral and autoimmune) can impair the ability of the liver to metabolise bilirubin resulting in jaundice.

**Posthepatic** causes of jaundice block the flow of bile through the biliary tree and into the small intestine, thereby leading to biliary congestion and the leakage of conjugated bilirubin into the systemic circulation. Causes include gallstone disease (e.g. common bile duct stone), pancreatic cancer, primary sclerosing cholangitis, primary biliary cholangitis and drug-induced cholestasis.

Read through the classical presentations table in the following section to develop an understanding of how the main differentials are classically present.

## Classical Presentations

| Differential | Classical Presentation |
|---|---|
| **Haemolytic Disorders** | Depending on the extent of haemolysis, patients may develop symptoms of anaemia (shortness of breath, fatigue and pallor). It may be precipitated by a recent infection (e.g. autoimmune haemolytic anaemia) or the patient may have a documented background of inherited haemolytic conditions (e.g. sickle cell disease, hereditary spherocytosis and G6PD deficiency). |
| **Gilbert Syndrome** | Well patients presenting with episodes of jaundice that typically occur when they are unwell (e.g. due to a viral infection). These episodes resolve spontaneously. It may also be an incidental finding on blood tests. |
| **Viral Hepatitis** | The acuity varies depending on the cause. Classically present in patients who have been in an endemic area or are from an at-risk population (e.g. IV drug users). **Hepatitis A**: Acute onset jaundice associated with fever and diarrhoea, and a recent history of eating potentially contaminated food. **Hepatitis B**: Can have both acute and chronic presentations. **Hepatitis C**: Often asymptomatic and may be incidentally noted on blood tests. |
| **Alcoholic Hepatitis** | Gradual onset right upper quadrant pain and jaundice in patients with a background of alcohol excess. |

| | |
|---|---|
| **Autoimmune Hepatitis** | Relatively acute onset right upper quadrant pain and jaundice that classically occurs in young women who may have a background of other autoimmune diseases. |
| **Hepatocellular Carcinoma** | Progressive jaundice associated with weight loss and loss of appetite. It is more common in patients with a background of chronic liver disease. |
| **Decompensated Chronic Liver Disease** | Patients with a background of chronic liver disease presenting with abdominal distension (ascites), worsening peripheral oedema, breathlessness (due to pulmonary oedema) and jaundice. There may be evidence of triggers for decompensation, such as recent alcohol intake, gastrointestinal bleeding or an infection. |
| **Gallstone Disease** | **Biliary Colic**: Intermittent epigastric and right upper quadrant pain that is worse after eating a fatty meal.<br>**Cholecystitis**: Persistent right upper quadrant pain associated with nausea, vomiting and a fever. Patients may have a preceding history of biliary colic.<br>**Acute Cholangitis**: Characterised by persistent right upper quadrant pain, jaundice and a fever (Charcot's triad). Patients are usually very unwell and require urgent intervention. |
| **Pancreatic Cancer** | Progressive painless jaundice associated with weight loss and loss of appetite. |
| **PSC and PBC** | Progressive painless jaundice that is often associated with pruritus due to the accumulation of bile salts in the skin. PSC is associated with ulcerative colitis and PBC often arises in patients with other autoimmune conditions (e.g. rheumatoid arthritis). |

The three main forms of viral hepatitis are transmitted via fae-cal-oral (hepatitis A) and bloodborne (hepatitis B and C) routes. Therefore, significant risk factors include recent travel to a viral hepatitis-endemic region, intravenous drug use and engaging in unprotected sexual intercourse with multiple partners. Furthermore, patients with viral hepatitis may be acutely unwell with a fever and other symptoms, such as diarrhoea.

# Assessment

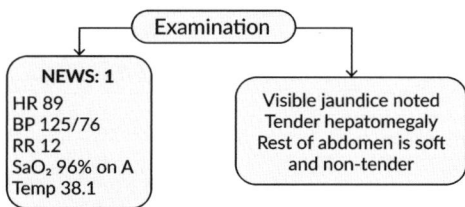

## *Observations*

Patients with infectious and inflammatory causes of jaundice such as viral hepatitis and biliary infections may have a **fever** and fea-tures of systemic upset (tachycardia and hypotension). If a patient has become profoundly anaemic due to an underlying haemolytic disorder, they may be **tachycardic**. Most chronic causes of jaun-dice (e.g. pancreatic cancer) are unlikely to cause any significant abnormalities in the patient's vital signs.

## *Examination*

**RUQ tenderness** may be noted in patients with biliary infections or hepatitis. In patients with a background of liver disease, many **features of chronic liver disease** may also be noted such as abdominal distension, spider naevi and caput medusae. A signifi-cant amount of weight loss may be a manifestation of an underlying malignancy (e.g. pancreatic cancer).

# Viral Hepatitis

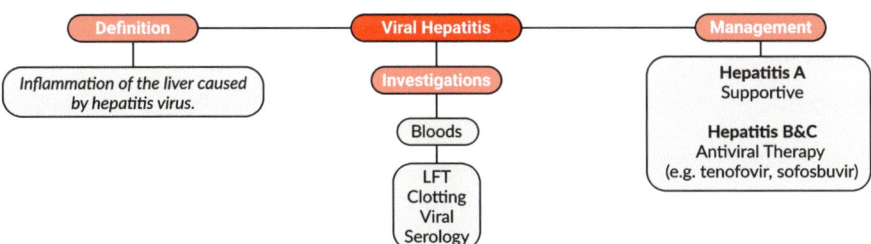

## Definition

Viral hepatitis is an umbrella term that refers to inflammation of the liver that is caused by hepatitis virus (A, B, C, D or E). Hepatitis A, B and C are the most common causes of viral hepatitis.

## Investigations

**LFT** is an important first-line blood test that will help determine the severity of viral hepatitis. It is likely to reveal a raised bilirubin along with a significantly raised AST and ALT. To assess whether the liver's synthetic function has been affected, a **clotting screen** should be sent — prothrombin time is a sensitive marker of deranged liver synthetic function. **Viral serology** will allow the viral hepatitis status of the patient to be determined.

## Management

Hepatitis A usually causes a mild and self-limiting illness that resolves without intervention. Advice should be provided about **symptomatic management**. Hepatitis B may be cleared by the patient; however, chronic infection requires treatment with **antiviral agents**, such as tenofovir and peginterferon alfa. Hepatitis C virus causes chronic infection and is also treated with antiviral agents, such as sofosbuvir.

# Bridge Box

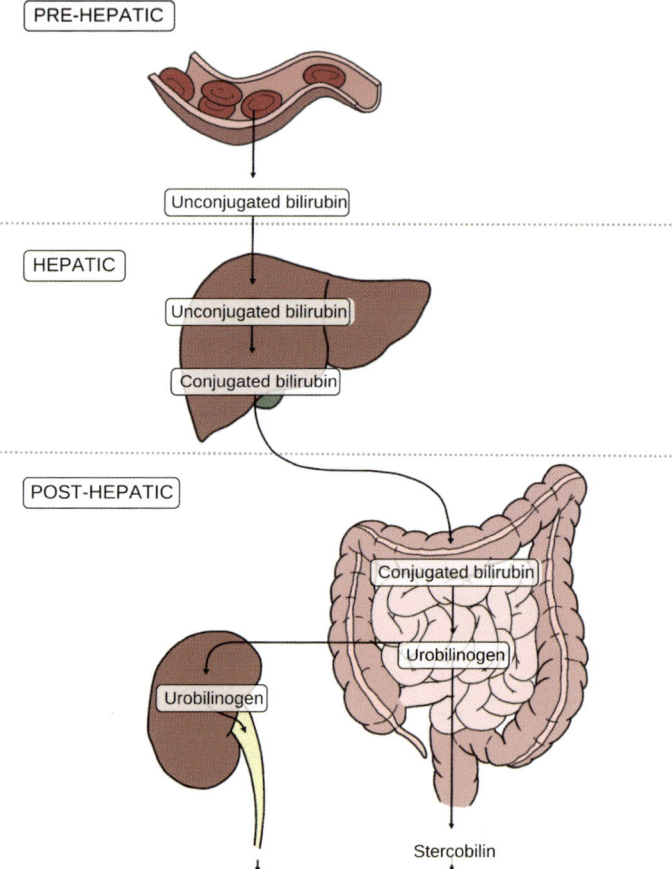

A clear understanding of bilirubin metabolism will help you make sense of the investigations that are often requested in patients presenting with jaundice. Unconjugated bilirubin is a breakdown product of heme which is released by dying red blood cells. This unconjugated bilirubin will then get transported to the liver where it gets conjugated by UDP glucuronyltransferase to form conjugated bilirubin. The conjugated bilirubin is then excreted into the bile canaliculi and makes its way into the small intestine. Within the intestines, it will be further metabolised by colonic bacteria into urobilinogen. This is a water-soluble compound that is reabsorbed into the circulation and excreted by the kidneys. The urobilinogen that is not reabsorbed and, hence, remains in the intestines is referred to as stercobilinogen. Stercobilinogen can then be oxidised to stercobilin which gives faeces its brown colour.

# Chapter 12

# Right Upper Quadrant Pain

Right upper quadrant pain is a common presentation that often requires referral to the surgical team. A basic understanding of the anatomy of the region can help determine which differentials are most likely.

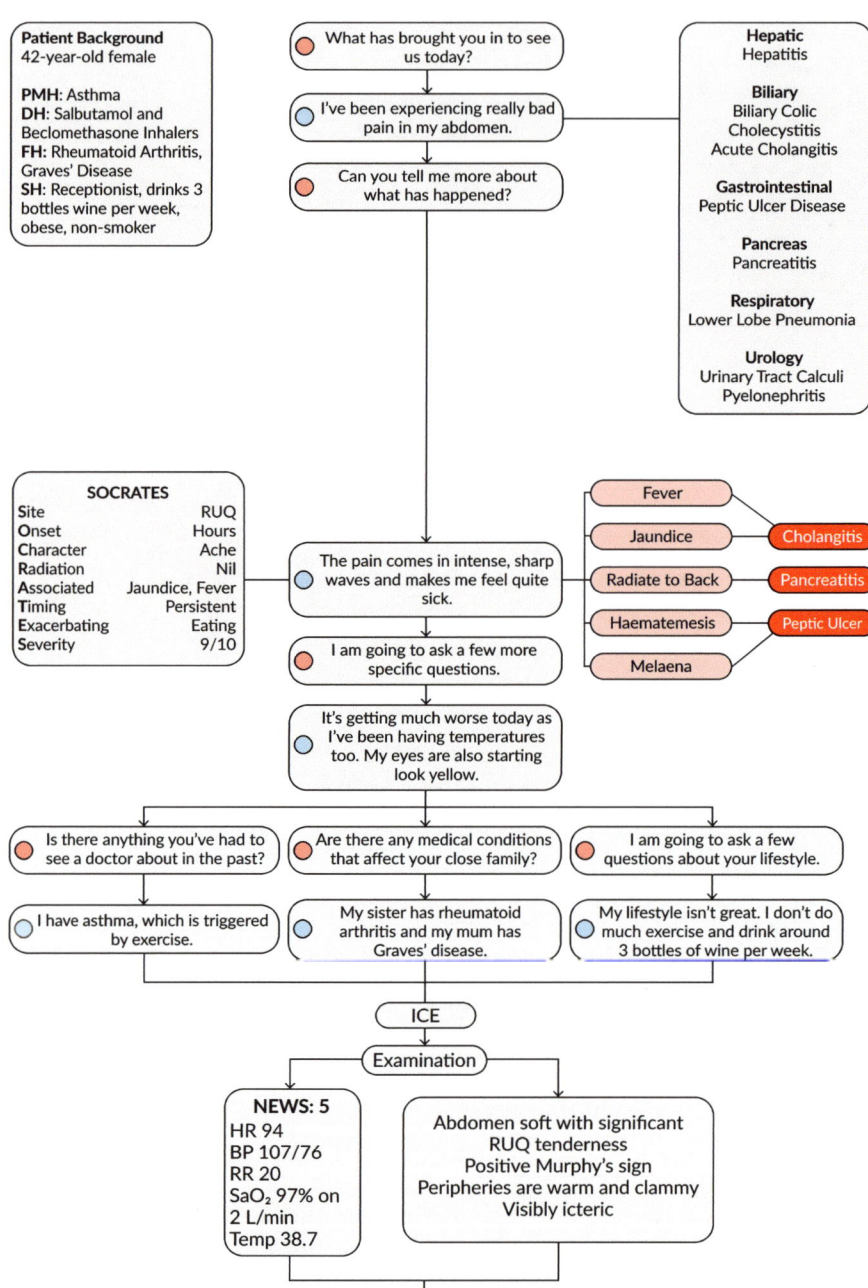

**Patient Background**
42-year-old female

**PMH:** Asthma
**DH:** Salbutamol and Beclomethasone Inhalers
**FH:** Rheumatoid Arthritis, Graves' Disease
**SH:** Receptionist, drinks 3 bottles wine per week, obese, non-smoker

What has brought you in to see us today?

I've been experiencing really bad pain in my abdomen.

Can you tell me more about what has happened?

**Hepatic**
Hepatitis

**Biliary**
Biliary Colic
Cholecystitis
Acute Cholangitis

**Gastrointestinal**
Peptic Ulcer Disease

**Pancreas**
Pancreatitis

**Respiratory**
Lower Lobe Pneumonia

**Urology**
Urinary Tract Calculi
Pyelonephritis

**SOCRATES**
| | |
|---|---|
| Site | RUQ |
| Onset | Hours |
| Character | Ache |
| Radiation | Nil |
| Associated | Jaundice, Fever |
| Timing | Persistent |
| Exacerbating | Eating |
| Severity | 9/10 |

The pain comes in intense, sharp waves and makes me feel quite sick.

I am going to ask a few more specific questions.

Fever

Jaundice — Cholangitis

Radiate to Back — Pancreatitis

Haematemesis — Peptic Ulcer

Melaena

It's getting much worse today as I've been having temperatures too. My eyes are also starting look yellow.

Is there anything you've had to see a doctor about in the past?

Are there any medical conditions that affect your close family?

I am going to ask a few questions about your lifestyle.

I have asthma, which is triggered by exercise.

My sister has rheumatoid arthritis and my mum has Graves' disease.

My lifestyle isn't great. I don't do much exercise and drink around 3 bottles of wine per week.

ICE

Examination

**NEWS: 5**
HR 94
BP 107/76
RR 20
SaO$_2$ 97% on 2 L/min
Temp 38.7

Abdomen soft with significant RUQ tenderness
Positive Murphy's sign
Peripheries are warm and clammy
Visibly icteric

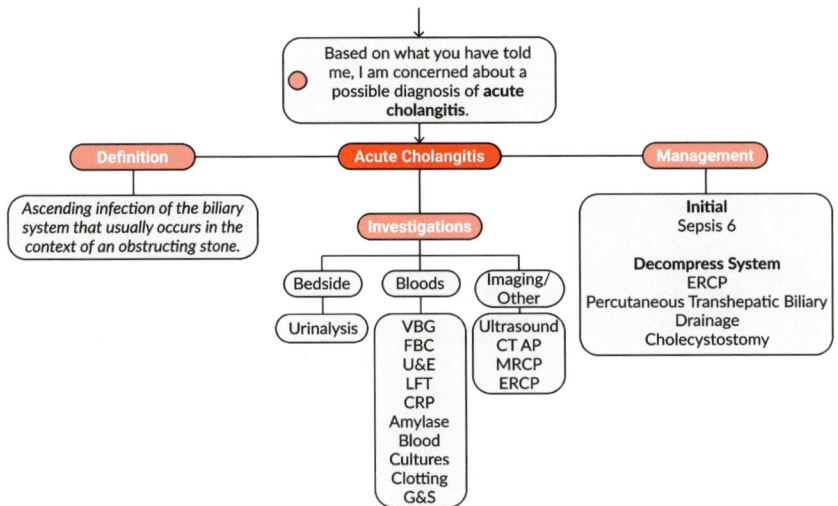

# Patient Background

**Patient Background**
42-year-old female

**PMH**: Asthma
**DH**: Salbutamol and Beclomethasone Inhalers
**FH**: Rheumatoid Arthritis, Graves' Disease
**SH**: Receptionist, drinks 3 bottles wine per week, obese, non-smoker

The **age** and **sex** of the patient can be used to assess the probability of a patient having certain causes of RUQ pain, for example, gallstone disease (biliary colic, cholecystitis and cholangitis) most commonly occurs in overweight and obese women who are over the age of 40 years. Patients with a background of **alcohol excess** may develop alcoholic hepatitis and are at increased risk of developing pancreatitis. Furthermore, the patient's use of regular and over-the-counter medications should be reviewed as certain common medications can cause gastric erosions and ulcers (e.g. **NSAIDs**).

# Differential Diagnosis

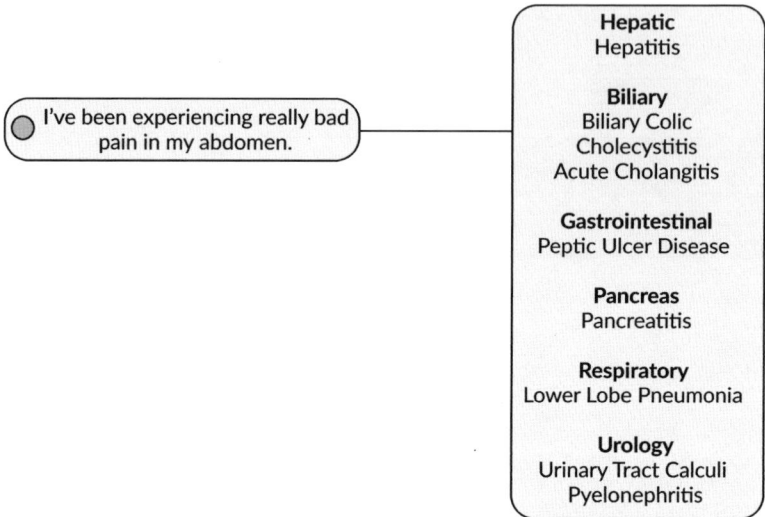

I've been experiencing really bad pain in my abdomen.

**Hepatic**
Hepatitis

**Biliary**
Biliary Colic
Cholecystitis
Acute Cholangitis

**Gastrointestinal**
Peptic Ulcer Disease

**Pancreas**
Pancreatitis

**Respiratory**
Lower Lobe Pneumonia

**Urology**
Urinary Tract Calculi
Pyelonephritis

The various causes of RUQ pain can be divided based on the organ or system affected. The main organs that spring to mind when considering the RUQ are the liver, biliary tree and pancreas. It is important to remember, however, that the right ureter and kidney and the base of the right lung lie near this area and diseases affecting these organs may also present with RUQ pain.

The main **hepatic** causes are the various forms of **hepatitis** (viral, alcoholic and autoimmune). They are likely to present with subacute RUQ pain associated with other features of systemic upset. It is important to screen for risk factors, such as living in an area where viral hepatitis is endemic, unsafe sex and intravenous drug use.

The **biliary** causes of RUQ pain exist on a spectrum. Gallstones are very common and usually do not cause any significant symptoms. A gallstone may transiently get stuck in a duct causing intermittent RUQ pain that is worse after eating a fatty meal (**biliary colic**). The presence of gallstones within the gallbladder also predisposes to infection (**cholecystitis**). If a gallstone obstructs the flow of bile along the common bile duct, it can subsequently become infected resulting in Charcot's triad of features (RUQ pain, jaundice and fever). Gallstones can also get stuck in the pancreatic duct causing gallstone **pancreatitis**. The other common cause of pancreatitis is alcohol excess.

The right lower lobe of the **lung** lies in close proximity to the liver and biliary system, so lung conditions such as pneumonia and (more rarely) PE may present with RUQ pain though you would expect to also see features of respiratory disease (e.g. tachypnoea and cough).

In some cases, diseases affecting the **right kidney** could present with RUQ pain though this is more likely to be described as right flank pain. Such causes include **renal colic** and **pyelone-phritis**. Urinalysis is a simple and useful investigation to screen for these diseases.

## SOCRATES

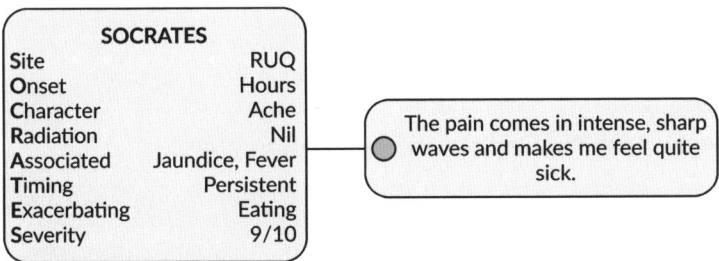

| SOCRATES | |
|---|---|
| Site | RUQ |
| Onset | Hours |
| Character | Ache |
| Radiation | Nil |
| Associated | Jaundice, Fever |
| Timing | Persistent |
| Exacerbating | Eating |
| Severity | 9/10 |

The pain comes in intense, sharp waves and makes me feel quite sick.

There are a few patterns of symptoms that are worth keeping at the back of your mind while you explore SOCRATES in a patient presenting with RUQ pain.

- **Site**: It is worth enquiring specifically about where the pain is worst. A patient with urinary tract calculi or pyelonephritis will likely describe the pain as being primarily in their right flank.
- **Onset**
  - **Rapid Onset**: Urinary tract calculi
  - **Subacute Onset**: Hepatitis, gallstone disease, peptic ulcer disease, pancreatitis, lower lobe pneumonia and pyelonephritis
- **Character**: Most causes of RUQ pain will give rise to a **dull** pain except for lower lobe pneumonia which may cause pleuritic pain.

- **Radiation**
  - **To Shoulder Tip**: Hepatitis, cholecystitis and acute cholangitis
  - **To Back**: Pancreatitis
  - **To Groin**: Urinary tract calculi
- **Associated Symptoms**
  - **Change in Bowel Habit**: Gallstone disease (steatorrhoea) and peptic ulcer disease (melaena)
  - **Jaundice**: Hepatitis and gallstone disease
  - **Shortness of Breath**: Pneumonia
  - **Dysuria**: Urinary tract calculi and pyelonephritis
- **Timing**
  - **Persistent**: Hepatitis, cholecystitis, cholangitis, lower lobe pneumonia and pyelonephritis
  - **Waxing and Waning**: Urinary tract calculi and biliary colic
  - **Intermittent**: Peptic ulcer disease
- **Exacerbating**
  - **After Meals**: Biliary colic and peptic ulcer disease
- **Severity**
  - **Very Severe**: Renal colic and pancreatitis

Read through the classical presentations table in the following section to develop an understanding of how the main differentials are classically present.

## Classical Presentations

| Differential | Classical Presentation |
|---|---|
| **Hepatitis** | Right upper quadrant discomfort associated with jaundice. The acuity and presence of other symptoms (e.g. fever) depend on the underlying cause (e.g. viral hepatitis, alcoholic hepatitis or autoimmune hepatitis). |
| **Biliary Colic** | Intermittent epigastric and right upper quadrant pain that is worse after eating a fatty meal. |

| | |
|---|---|
| **Cholecystitis** | Persistent right upper quadrant pain associated with nausea, vomiting and a fever. Patients may have a preceding history of biliary colic. |
| **Acute Cholangitis** | Characterised by persistent right upper quadrant pain, jaundice and a fever (Charcot's triad). Patients are usually very unwell and require urgent intervention. |
| **Peptic Ulcer Disease** | Chronic history of burning epigastric pain that may occur at the time of a meal (gastric ulcer) or a few hours afterwards (duodenal ulcer). If the ulcer is bleeding, the patient may also describe melaena. |
| **Pancreatitis** | Gradual onset severe epigastric pain associated with nausea and vomiting. Patients may have a history of alcohol excess or known gallstones. |
| **Lower Lobe Pneumonia** | Gradual onset chest discomfort, shortness of breath and cough productive of yellow-green sputum. May be accompanied by a fever and lethargy. |
| **Urinary Tract Calculi** | Waxing and waning unilateral loin pain that may radiate towards the groin. The pain can be incredibly intense and cause nausea and vomiting. Patients may also experience dysuria. Accompanying features of sepsis are a red flag symptom that may be suggestive of an infected and obstructed urinary tract. |
| **Pyelonephritis** | Unilateral loin pain that may be associated with dysuria and urinary frequency. Patients may also be systemically unwell with a fever. |

# Red Flags

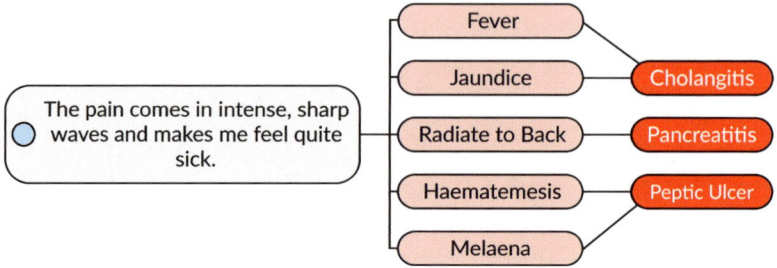

Acute cholangitis can lead to rapidly worsening sepsis that requires decompression of the biliary system. The main features of acute cholangitis are summarised as **Charcot's triad** (fever, jaundice and RUQ pain). A history of intense pain that **radiates to the back** is suggestive of pancreatitis. Though most cases of pancreatitis can be managed with fluid resuscitation and analgesia or removal of an offending stone, it can lead to an overwhelming systemic inflammatory response that can cause multi-organ failure. It is, therefore, important to identify and treat acute pancreatitis effectively.

Patients who are unwell with sepsis or who are simply in a lot of pain may appear **tachypnoeic**, however, it may also be suggestive of a lower lobe pneumonia, especially when accompanied by desaturation. Peptic ulcers are very common, however, the presence of **haematemesis** or **melaena** associated with severe RUQ pain may be suggestive of a bleeding peptic ulcer that could also be at risk of perforating.

# Assessment

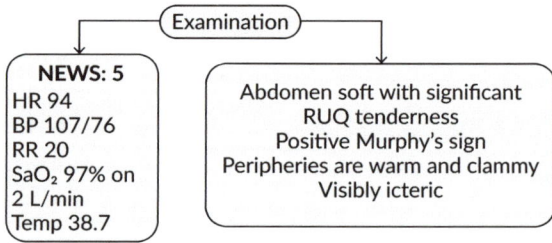

## *Observations*

Patients with infectious or inflammatory conditions (e.g. hepatitis, cholecystitis, cholangitis, pancreatitis, pneumonia and pyelonephritis) may have developed a **fever** and other features of systemic inflammation (e.g. tachycardia and hypotension). Respiratory diseases like PE and pneumonia are more likely to cause **tachypnoea** and **hypoxia**, however, this may also be a manifestation of severe sepsis or severe pancreatitis (due to acute respiratory distress syndrome).

## *Examination*

**Murphy's sign** is a useful test of gallbladder inflammation and may be suggestive of cholecystitis or cholangitis. Patients with cholangitis and hepatitis may be **visibly icteric**. If patients have a **rigid and exquisitely tender abdomen** in the context of previous RUQ or epigastric pain, a perforated peptic ulcer should be considered. Patients with pyelonephritis, on the other hand, may demonstrate **renal angle tenderness** and may also be tender in the suprapubic region due to a lower urinary tract infection. In cases of haemorrhagic pancreatitis, **Grey Turner** and **Cullen's signs** may be noted (though this is rare). The chest should also be auscultated as part of the assessment, as right **basal crepitations** may be heard in patients with pneumonia.

# Acute Cholangitis

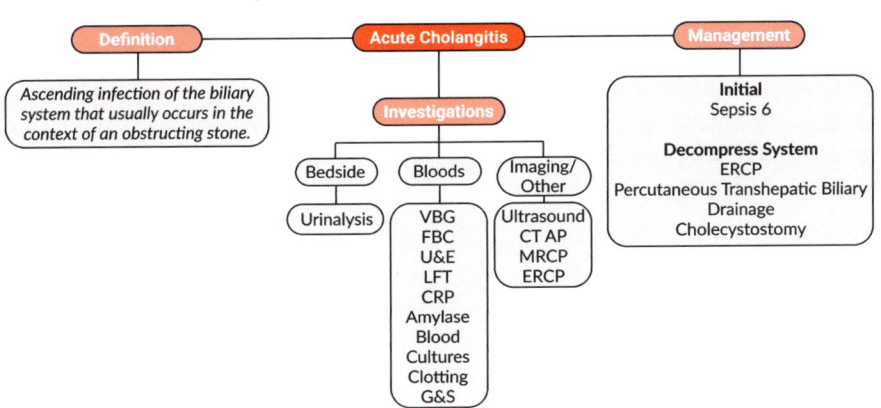

## Definition

Acute cholangitis (also known as ascending cholangitis) is a serious infection of the biliary tree that usually occurs secondary to an obstructing gallstone. It can lead to severe sepsis.

## Investigations

At the bedside, **urinalysis** can be useful in demonstrating evidence of biliary obstruction. This will be evidenced by a negative urobilinogen which suggests that bile is not flowing into the intestines. A **VBG** provides useful early information that can help determine the severity of the infection — lactic acidosis would indicate severe infection and the bilirubin can also be quantified. The inflammatory markers are likely to be raised (**FBC** and **CRP**) and the **LFT** is likely to show an obstructive pattern (raised ALP and GGT). As the infection can ascend and spread into the circulation through the liver, **blood cultures** should be taken as this can allow identification of the organism and its sensitivities. A patient with acute cholangitis is likely to require some form of intervention to decompress the obstructed biliary system so a **clotting screen** and **G&S** should also be taken during the initial work-up.

As acute pancreatitis is a reasonable differential diagnosis, the serum **amylase** level should also be checked — it is likely to be somewhat raised with most causes of RUQ pain, however, it will be significantly elevated in pancreatitis.

An **abdominal ultrasound** scan can demonstrate a dilated common bile duct. In many cases, a **CT abdomen and pelvis with contrast** will be requested to better delineate the anatomy and plan surgical intervention. An **MRCP** (magnetic resonance cholangiopancreatography) is a specialised form of MRI that better visualises the biliary tree and an **ERCP** (endoscopic retrograde cholangiopancreatography) has both diagnostic and therapeutic applications — it can be used to inject dye into the biliary tree to locate and remove the obstructing stone.

## *Management*

A patient with acute cholangitis is likely to be systemically unwell so should be managed in accordance with the **sepsis 6** protocol (administer broad-spectrum antibiotics, oxygen and IV fluids). The obstructed system will then need to be urgently decompressed to gain control of the source of the infection. This can be achieved via an **ERCP**, **percutaneous transhepatic biliary drainage** or a **cholecystostomy**.

# Bridge Box

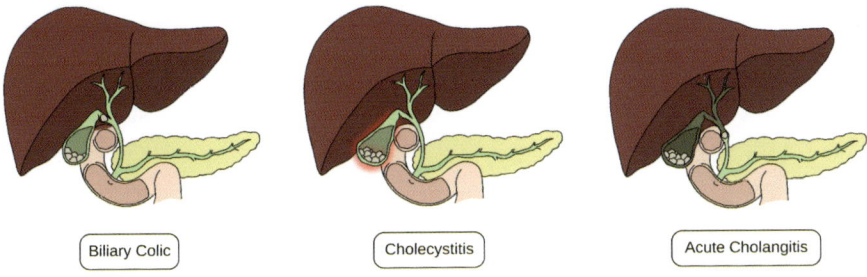

Biliary Colic

Cholecystitis

Acute Cholangitis

Gallstone-related causes of RUQ pain.

# Chapter 13

# Iliac Fossa Pain

Abdominal pain is an extremely common presentation, and often the site of the pain can provide important clues about the underlying cause. Iliac fossa pain has a similar range of differentials on both sides given the bilateral representation of several organs. There are, however, a few causes that are specific to one side.

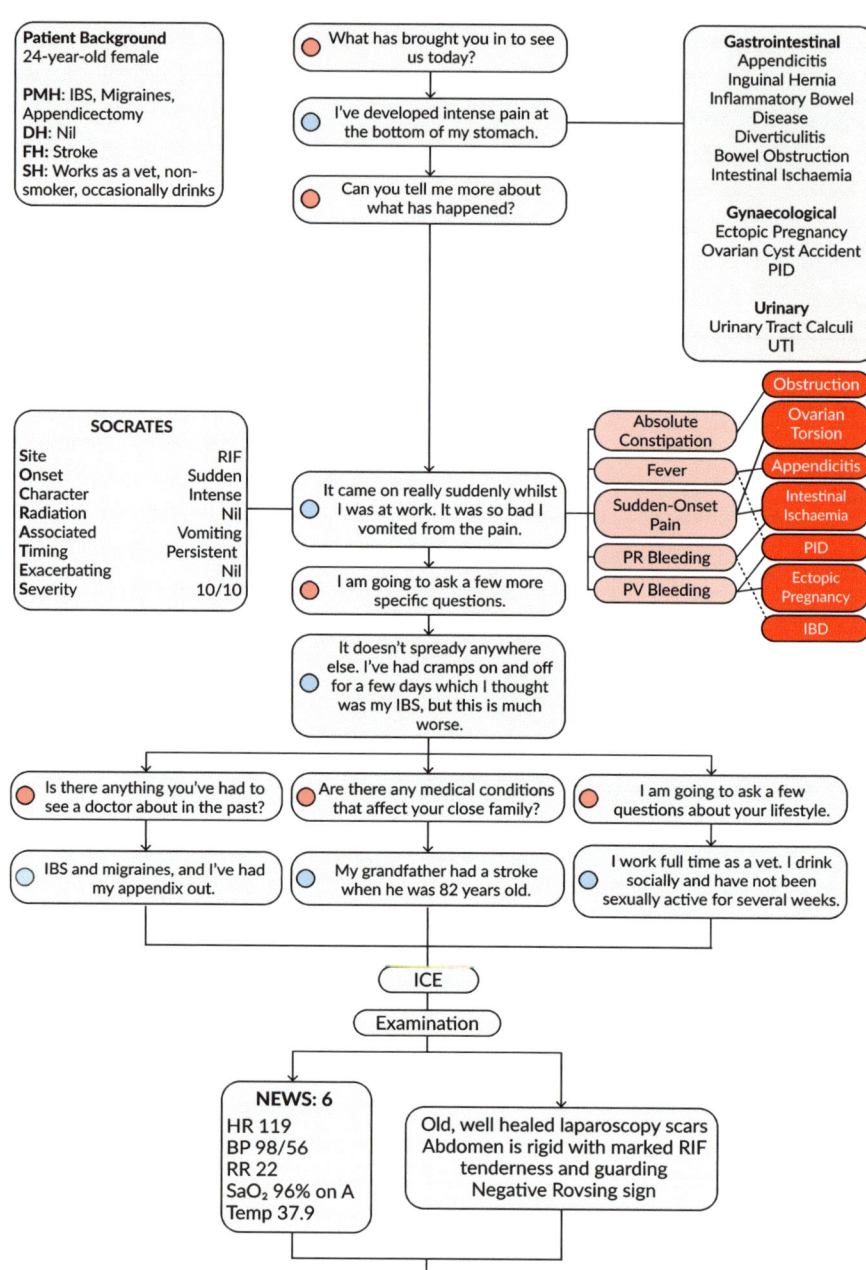

**Patient Background**
24-year-old female

**PMH:** IBS, Migraines, Appendicectomy
**DH:** Nil
**FH:** Stroke
**SH:** Works as a vet, non-smoker, occasionally drinks

What has brought you in to see us today?

I've developed intense pain at the bottom of my stomach.

Can you tell me more about what has happened?

**Gastrointestinal**
Appendicitis
Inguinal Hernia
Inflammatory Bowel Disease
Diverticulitis
Bowel Obstruction
Intestinal Ischaemia

**Gynaecological**
Ectopic Pregnancy
Ovarian Cyst Accident
PID

**Urinary**
Urinary Tract Calculi
UTI

**SOCRATES**

| | |
|---|---|
| Site | RIF |
| Onset | Sudden |
| Character | Intense |
| Radiation | Nil |
| Associated | Vomiting |
| Timing | Persistent |
| Exacerbating | Nil |
| Severity | 10/10 |

It came on really suddenly whilst I was at work. It was so bad I vomited from the pain.

I am going to ask a few more specific questions.

Absolute Constipation

Fever

Sudden-Onset Pain

PR Bleeding

PV Bleeding

Obstruction

Ovarian Torsion

Appendicitis

Intestinal Ischaemia

PID

Ectopic Pregnancy

IBD

It doesn't spready anywhere else. I've had cramps on and off for a few days which I thought was my IBS, but this is much worse.

Is there anything you've had to see a doctor about in the past?

Are there any medical conditions that affect your close family?

I am going to ask a few questions about your lifestyle.

IBS and migraines, and I've had my appendix out.

My grandfather had a stroke when he was 82 years old.

I work full time as a vet. I drink socially and have not been sexually active for several weeks.

ICE

Examination

**NEWS: 6**

HR 119
BP 98/56
RR 22
SaO₂ 96% on A
Temp 37.9

Old, well healed laparoscopy scars
Abdomen is rigid with marked RIF tenderness and guarding
Negative Rovsing sign

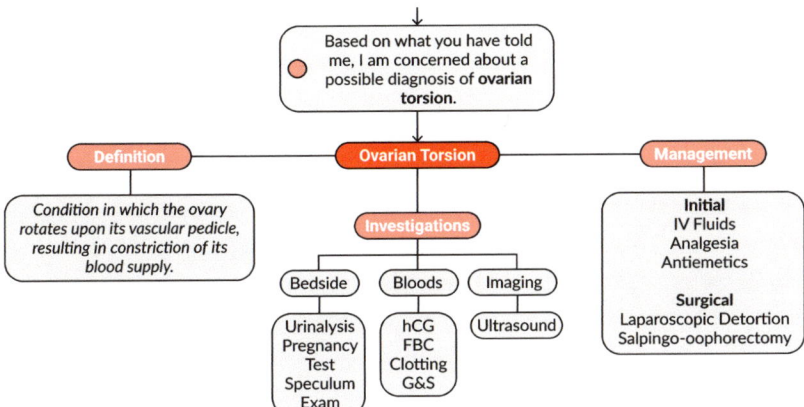

# Patient Background

**Patient Background**
24-year-old female

**PMH**: IBS, Migraines, Appendicectomy
**DH**: Nil
**FH**: Stroke
**SH**: Works as a vet, non-smoker, occasionally drinks

The **sex** of the patient is important to consider as diseases affecting the female reproductive organs are common causes of lower abdominal pain (e.g. ovarian cyst accident). Furthermore, **younger** women are more likely to develop most causes of acute abdominal pain related to the female reproductive organs. When assessing a transgender patient with abdominal pain, you should sensitively enquire about their operative history. For example, it is important to establish whether a transgender man still has ovaries as this may affect their differential diagnosis. Transgender people are known to be at increased risk of poor physical and mental health outcomes, in part due to misdiagnosis and a poor understanding, among healthcare professionals, of the specific health concerns that affect the transgender community.

A background of **gynaecological diseases** (e.g. heavy menstrual bleeding and fibroids) may suggest that further investigations tailored towards gynaecological causes are warranted. A patient's **prior surgical history** will help rule out certain diagnoses (e.g. previous appendicectomy) and increase the risk of other diagnoses (e.g. small bowel obstruction).

## Differential Diagnosis

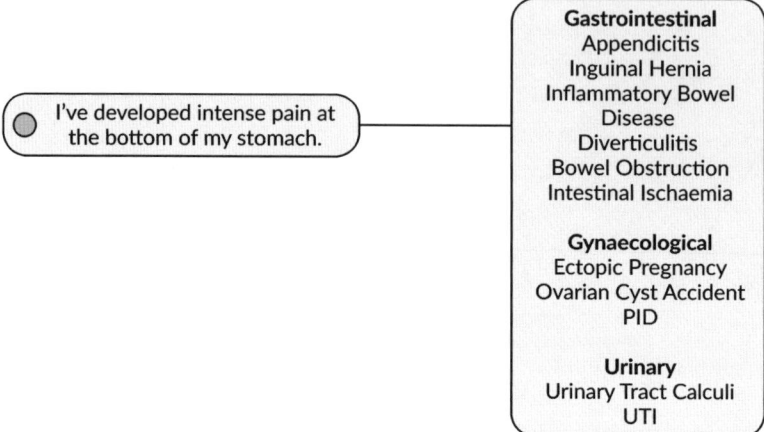

It is easiest to think of the potential causes of RIF pain by going through the organs that lie in that anatomical space.

The main **gastrointestinal** causes to consider are appendicitis, inguinal hernia, inflammatory bowel disease (Crohn's disease has a predilection for affecting the terminal ileum), bowel obstruction and intestinal ischaemia.

When assessing women and some transgender men, you should ask questions pertaining to gynaecological symptoms, such as irregular periods, abnormal vaginal discharge and dyspareunia. This will help identify **gynaecological** causes, such as ectopic pregnancy, ovarian cyst accidents and pelvic inflammatory disease (PID). Some patients with chronic conditions such as fibroids or endometriosis may present to A&E with a particularly severe episode of pain that cannot be managed at home.

Urinary tract calculi and UTIs are common **urinary** conditions that can also present with RIF pain.

# SOCRATES

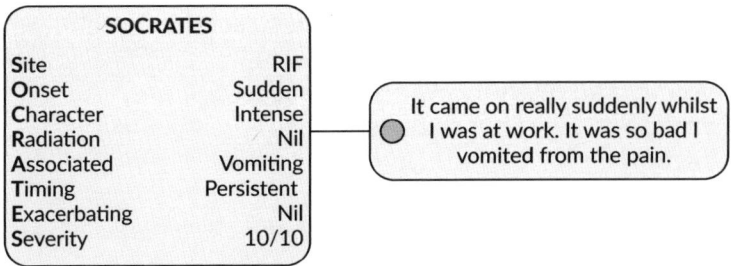

| SOCRATES | |
|---|---|
| Site | RIF |
| Onset | Sudden |
| Character | Intense |
| Radiation | Nil |
| Associated | Vomiting |
| Timing | Persistent |
| Exacerbating | Nil |
| Severity | 10/10 |

*It came on really suddenly whilst I was at work. It was so bad I vomited from the pain.*

There are a few patterns of symptoms that are worth keeping at the back of your mind while you explore SOCRATES in a patient presenting with iliac fossa pain.

- **Site**
  - **Usually Right**: Appendicitis
  - **Usually Left**: Diverticulitis
  - **Either Side**: Inguinal hernia, inflammatory bowel disease, bowel obstruction, intestinal ischaemia, ectopic pregnancy, ovarian cyst accident, ovarian torsion, PID, urinary tract calculi and UTI
- **Onset**
  - **Sudden**: Ovarian torsion, urinary tract calculi, intestinal ischaemia, ovarian cyst accident and incarcerated hernia
  - **Gradual**: Appendicitis, inflammatory bowel disease, diverticulitis, bowel obstruction, PID, ectopic pregnancy and UTI
- **Character**
  - **Intense**: Ovarian torsion and urinary tract calculi
  - **Dull**: Appendicitis, inflammatory bowel disease, diverticulitis, ectopic pregnancy, UTI, bowel obstruction, incarcerated hernia and intestinal ischaemia
- **Radiation**
  - **Loin to Groin**: Urinary tract calculi
  - **Umbilical to RIF**: Appendicitis
- **Associated Symptoms**
  - **Vaginal Discharge and Irregular Bleeding**: PID and ectopic pregnancy
  - **Dysuria**: UTI and urinary tract calculi

- ○ **Diarrhoea and PR Bleeding**: Inflammatory bowel disease, diverticulitis and intestinal ischaemia
- ○ **Abdominal Distension**: Bowel obstruction
- **Timing**
  - ○ **Waxing and Waning**: Urinary tract calculi
  - ○ **Persistent**: All other causes
- **Exacerbating**
  - ○ **Sex**: PID
  - ○ **Eating**: Intestinal ischaemia (*'gut claudication'*)
- **Severity**
  - ○ **Very Severe**: Urinary tract calculi and ovarian torsion

Read through the classical presentations table in the following section to develop an understanding of how the main differentials are classically present.

## Classical Presentations

| Differential | Classical Presentation |
|---|---|
| **Appendicitis** | Subacute onset epigastric pain that eventually radiates to the right iliac fossa. Associated with nausea, vomiting and diarrhoea. May also cause systemic upset (fever). |
| **Inguinal Hernia (Incarcerated)** | Sudden onset severe abdominal pain with an irreducible lump emerging from the inguinal canal (into the scrotum in men). If it is causing an obstruction, patients may also be vomiting and be unable to pass faeces or flatus. |
| **Inflammatory Bowel Disease** | Crohn's disease tends to present with subacute onset RIF pain associated with diarrhoea (due to terminal ileitis). There may be a background of episodic diarrhoea and systemic upset. Ulcerative colitis is more commonly associated with rectal bleeding. |
| **Diverticulitis** | Gradual onset left iliac fossa pain which may be associated with diarrhoea and rectal bleeding. Patients may also have a fever. |

| | |
|---|---|
| **Bowel Obstruction** | Subacute onset generalised abdominal pain associated with absolute constipation and vomiting. Patients may have a history of previous abdominal surgery. |
| **Intestinal Ischaemia** | **Acute Mesenteric Ischaemia**: Sudden onset generalised abdominal pain associated with hypotension and a relatively normal abdominal examination. **Chronic Mesenteric Ischaemia**: Gradual onset abdominal pain that occurs soon after eating (sometimes referred to as gut claudication). **Ischaemic Colitis**: Sudden onset left-sided abdominal pain associated with rectal bleeding. |
| **Ectopic Pregnancy** | Acute onset iliac fossa pain associated with abnormal vaginal bleeding in a woman of fertile age. It is often associated with nausea and vomiting, and they may mention that their period is delayed. |
| **Ovarian Cyst Accident** | Sudden onset iliac fossa pain in a patient that is systemically well. The pain resolves spontaneously and there may have been some preceding, milder iliac fossa discomfort from the presence of the cyst. |
| **Pelvic Inflammatory Disease** | Gradual onset iliac fossa and suprapubic pain associated with abnormal vaginal discharge and, sometimes, irregular menstrual bleeding. Patients may sometimes be systemically unwell with a fever. |
| **Ovarian Torsion** | Sudden onset severe iliac fossa pain associated with nausea and vomiting. Fails to resolve with simple analgesia. |

| Urinary Tract Calculi | Waxing and waning unilateral loin pain that may radiate towards the groin. The pain can be incredibly intense and cause nausea and vomiting. Patients may also experience dysuria. Accompanying features of sepsis are a red flag symptom that may be suggestive of an infected and obstructed urinary tract. |
| :---: | :--- |
| UTI | Gradual onset lower abdominal pain, dysuria and urinary frequency. Patients may describe their urine as being cloudy and foul-smelling. If the infection ascends towards the kidneys, it can cause loin pain. |

# Red Flags

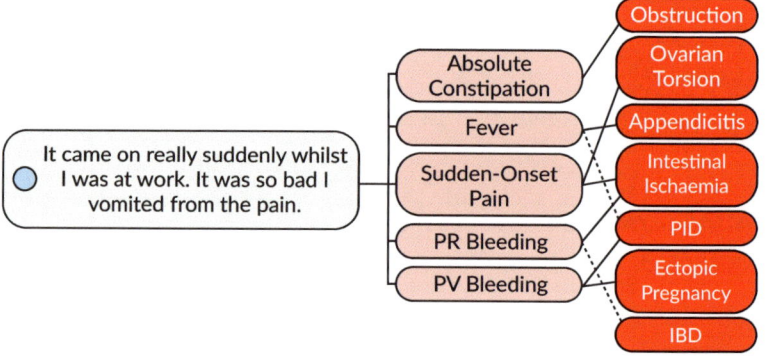

Some of the causes of RIF pain are dangerous and can lead to significant organ damage if not dealt with promptly. Patients with abdominal pain, persistent vomiting and **absolute constipation** (no faeces or flatus) should be managed as bowel obstruction pending further investigation. The presence of a **fever** in the context of severe RIF pain is suggestive of infective or inflammatory pathology (e.g. appendicitis and PID). **Sudden onset pain** is usually associated with ovarian torsion and intestinal ischaemia where the underlying pathophysiological mechanism is discrete and abrupt (e.g. twisting of the ligaments and arterial occlusion by an embolus). **Rectal bleeding** is also associated with intestinal ischaemia and is a common feature in patients with inflammatory bowel disease (especially ulcerative colitis). It may also be noted in some cases of appendicitis. **Vaginal bleeding** is associated with concerning gynaecological causes of RIF pain including ectopic pregnancy and PID.

# Assessment

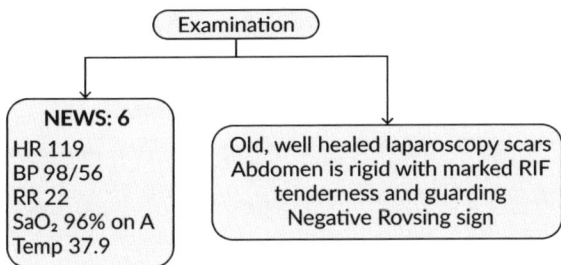

## *Observations*

Patients with inflammatory and infectious conditions (e.g. appendicitis and PID) may be noted to have a **fever** and will likely have other evidence of systemic upset. **Tachycardia** and **tachypnoea** are common features of any patient that is in significant pain.

## *Examination*

Upon inspection, the presence of **surgical scars** suggests that the patient may have adhesions which can cause bowel obstruction. Other features of bowel obstruction include a **distended abdomen** with **absent** or **tinkling bowel sounds**. On the other hand, the presence of the scars may suggest that the patient has already had organs removed that may otherwise be considered in the generation of differentials (e.g. appendicectomy and cholecystectomy). The presence of **guarding** and **rebound tenderness** is suggestive of peritonism which is usually associated with inflammatory and infectious conditions such as appendicitis and inflammatory bowel disease but may also be seen in ectopic pregnancy and PID. Intestinal ischaemia, though very painful, may yield a relatively normal abdominal examination (pain out of proportion with examination findings).

# Ovarian Torsion

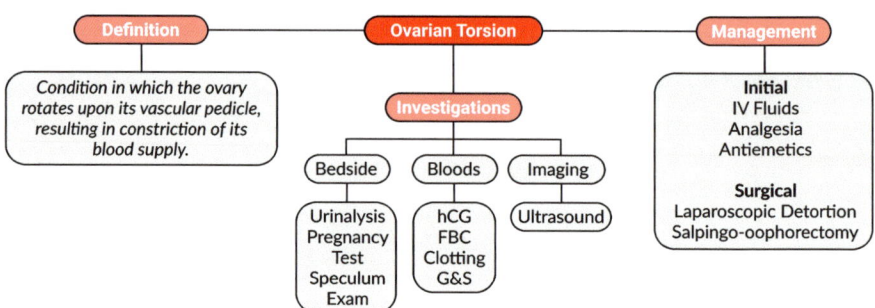

## *Definition*

Ovarian torsion is a condition in which the ovary rotates upon its vascular pedicle. The ensuing constriction of its blood supply can lead to the ovary becoming necrotic, so it requires prompt identification and management.

## *Investigations*

At the bedside, **urinalysis** and a **pregnancy test** are key investigations as they can help distinguish ovarian torsion from other differentials (UTI and ectopic pregnancy). Similarly, a speculum examination will help investigate PID as a possible alternative diagnosis. A **serum hCG** should be requested as ectopic pregnancy is a plausible alternative diagnosis and management is guided, in part, by the serum hCG concentration. As the patient will likely require surgical intervention, a **clotting screen** and **G&S** should be sent. A **transvaginal ultrasound scan** is the imaging modality of choice in suspected ovarian torsion and will likely reveal an enlarged and oedematous ovary which may also demonstrate '*whirlpool sign*' (caused by the twisted vascular pedicle).

### Management

The initial management of ovarian torsion involves resuscitating the patient with IV fluids and controlling their pain and nausea. Subsequent surgical intervention may involve **detortion** of the ovary or a **salpingo-oophorectomy** (removal of the affected ovary and fallopian tube).

## Bridge Box

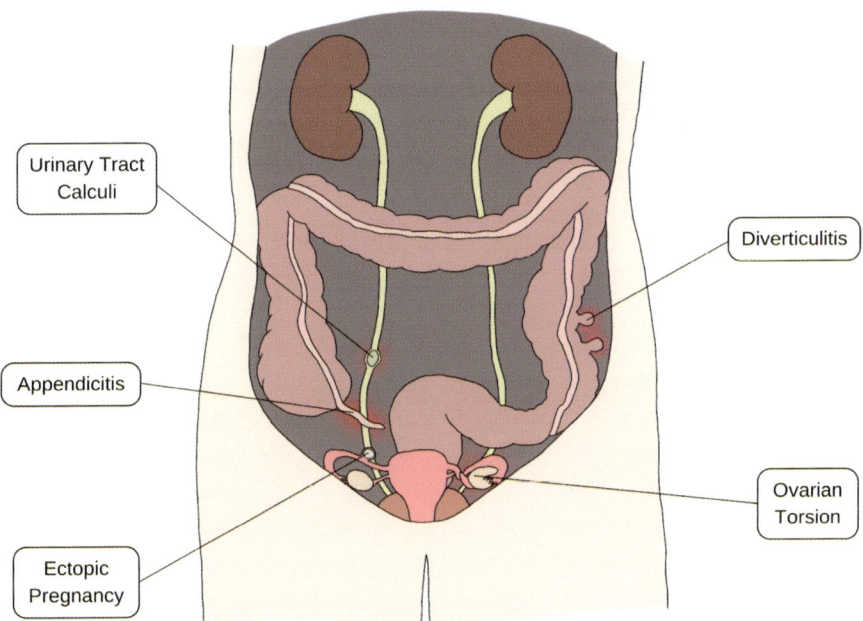

Differentials for iliac fossa pain.

# Chapter 14

# Dysuria

Painful urination is a common and troubling system that can cause significant disruption to a patient's life. Much of the time, it can be managed with simple treatments in primary care, however, there are a few serious causes that require further investigation.

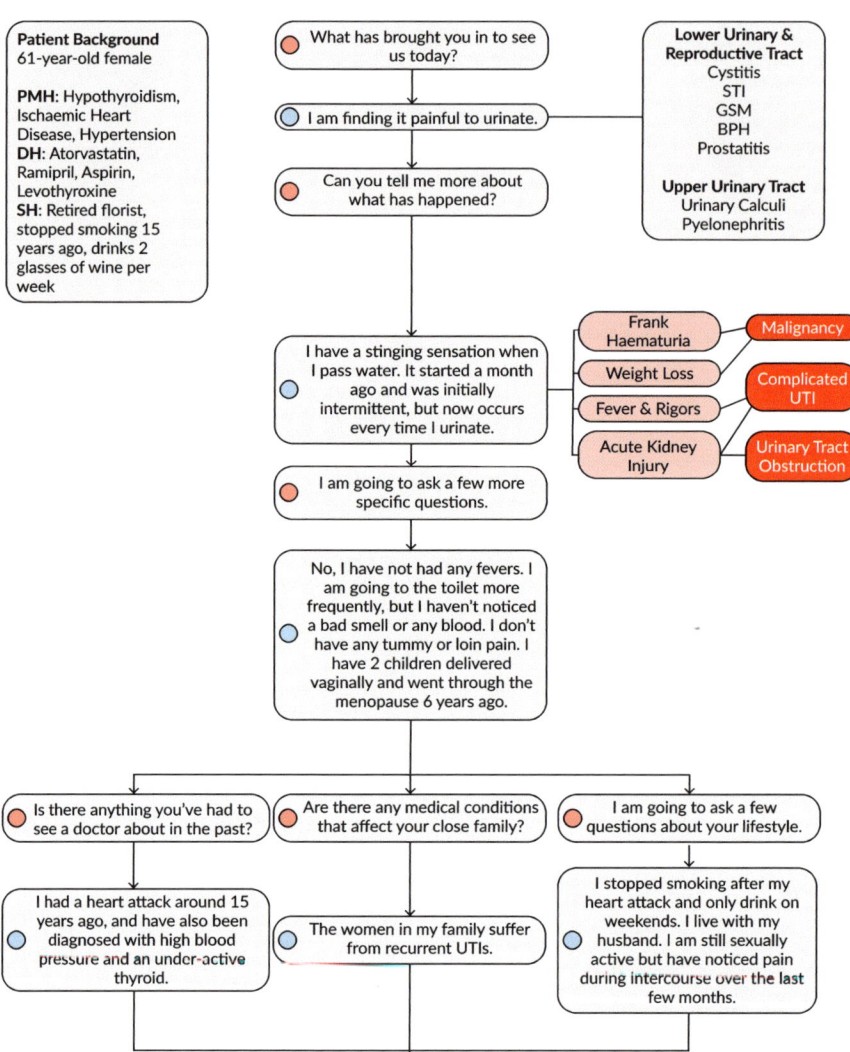

**Patient Background**
61-year-old female

**PMH**: Hypothyroidism, Ischaemic Heart Disease, Hypertension
**DH**: Atorvastatin, Ramipril, Aspirin, Levothyroxine
**SH**: Retired florist, stopped smoking 15 years ago, drinks 2 glasses of wine per week

What has brought you in to see us today?

I am finding it painful to urinate.

Can you tell me more about what has happened?

**Lower Urinary & Reproductive Tract**
Cystitis
STI
GSM
BPH
Prostatitis

**Upper Urinary Tract**
Urinary Calculi
Pyelonephritis

I have a stinging sensation when I pass water. It started a month ago and was initially intermittent, but now occurs every time I urinate.

Frank Haematuria — Malignancy

Weight Loss — Complicated UTI

Fever & Rigors

Acute Kidney Injury — Urinary Tract Obstruction

I am going to ask a few more specific questions.

No, I have not had any fevers. I am going to the toilet more frequently, but I haven't noticed a bad smell or any blood. I don't have any tummy or loin pain. I have 2 children delivered vaginally and went through the menopause 6 years ago.

Is there anything you've had to see a doctor about in the past?

Are there any medical conditions that affect your close family?

I am going to ask a few questions about your lifestyle.

I had a heart attack around 15 years ago, and have also been diagnosed with high blood pressure and an under-active thyroid.

The women in my family suffer from recurrent UTIs.

I stopped smoking after my heart attack and only drink on weekends. I live with my husband. I am still sexually active but have noticed pain during intercourse over the last few months.

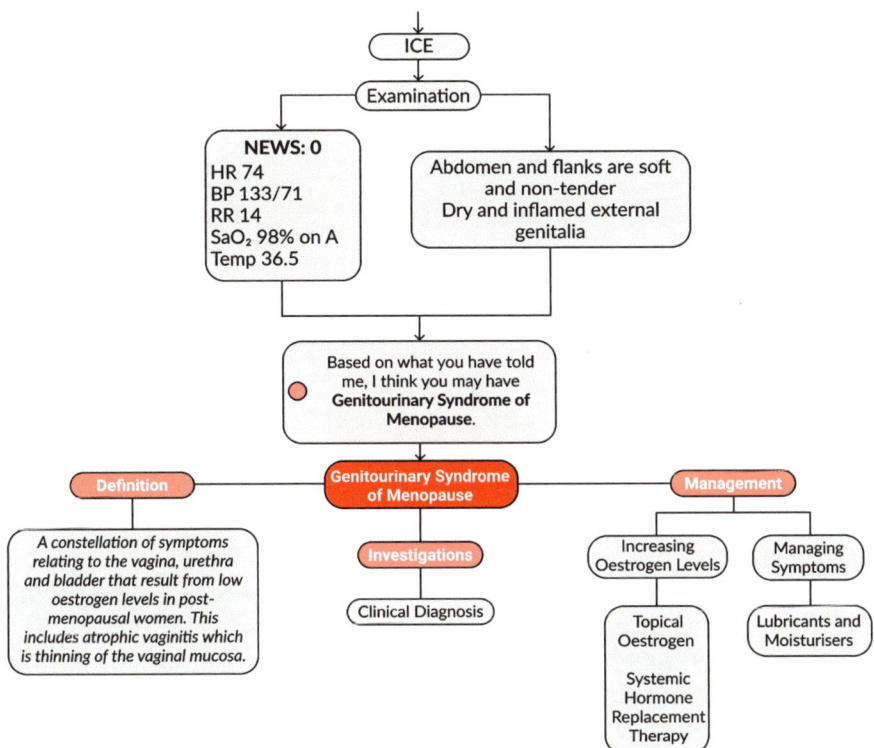

# Patient Background

**Patient Background**
61-year-old female

**PMH**: Hypothyroidism, Ischaemic Heart Disease, Hypertension
**DH**: Atorvastatin, Ramipril, Aspirin, Levothyroxine
**SH**: Retired florist, stopped smoking 15 years ago, drinks 2 glasses of wine per week

With dysuria, the age and sex of the patient can help assess the likelihood of the various differentials. **Women** are at increased risk of developing UTIs due to their shorter urethra. Furthermore, **older men** are more likely to develop lower urinary tract symptoms secondary to prostate enlargement. On the other hand, **younger patients** are at greater risk of contracting sexually transmitted infections (STIs).

## Differential Diagnosis

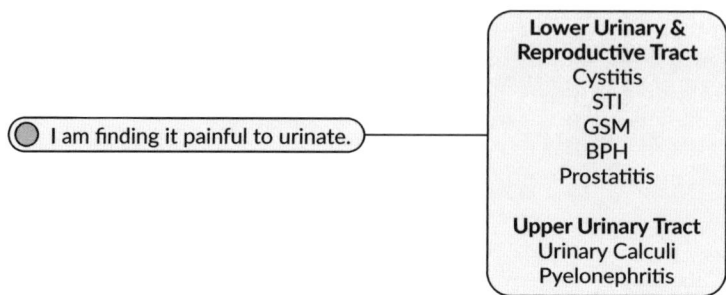

The causes of dysuria can be broadly divided into those relating to the lower urinary tract and upper urinary tract. Common causes of dysuria affecting the lower urinary tract include cystitis (lower urinary tract infection), STIs and genitourinary syndrome (previously known as atrophic vaginitis).

Older patients, in particular, are at greater risk of developing **urinary retention** which, in turn, can cause dysuria. Common factors that contribute to the development of urinary retention in this age group include **prostate enlargement** and **constipation**.

Causes of dysuria originating from the upper urinary tract include **urinary tract calculi** and **pyelonephritis**.

Read through the classical presentations table in the following section to develop an understanding of how the main differentials are classically present.

## Classical Presentations

| Differential | Classical Presentation |
|---|---|
| **Cystitis** | Gradual onset lower abdominal pain, dysuria and urinary frequency. Patients may describe their urine as being cloudy and foul-smelling. |
| **STI** | Gradual onset lower abdominal or scrotal discomfort associated with dysuria and urinary frequency. Patients may also note abnormal vaginal or penile discharge. |

| Genitourinary Syndrome of Menopause | Vaginal dryness associated with dyspareunia and dysuria. Patients may also have other menopausal symptoms such as hot flushes and mood swings. |
|---|---|
| Benign Prostatic Hyperplasia | Occurs in older men and presents with **storage** symptoms (frequency, urgency, nocturia and dysuria) and **voiding** symptoms (hesitancy, incomplete emptying, poor stream and straining). |
| Prostatitis | Dysuria associated with pain upon defecation. Patients may also have penile discharge. |
| Urinary Tract Calculi | Waxing and waning unilateral loin pain that may radiate towards the groin. The pain can be incredibly intense and cause nausea and vomiting. Patients may also experience dysuria. Accompanying features of sepsis are a red flag symptom that may be suggestive of an infected and obstructed urinary tract. |
| Pyelonephritis | Unilateral loin pain that may be associated with dysuria and urinary frequency. Patients may also be systemically unwell with a fever. |

# Red Flags

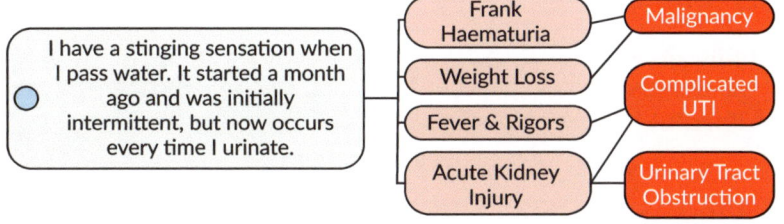

Most cases of dysuria are mild and can be managed with simple treatments as an outpatient, such as antibiotics and analgesia. There are a few features in the clinical history and diagnostic work-up, however, that should raise concern.

Malignancies of the urinary tract (bladder, ureters and kidneys) can cause **frank haematuria** and may be associated with other systemic symptoms such as **weight loss**. Classically, however, haematuria due to malignancy is *painless*.

UTIs can ascend the urinary tract and cause systemic upset which manifests with **fevers and rigors**. Furthermore, pyelonephritis and the organ hypoperfusion associated with sepsis can lead to **acute kidney injury** (manifesting with a raised urea and creatinine on the blood tests). In patients with loin to groin pain suggestive of a urinary tract calculus, the presence of a **fever** and/or **acute kidney injury** are red flag signs suggestive of an infected and obstructed system that requires urgent urology discussion for decompression.

## Assessment

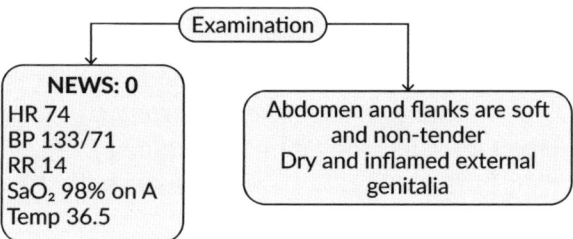

## *Observations*

In infectious causes of dysuria (e.g. UTI and STI), some patients may, if severe, show signs of sepsis (**fever, hypotension** and **tachycardia**).

## *Examination*

**Lower abdominal discomfort** is suggestive of an inflamed or irritated bladder, or female reproductive tract. Patients with pyelonephritis may demonstrate **renal angle tenderness**. In cases of urinary retention, a **palpable, enlarged bladder** may be noted. Dysuria may also arise due to genital abnormalities such as genitourinary syndrome of menopause, in which case the **external genitalia may appear dry and inflamed**.

# Genitourinary Syndrome of Menopause

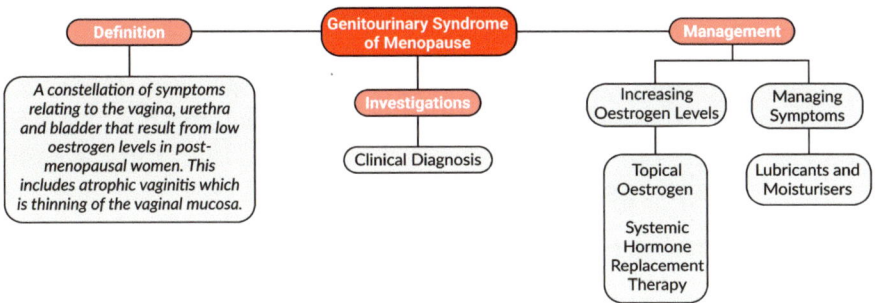

## *Definition*

Previously known as atrophic vaginitis, GSM is a constellation of symptoms relating to the vagina, urethra and bladder that result from low oestrogen levels in postmenopausal women. Without the influence of oestrogen, the vaginal mucosa becomes thin and fragile leading to symptoms, such as dyspareunia, postmenopausal bleeding and dysuria.

## *Investigations*

At the bedside, simple investigations that can help determine the likelihood of alternate diagnoses include **urinalysis**, which will likely be positive for leucocytes and nitrites in infectious causes of dysuria, and positive for blood in the case of urinary tract calculi. If there is any concern about urinary retention, a **post-void bladder scan** can be performed to check the residual volume.

Often GSM and UTIs present with relatively mild symptoms and, hence, do not warrant blood tests. If patients with atrophic vaginitis are presenting with postmenopausal bleeding in addition to dysuria, an **FBC** may be appropriate to assess the extent of the blood loss.

GSM is largely a clinical diagnosis and does not require imaging. In patients presenting with postmenopausal bleeding, however, an **ultrasound scan** should be arranged to check for endometrial hyperplasia and cancer.

## Management

The management of GSM can include non-hormonal agents for symptomatic relief (e.g. lubricants and moisturisers). As the changes arise due to the absence of oestrogen, **topical and systemic oestrogens** can be used to effectively manage the condition.

## Bridge Box

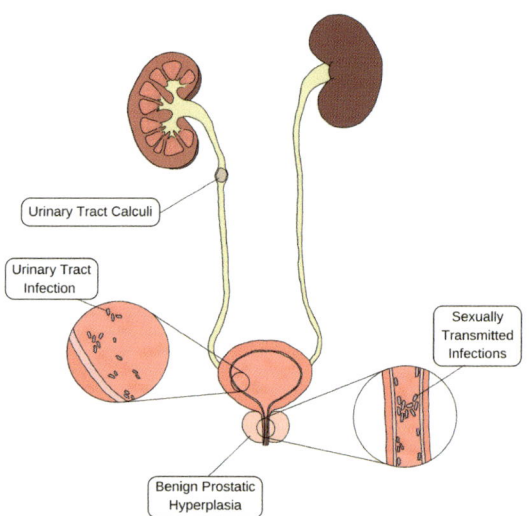

Differentials for dysuria.

# Chapter 15

# Polyuria

Polyuria is the production of excess urine. It can be a troubling and disruptive symptom and is commonly encountered in primary care.

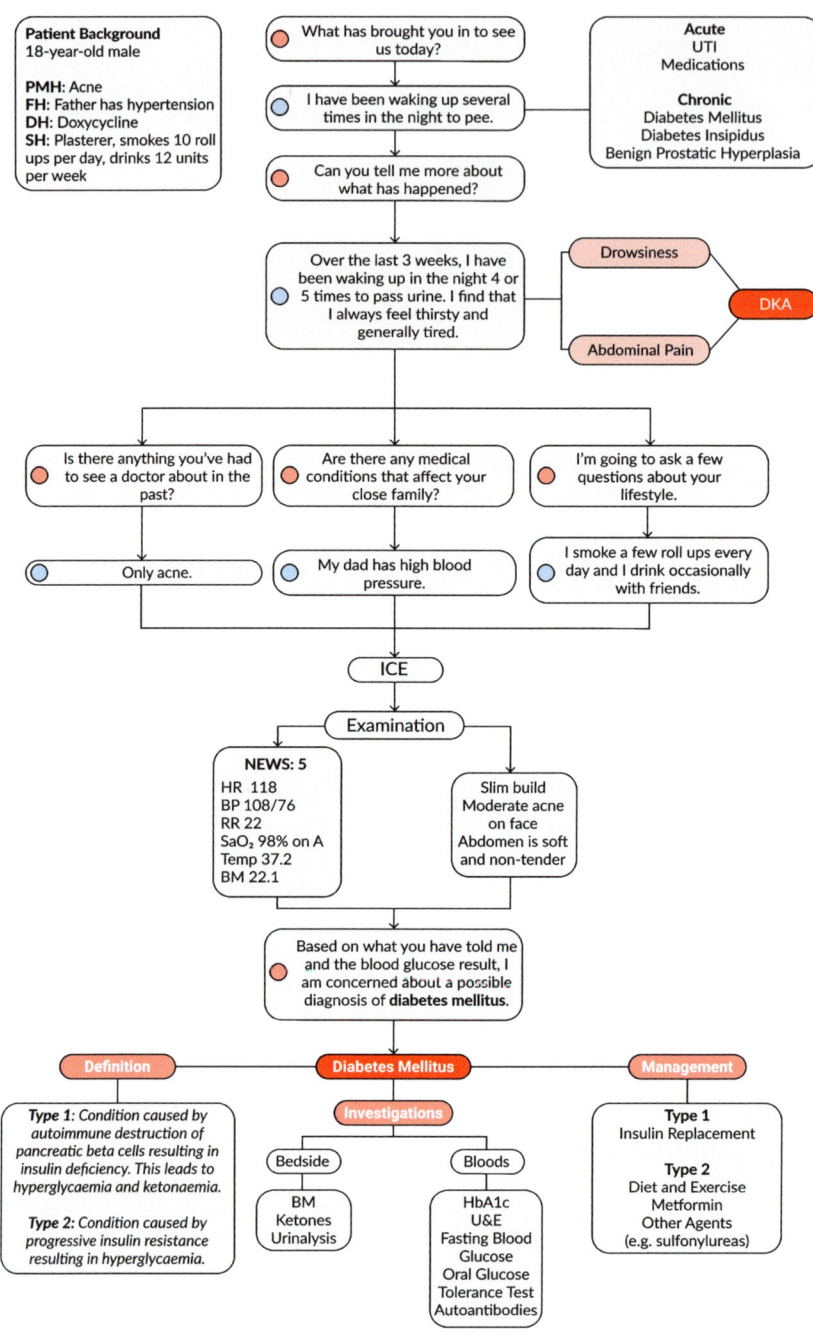

**Patient Background**
18-year-old male

**PMH:** Acne
**FH:** Father has hypertension
**DH:** Doxycycline
**SH:** Plasterer, smokes 10 roll ups per day, drinks 12 units per week

What has brought you in to see us today?

I have been waking up several times in the night to pee.

Can you tell me more about what has happened?

Over the last 3 weeks, I have been waking up in the night 4 or 5 times to pass urine. I find that I always feel thirsty and generally tired.

**Acute**
UTI
Medications

**Chronic**
Diabetes Mellitus
Diabetes Insipidus
Benign Prostatic Hyperplasia

Drowsiness

Abdominal Pain

DKA

Is there anything you've had to see a doctor about in the past?

Are there any medical conditions that affect your close family?

I'm going to ask a few questions about your lifestyle.

Only acne.

My dad has high blood pressure.

I smoke a few roll ups every day and I drink occasionally with friends.

ICE

Examination

**NEWS: 5**
HR 118
BP 108/76
RR 22
SaO$_2$ 98% on A
Temp 37.2
BM 22.1

Slim build
Moderate acne on face
Abdomen is soft and non-tender

Based on what you have told me and the blood glucose result, I am concerned about a possible diagnosis of **diabetes mellitus**.

**Definition**

**Diabetes Mellitus**

**Management**

*Type 1*: Condition caused by autoimmune destruction of pancreatic beta cells resulting in insulin deficiency. This leads to hyperglycaemia and ketonaemia.

*Type 2*: Condition caused by progressive insulin resistance resulting in hyperglycaemia.

**Investigations**

Bedside

BM
Ketones
Urinalysis

Bloods

HbA1c
U&E
Fasting Blood Glucose
Oral Glucose Tolerance Test
Autoantibodies

**Type 1**
Insulin Replacement

**Type 2**
Diet and Exercise
Metformin
Other Agents
(e.g. sulfonylureas)

# Patient Background

> **Patient Background**
> 18-year-old male
>
> **PMH:** Acne
> **FH:** Father has hypertension
> **DH:** Doxycycline
> **SH:** Plasterer, smokes 10 roll
> ups per day, drinks 12 units
> per week

The age of the patient can provide an insight into the likely causes of polyuria. Typically, a relatively acute history of polyuria in **younger patients** is more likely to be in keeping with UTIs and STIs. On the other hand, a more chronic history of frequent urination in **older men** is more likely sugges-tive of a prostate-related issue such as benign prostatic hyperpla-sia or prostate cancer.

The drug history may allude to potential precipitants of polyuria. Patients who are started on **diuretics** should be counselled on the fact that they will be needing to urinate more frequently, however, when used for indications other than fluid overload (e.g. indapam-ide for hypertension and acetazolamide for idiopathic intracranial hypertension), the mechanism of action of the drug may not have been clearly explained to the patient.

# Differential Diagnosis

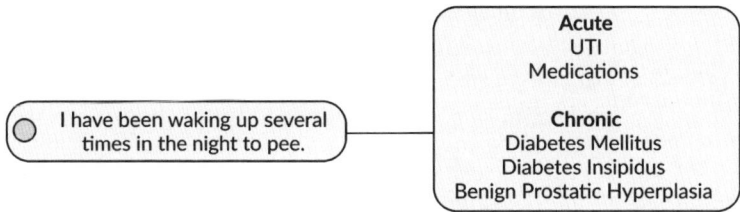

The differentials can be divided based on the acuity of the presen-tation. Patients who have a **UTI** or an **STI** or who have developed polyuria secondary to a **drug** are likely to present with a relatively short history of polyuria. In the case of a UTI, patients may add that their urine is foul-smelling and cloudy and that it *'burns'* when they pass urine.

A more prolonged history of polyuria may be suggestive of an underlying chronic condition, such as **diabetes mellitus** and, more rarely, **diabetes insipidus**. Both conditions will be associated with **polydipsia** and may also feature **weight loss** and **fatigue**. In older men, **benign prostatic hyperplasia (BPH)** is a common cause of polyuria. It is important to ask about **lower urinary tract symptoms** which can be remembered using the mnemonic *FUND HIPS*:

- **F**requency
- **U**rgency
- **N**octuria
- **D**ysuria
- **H**esitancy
- **I**ncomplete Emptying
- **P**oor Stream
- **S**training

Read through the classical presentations table in the following section to develop an understanding of how the main differentials are classically present.

## Classical Presentations

| Differential | Classical Presentation |
|---|---|
| UTI | Gradual onset lower abdominal pain, dysuria and urinary frequency. Patients may describe their urine as being cloudy and foul-smelling. If the infection ascends towards the kidneys, it can cause loin pain. |
| **Medication Side Effect** | Occurs in patients who are taking diuretics (e.g. loop diuretics, thiazide diuretics, aldosterone antagonists and carbonic anhydrase inhibitors). |
| **Diabetes Mellitus** | **Type 1 Diabetes Mellitus**: Presenting in young people with a history of polyuria and nocturia. They may describe some weight loss and trouble gaining weight. They may present acutely with diabetic ketoacidosis.<br>**Type 2 Diabetes Mellitus**: Presenting in adults with polyuria and nocturia. Patients are often overweight and there may be a family history. |

| Diabetes Insipidus | Patients will develop polyuria and polydipsia. There may be a clear precipitant, such as a brain injury or causative medication (e.g. lithium). |
|---|---|
| Benign Prostatic Hyperplasia | Occurs in older men and presents with **storage** symptoms (frequency, urgency, nocturia and dysuria) and **voiding** symptoms (hesitancy, incomplete emptying, poor stream and straining). |

## Red Flags

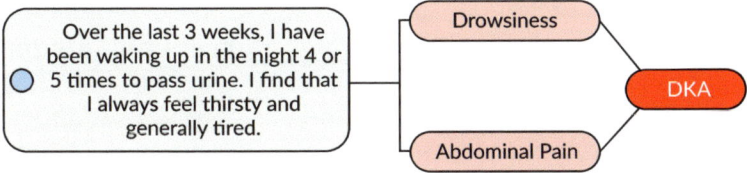

Young patients with type 1 diabetes mellitus may present for the first time with diabetic ketoacidosis (DKA). In such cases, they may also complain of **abdominal pain** and, if severe, they may appear **drowsy**.

Though it is less common than BPH, **prostate cancer** may also present for the first time with polyuria. Possible associated symptoms include **haematuria** and **haematospermia**.

## Assessment

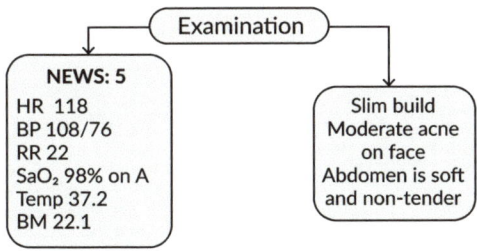

## Observations

The observations alone are unlikely to reveal much useful information in a patient presenting with polyuria. The main exception is a complicated UTI which may cause a **fever**, confusion and systemic upset, especially in frail patients. Patients with DKA may be profoundly dehydrated which manifests with **hypotension** and **tachycardia**.

## Examination

Abdominal examination will likely provide some useful clues in all age groups presenting with polyuria. **Suprapubic tenderness** would be in keeping with a diagnosis of UTI. If there is a **palpably enlarged bladder** that may be tender, it could be suggestive of chronic urinary retention secondary to an obstruction at the prostatic urethra. Chronic retention can lead to overflow incontinence which may, paradoxically, present as polyuria as patients in chronic retention do not usually feel significant discomfort.

　　If a prostatic issue is suspected, a **digital rectal examination** should be performed. This may reveal a **smoothly enlarged prostate with a palpable central sulcus** in BPH or a **craggy, irregularly enlarged prostate** in prostate cancer.

# Diabetes Mellitus

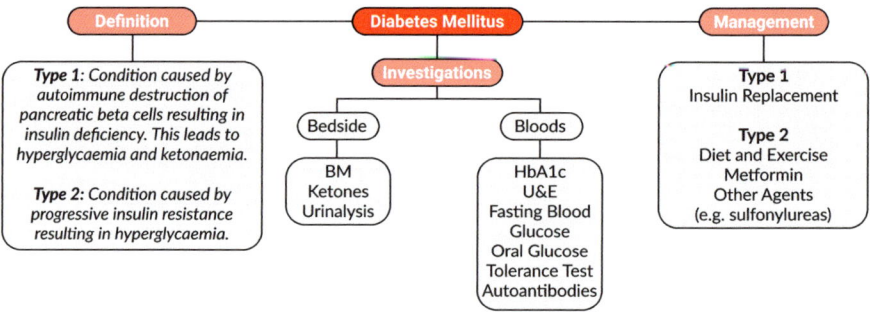

## Definition

Diabetes mellitus refers to a condition in which either a lack of insulin (type 1) or insulin resistance leads to hyperglycaemia. Persistently elevated blood sugar levels can lead to micro- and macrovascular damage (e.g. myocardial infarction, retinopathy and nephropathy).

## Investigations

At the bedside, measuring **capillary glucose and ketones** are useful initial investigations to perform. A random capillary glucose that is over 11.1 mmol/l in a symptomatic patient is suggestive of a diagnosis of diabetes mellitus. A **urine dipstick** is another simple but effective investigation as it will likely demonstrate glycosuria.

A formal diagnosis of diabetes mellitus can be made using **HbA1c** which measures the glycation of haemoglobin and gauges blood sugar levels over the preceding 3 months. A value over 48 mmol/mol in a symptomatic patient is considered diagnostic of diabetes mellitus. A diagnosis can also be made by measuring **fasting blood glucose** or performing an **oral glucose tolerance test**. A panel of antibodies (**anti-islet cell** and **anti-GAD**) will also facilitate a diagnosis of type 1 diabetes mellitus.

## Management

The management of **type 1 diabetes mellitus** focuses on replacing insulin in as physiological a manner as possible. This often involves starting with a basal-bolus regimen and teaching the patient to carbohydrate count to allow them to estimate their insulin requirements as accurately as possible. Some patients may have insulin pumps that deliver a steady infusion of insulin throughout the day and allows them to deliver boluses at mealtimes.

**Type 2 diabetes mellitus** is initially managed with a combination of diet and exercise, and oral agents (e.g. metformin, sulfonylureas and gliptins). In some cases, insulin will also be used.

# Bridge Box

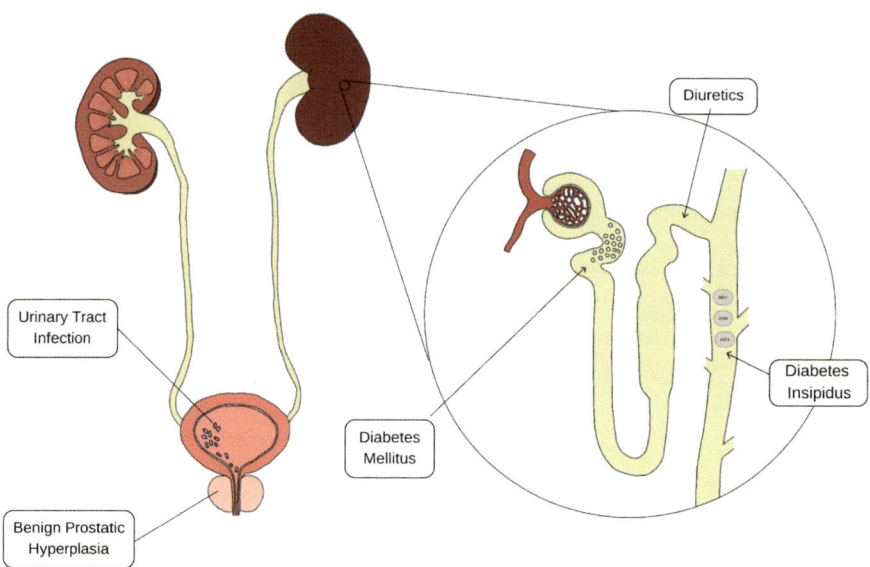

Polyuria can result either from irritation and obstruction of the urinary tract or from interference with the kidneys' reabsorptive mechanisms. Common causes of irritation and obstruction of the urinary tract include urinary tract infections and prostate enlargement, respectively. The elevated serum glucose concentration in patients with undiagnosed diabetes mellitus exceeds the capacity of the proximal tubule to reabsorb the glucose. The presence of glucose within the filtrate creates an osmotic gradient which draws more water into the tubule resulting in increased urine output. Diuretics usually work by blocking various transporters that are responsible for the reabsorption of sodium into the circulation (loop diuretics target the Na/K/Cl triple transporter in the ascending limb of the loop of Henle and thiazide diuretics target the Na/Cl transporter in the distal convoluted tubule). Like glucose, the increased level of sodium within the urinary filtrate draws more water into the tubule resulting in diuresis. ADH acts on the epithelial cells of the collecting duct to increase water reabsorption in response to various physiological changes (e.g. decrease in blood pressure). In diabetes insipidus, patients either fail to produce ADH (central) or their kidneys fail to respond to ADH (nephrogenic).

# Chapter 16

# Constipation

Most people will become constipated at some point in their lives, but this normally improves with simple lifestyle changes. In some cases, the cause of constipation is more complex and requires further investigation and management.

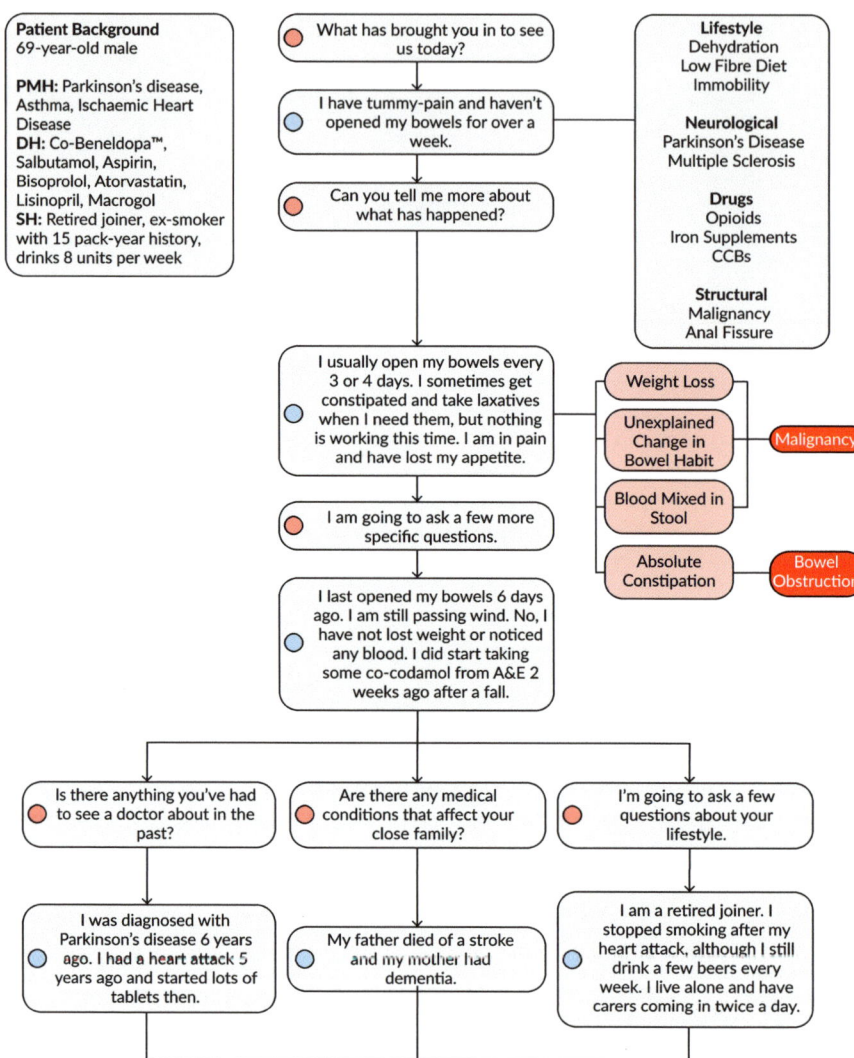

**Patient Background**
69-year-old male

**PMH:** Parkinson's disease,
Asthma, Ischaemic Heart
Disease
**DH:** Co-Beneldopa™,
Salbutamol, Aspirin,
Bisoprolol, Atorvastatin,
Lisinopril, Macrogol
**SH:** Retired joiner, ex-smoker
with 15 pack-year history,
drinks 8 units per week

What has brought you in to see us today?

I have tummy-pain and haven't opened my bowels for over a week.

Can you tell me more about what has happened?

**Lifestyle**
Dehydration
Low Fibre Diet
Immobility

**Neurological**
Parkinson's Disease
Multiple Sclerosis

**Drugs**
Opioids
Iron Supplements
CCBs

**Structural**
Malignancy
Anal Fissure

I usually open my bowels every 3 or 4 days. I sometimes get constipated and take laxatives when I need them, but nothing is working this time. I am in pain and have lost my appetite.

Weight Loss

Unexplained Change in Bowel Habit

Blood Mixed in Stool

Malignancy

I am going to ask a few more specific questions.

Absolute Constipation

Bowel Obstruction

I last opened my bowels 6 days ago. I am still passing wind. No, I have not lost weight or noticed any blood. I did start taking some co-codamol from A&E 2 weeks ago after a fall.

Is there anything you've had to see a doctor about in the past?

Are there any medical conditions that affect your close family?

I'm going to ask a few questions about your lifestyle.

I was diagnosed with Parkinson's disease 6 years ago. I had a heart attack 5 years ago and started lots of tablets then.

My father died of a stroke and my mother had dementia.

I am a retired joiner. I stopped smoking after my heart attack, although I still drink a few beers every week. I live alone and have carers coming in twice a day.

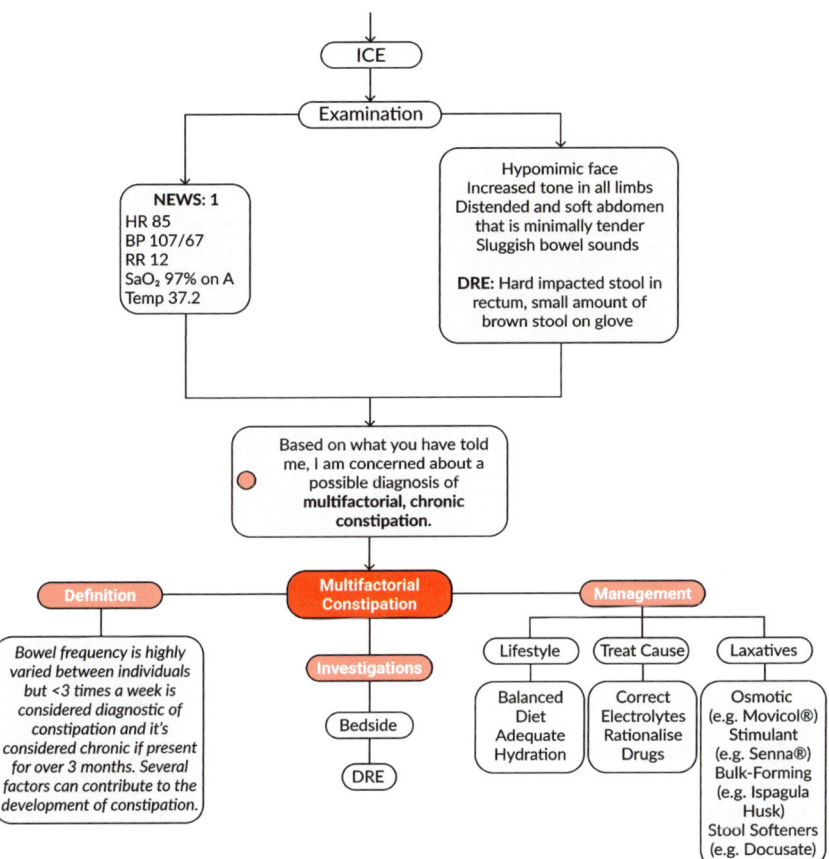

# Patient Background

**Patient Background**
69-year-old male

**PMH:** Parkinson's disease, Asthma, Ischaemic Heart Disease
**DH:** Co-Beneldopa™, Salbutamol, Aspirin, Bisoprolol, Atorvastatin, Lisinopril, Macrogol
**SH:** Retired joiner, ex-smoker with 15 year-pack history, drinks 8 units per week

Constipation can affect patients of **any age**, however, it tends to be particularly common in elderly patients. Immobility is an important lifestyle factor that contributes to the development of constipation, so patients who are particularly frail or those that have conditions that **limit their mobility** (e.g. osteoarthritis) are more likely to develop constipation. It is worth noting any **neurological conditions**, such as

Parkinson's disease and multiple sclerosis, that may impair gastro-intestinal motility and cause difficulty mobilising. There are many **drugs** that can contribute to a patient becoming constipated, so the patient's regular medications should also be screened.

## Differential Diagnosis

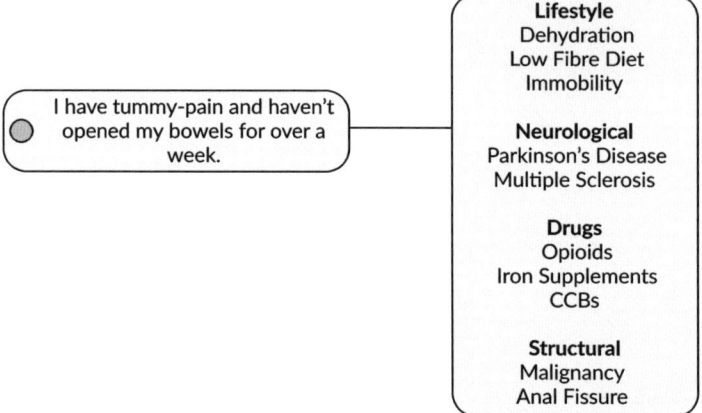

The causes of constipation can be divided into lifestyle, neurologi-cal, drug-related and structural. Of these, lifestyle causes are most common and usually relatively easy to treat. Patients should be asked about their **fluid intake** and their usual **diet**, as well as their **mobility**. Any neurological condition that impairs a patient's mobil-ity increases the risk of constipation, but two relatively common conditions that are strongly associated with constipation due to abnormalities in intestinal motility and impaired mobility include **Parkinson's disease** and **multiple sclerosis**.

The common drug classes that tend to lead to constipation are **opioids**, **iron supplements** and **calcium channel blockers**, so patients should be asked about any recent changes to their medi-cations. **Malignancy** (i.e. colorectal cancer) is a concerning struc-tural cause that should be considered, particularly in older patients presenting with constipation. **Anal fissures** are common and can cause intense anal pain during defecation which makes patients reluctant to go to the toilet resulting in a vicious cycle of constipa-tion and worsening fissures.

Read through the classical presentations table in the following section to develop an understanding of how the main differentials are classically present.

## Classical Presentations

| Differential | Classical Presentation |
|---|---|
| **Lifestyle Factors** | Gradual onset of hard stools and infrequent bowel motions in patients who are known to have a diet that is low in fibre, poor fluid intake and reduced mobility. |
| **Parkinson's Disease** | Gradual onset history of worsening mobility. Classically presenting with bradykinesia, rigidity, postural instability and a stooped, shuffling gait. Subsequent autonomic dysfunction can lead to constipation and urinary incontinence. |
| **Multiple Sclerosis** | Classically presents with two or more episodes of acute neurological defects (e.g. optic neuritis) and can follow a relapsing–remitting, primary progressive or secondary progressive pattern. Can progress to limit mobility and affect bladder and bowel function. |
| **Drug-Induced** | Common causes include iron supplements, calcium channel blockers and opioid analgesia. |
| **Colorectal Cancer** | Gradual onset of worsening constipation that may be associated with rectal bleeding and unintentional weight loss. May sometimes present with bowel obstruction secondary to a malignant stricture. May be identified after incidentally noting iron deficiency anaemia on a routine blood test. |

| | |
|---|---|
| **Anal Fissure** | Tearing pain around the anal opening when attempting to pass a bowel motion. Stools may be streaked in blood or fresh blood may be evident upon wiping with toilet paper. |

## Red Flags

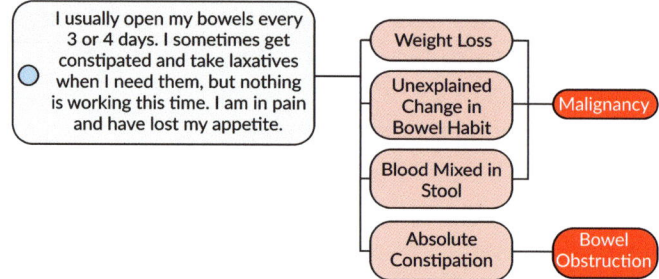

The main acutely concerning causes and consequences of constipation are malignancy (colorectal cancer) and bowel obstruction. Older patients with **altered bowel habits** should be asked about the presence of **blood in the stool** and whether they have **unintentionally lost weight** recently. These features are associated with malignancy. Patients with bowel obstruction tend to present acutely with **absolute constipation** (no faeces or flatus), abdominal distension and vomiting. It is worth noting that vomiting may not always be a prominent feature of bowel obstruction, especially when the transition point is in the distal large bowel.

## Assessment

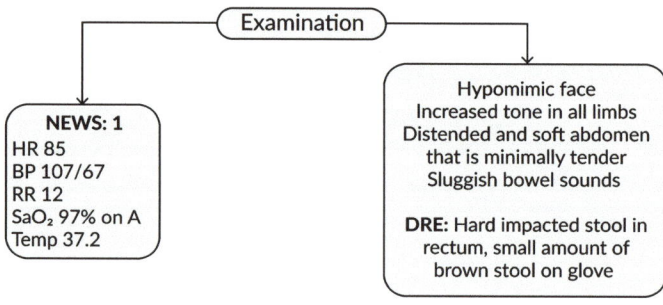

## *Observations*

Constipation tends to present with a chronic history, and, in these cases, it is unlikely to cause any significant changes in the patient's observations.

## *Examination*

It is very unlikely that constipation will be the presenting feature of a neurological condition, however, you may note the **degree of physical impairment** that has been caused by the neurological condition (e.g. resting tremor and spasticity). In cases of bowel obstruction, the abdomen is likely to be **distended** with a **resonant percussion note** and **tinkling or absent bowel sounds**. The patient may also be complaining of generalised abdominal discomfort. A **DRE** is often appropriate in evaluating a patient with chronic constipation because it may reveal hard stool in the rectum.

## Multifactorial Chronic Constipation

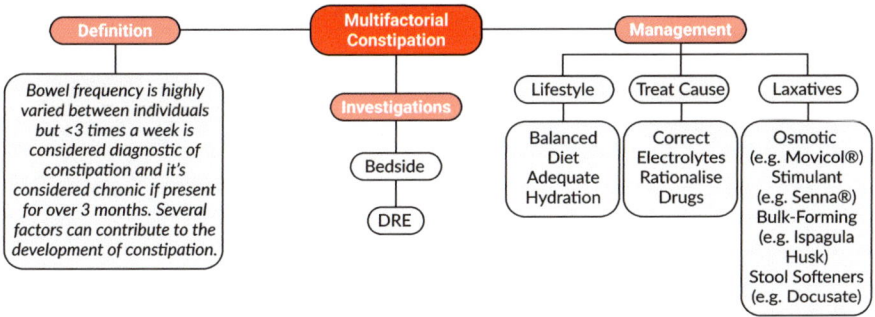

## *Definition*

Bowel frequency has a relatively broad range that is considered normal, and it is important to establish what the patient considers to be normal before making a diagnosis of constipation. Generally speaking, a bowel frequency of fewer than 3 times per week for longer than 3 months is considered diagnostic of chronic constipation. Often, several factors will contribute to the development of constipation.

## *Investigations*

Constipation can usually be diagnosed clinically, but a DRE may be performed to determine if there is hard stool within the rectum. Occasionally, some blood tests may be sent to determine whether there are any underlying medical causes of constipation (e.g. TFT for hypothyroidism and bone profile for hypercalcaemia). If a patient has developed bowel obstruction secondary to constipation or if the diagnosis is uncertain, an **abdominal X-ray** or **CT abdomen and pelvis** may be performed.

## *Management*

Often, simple **lifestyle changes** such as eating a balanced diet and increasing fluid intake can help resolve the symptoms of constipation. If a clear underlying precipitant is identified (e.g. hypercalcaemia and opioids) these should be attended to accordingly. There is an array of **laxatives** that can be used to help the patient establish a normal bowel habit. If the DRE reveals hard, impacted stool within the rectum, suppositories and enemas should be considered in addition to oral laxatives to help loosen the stools.

# Bridge Box

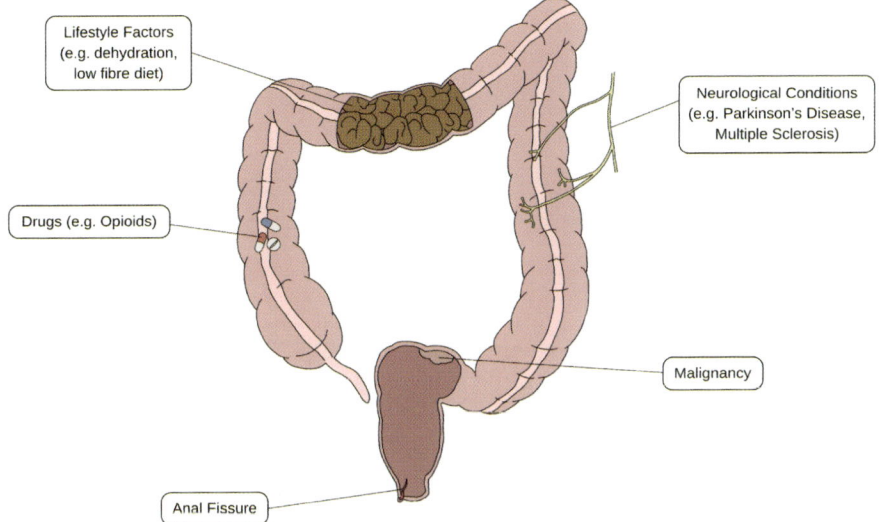

Lifestyle Factors
(e.g. dehydration,
low fibre diet)

Neurological Conditions
(e.g. Parkinson's Disease,
Multiple Sclerosis)

Drugs (e.g. Opioids)

Malignancy

Anal Fissure

Causes of constipation.

# Chapter 17

# Diarrhoea

Most people will experience a bout of diarrhoea at some point and most cases will resolve spontaneously. Severe and/or chronic diarrhoea, however, may be suggestive of a serious underlying condition that can be very debilitating if not attended to promptly.

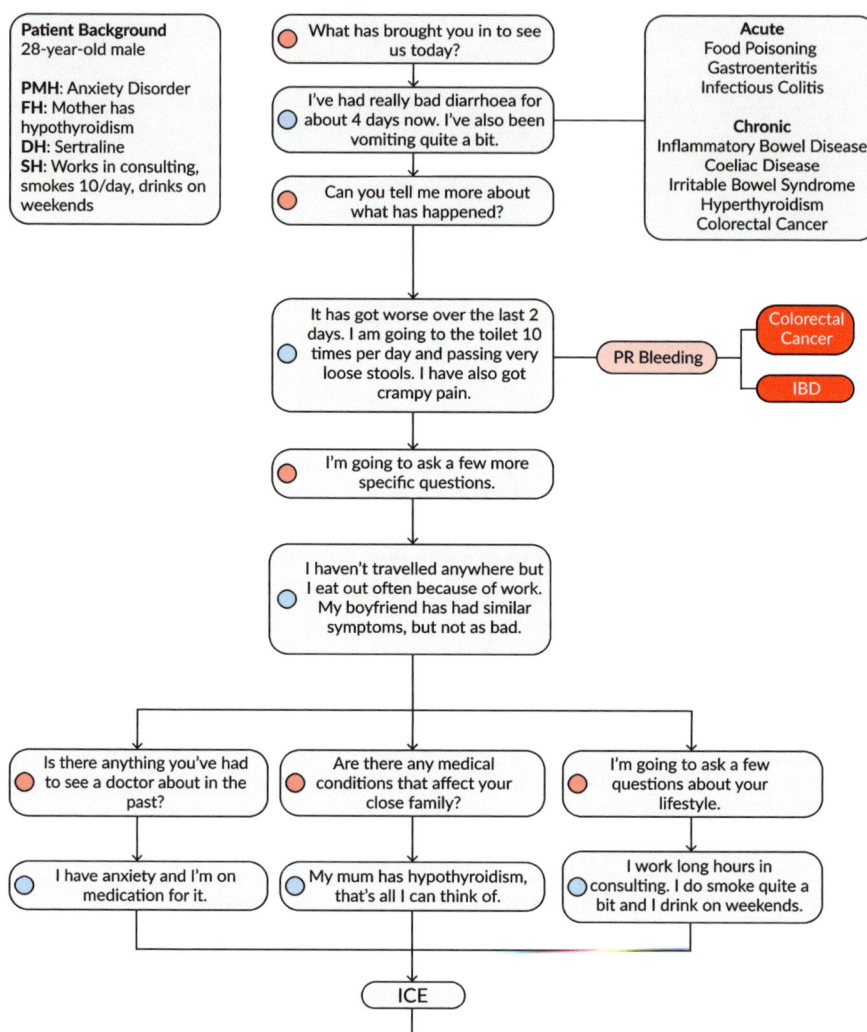

**Patient Background**
28-year-old male

**PMH:** Anxiety Disorder
**FH:** Mother has hypothyroidism
**DH:** Sertraline
**SH:** Works in consulting, smokes 10/day, drinks on weekends

What has brought you in to see us today?

I've had really bad diarrhoea for about 4 days now. I've also been vomiting quite a bit.

Can you tell me more about what has happened?

**Acute**
Food Poisoning
Gastroenteritis
Infectious Colitis

**Chronic**
Inflammatory Bowel Disease
Coeliac Disease
Irritable Bowel Syndrome
Hyperthyroidism
Colorectal Cancer

It has got worse over the last 2 days. I am going to the toilet 10 times per day and passing very loose stools. I have also got crampy pain.

PR Bleeding

Colorectal Cancer

IBD

I'm going to ask a few more specific questions.

I haven't travelled anywhere but I eat out often because of work. My boyfriend has had similar symptoms, but not as bad.

Is there anything you've had to see a doctor about in the past?

Are there any medical conditions that affect your close family?

I'm going to ask a few questions about your lifestyle.

I have anxiety and I'm on medication for it.

My mum has hypothyroidism, that's all I can think of.

I work long hours in consulting. I do smoke quite a bit and I drink on weekends.

ICE

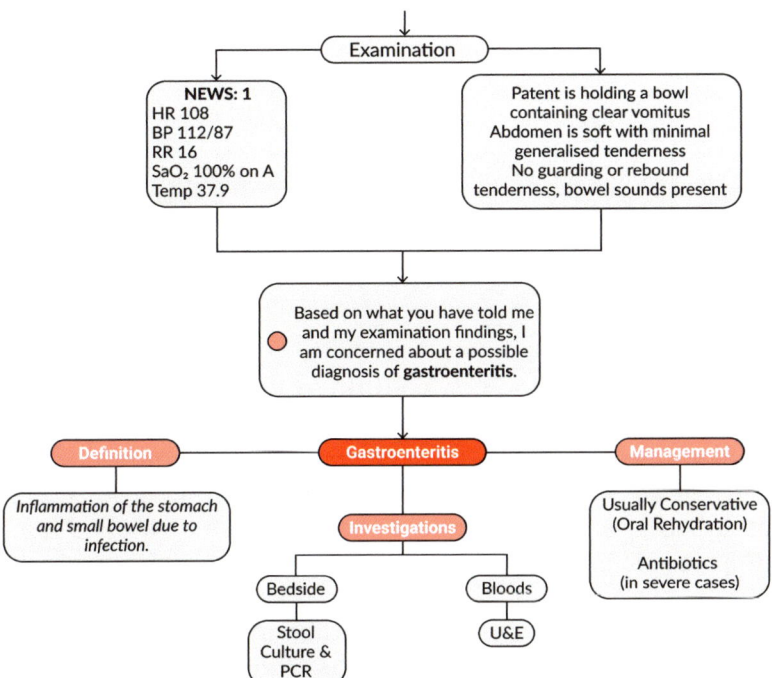

## Patient Background

**Patient Background**
28-year-old male

**PMH**: Anxiety Disorder
**FH**: Mother has hypothyroidism
**DH**: Sertraline
**SH**: Works in consulting, smokes 10/day, drinks on weekends

Infectious causes of diarrhoea (e.g. gastro-enteritis) can occur at any age, however, the causes of chronic diarrhoea tend to present more commonly in certain age groups. Inflammatory bowel disease and coeliac disease are more commonly present in **younger patients**. A subacute or chronic change in bowel habit in **older patients** should raise suspicion of a possible diagnosis of colorectal cancer. The patient's lifestyle and dietary habits can also reveal potential causes of diarrhoea (e.g. food poisoning from takeaway food).

# Differential Diagnosis

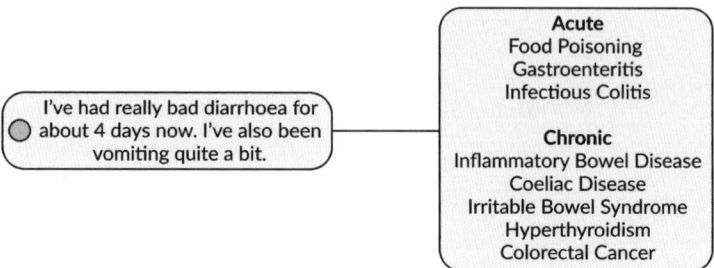

The causes of diarrhoea can be broadly categorised based on the duration of symptoms. Acute diarrhoea is usually suggestive of an infection or the effects of toxins from infectious agents (**food poisoning**, **gastroenteritis** and **infectious colitis**). It is, therefore, important to ask detailed questions about what the patient had eaten in the days leading up to their symptoms and whether they have any close contacts with similar symptoms. Asking about recent travel is also necessary as certain infectious agents are primarily found in endemic regions across the world (e.g. *Vibrio cholerae* and *Giardia lamblia*).

Chronic diarrhoea may be suggestive of an underlying disorder of the gastrointestinal tract (e.g. **inflammatory bowel disease** or **coeliac disease**). These are usually present in younger patients. **Irritable bowel syndrome** is largely a diagnosis of exclusion that may present with fluctuating episodes of diarrhoea and constipation associated with abdominal bloating. **Hyperthyroidism** increases the body's metabolic rate, thereby increasing gastrointestinal motility and manifesting as diarrhoea. A change in bowel habit in older patients should also be investigated further as it may be the presenting symptom of underlying **colorectal cancer**.

Read through the classical presentations table in the following section to develop an understanding of how the main differentials are classically present.

# Classical Presentations

| Differential | Classical Presentation |
|---|---|
| **Food Poisoning** | Acute onset diarrhoea and vomiting within hours of eating contaminated food. Usually caused by toxins produced by bacteria (e.g. *Staphylococcus aureus*). Symptoms usually subside within one day and vomiting is a prominent feature. |
| **Gastroenteritis** | Acute onset diarrhoea, vomiting and abdominal pain that is usually associated with recently eating an unusual meal. Patients often have close contact with similar symptoms. |
| **Infectious Colitis** | Explosive watery diarrhoea that often occurs in elderly hospital inpatients who have recently received a course of antibiotics (in particular, clindamycin, ciprofloxacin, co-amoxiclav and cephalosporins). |
| **Inflammatory Bowel Disease** | Crohn's disease tends to present with subacute onset RIF pain associated with diarrhoea (due to terminal ileitis). There may be a background of episodic diarrhoea and systemic upset. Ulcerative colitis is more commonly associated with rectal bleeding. |
| **Coeliac Disease** | Chronic history of diarrhoea that may be pale and difficult to flush away (steatorrhoea), and weight loss. May be associated with a vesicular rash on the extensor surfaces (dermatitis herpetiformis) and some patients may have a family history. |
| **Irritable Bowel Syndrome** | Chronic condition characterised by alternating spells of constipation and diarrhoea. Patients often complain of bloating and episodes may be triggered by stress. |

| | |
|---|---|
| **Hyperthyroidism** | Chronic history of anxiety, excessive sweating, palpitations, tremor, heat intolerance and diarrhoea. Some patients may even notice a midline enlargement in their neck. |
| **Colorectal Cancer** | Gradual onset of worsening constipation that may be associated with rectal bleeding and unintentional weight loss. May sometimes present with bowel obstruction secondary to a malignant stricture. May be identified after incidentally noting iron deficiency anaemia on a routine blood test. |

# Red Flags

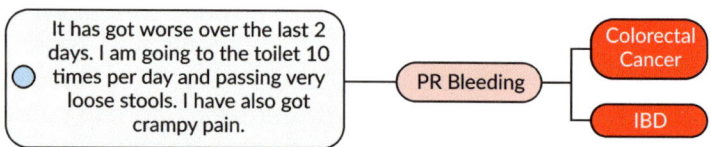

**PR bleeding** is a major red flag in the context of chronic diarrhoea as it may be suggestive of serious underlying pathology. In older patients, bleeding associated with new diarrhoea is highly suggestive of colorectal cancer. Acute bloody diarrhoea and abdominal pain in an elderly patient may be suggestive of ischaemic colitis. In younger patients, a subacute or chronic history of bloody diarrhoea may be suggestive of inflammatory bowel disease (in particular, ulcerative colitis), though it can also occur due to infectious causes of diarrhoea (e.g. shigellosis). It is worth noting that there is a second peak in the incidence of inflammatory bowel disease later in life (around 50–60 years).

# Assessment

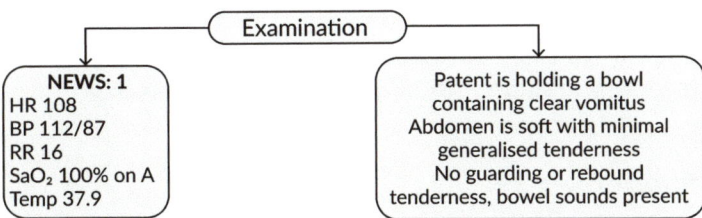

Examination

| NEWS: 1 | Patent is holding a bowl |
| HR 108 | containing clear vomitus |
| BP 112/87 | Abdomen is soft with minimal |
| RR 16 | generalised tenderness |
| SaO₂ 100% on A | No guarding or rebound |
| Temp 37.9 | tenderness, bowel sounds present |

## *Observations*

Patients presenting with acute diarrhoeal illnesses may be very dehydrated, and this may be reflected in their observations (**tachycardia** and **hypotension**). Infectious causes of diarrhoea may also cause a **fever**.

## *Examination*

Patients with acute diarrhoea should be examined while wearing gloves and gowns to reduce the risk of transmission. Most causes of diarrhoea will cause some **generalised abdominal discomfort**. Crohn's disease has a predilection to involve the terminal ileum, thereby causing **right iliac fossa tenderness**. In some lean patients with large colorectal tumours, it may be palpable upon examination of the abdomen. The fit of the patient's clothing may provide a crude indication of whether the patient has lost weight.

# Gastroenteritis

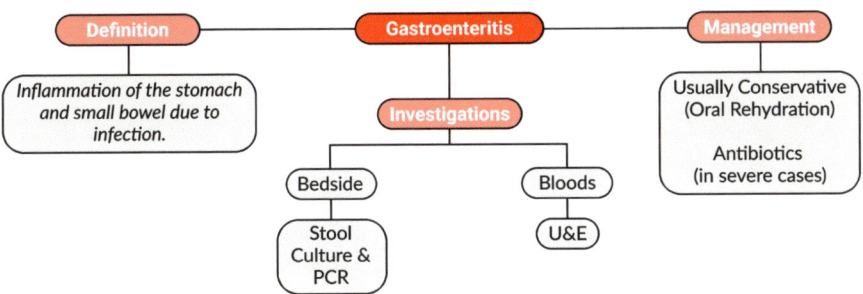

| Definition | Gastroenteritis | Management |
| Inflammation of the stomach and small bowel due to infection. | Investigations | Usually Conservative (Oral Rehydration) |
| | Bedside          Bloods | Antibiotics (in severe cases) |
| | Stool Culture & PCR     U&E | |

## Definition

Gastroenteritis refers to inflammation of the stomach and small bowel usually due to a viral infection. It differs from infectious colitis which refers to infection and inflammation of the colon.

## Investigations

Gastroenteritis is largely a clinical diagnosis and often viral — a **stool culture and PCR** is useful to identify the causative agent. If the patient has become particularly dehydrated due to the episode of gastroenteritis, they may have developed a pre-renal AKI, so their **U&E** should be checked.

## Management

As most cases of gastroenteritis are viral, they often resolve spontaneously over a few days. Patients should be encouraged to increase their oral fluid intake and use rehydration solutions. If a bacterial cause (e.g. *Campylobacter jejuni*) is suspected and the infection is severe, antibiotics may be considered (e.g. clarithromycin).

# Bridge Box

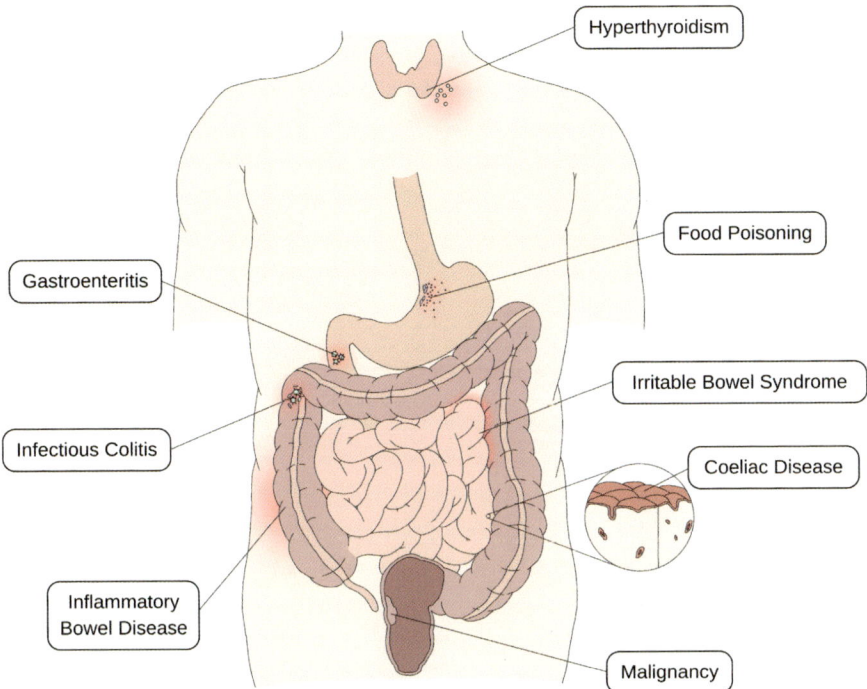

Differentials for diarrhoea.

# Chapter 18

# Rectal Bleeding

Rectal bleeding is a concerning symptom that can have a variety of causes. It is important to establish the nature of the bleeding to be able to delineate the potential underlying causes.

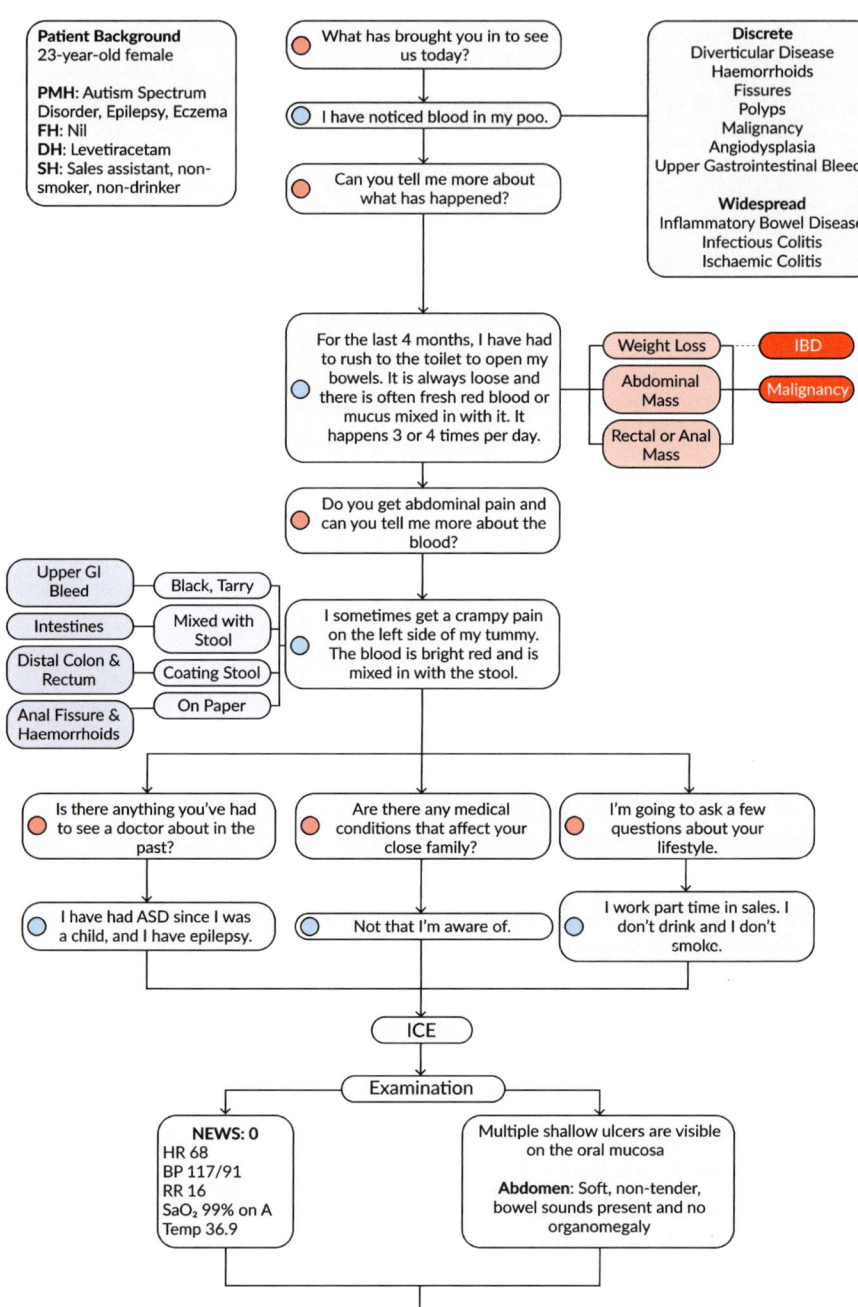

**Patient Background**
23-year-old female

**PMH:** Autism Spectrum Disorder, Epilepsy, Eczema
**FH:** Nil
**DH:** Levetiracetam
**SH:** Sales assistant, non-smoker, non-drinker

What has brought you in to see us today?

I have noticed blood in my poo.

Can you tell me more about what has happened?

**Discrete**
Diverticular Disease
Haemorrhoids
Fissures
Polyps
Malignancy
Angiodysplasia
Upper Gastrointestinal Bleeds

**Widespread**
Inflammatory Bowel Disease
Infectious Colitis
Ischaemic Colitis

For the last 4 months, I have had to rush to the toilet to open my bowels. It is always loose and there is often fresh red blood or mucus mixed in with it. It happens 3 or 4 times per day.

Weight Loss

Abdominal Mass

Rectal or Anal Mass

IBD

Malignancy

Do you get abdominal pain and can you tell me more about the blood?

Upper GI Bleed — Black, Tarry

Intestines — Mixed with Stool

Distal Colon & Rectum — Coating Stool

Anal Fissure & Haemorrhoids — On Paper

I sometimes get a crampy pain on the left side of my tummy. The blood is bright red and is mixed in with the stool.

Is there anything you've had to see a doctor about in the past?

Are there any medical conditions that affect your close family?

I'm going to ask a few questions about your lifestyle.

I have had ASD since I was a child, and I have epilepsy.

Not that I'm aware of.

I work part time in sales. I don't drink and I don't smoke.

ICE

Examination

**NEWS: 0**
HR 68
BP 117/91
RR 16
SaO₂ 99% on A
Temp 36.9

Multiple shallow ulcers are visible on the oral mucosa

**Abdomen:** Soft, non-tender, bowel sounds present and no organomegaly

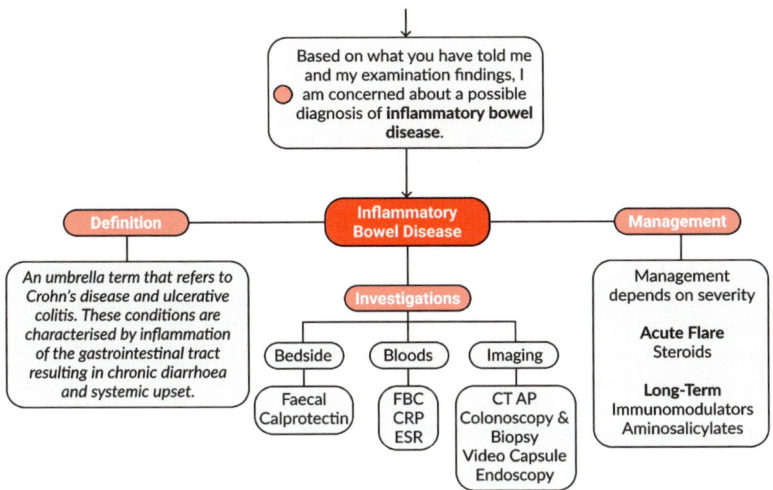

# Patient Background

**Patient Background**
23-year-old female

**PMH:** Autism Spectrum
Disorder, Epilepsy, Eczema
**FH:** Nil
**DH:** Levetiracetam
**SH:** Sales assistant, non-
smoker, non-drinker

The **age** of the patient can help assess the likelihood of the various differentials for rectal bleeding. Generally speaking, ischaemic colitis, diverticular bleeds and colorectal cancer are mainly seen in **older patients**. Some benign causes such as haemorrhoids and anal fissures can be seen at any age, and inflammatory bowel disease has a bimodal age of presentation (first peak at 15–25 years and a second, smaller peak at 40–70 years).

The drug history should be screened for any **anticoagulants** or **antiplatelets** that may increase the risk of bleeding.

# Differential Diagnosis

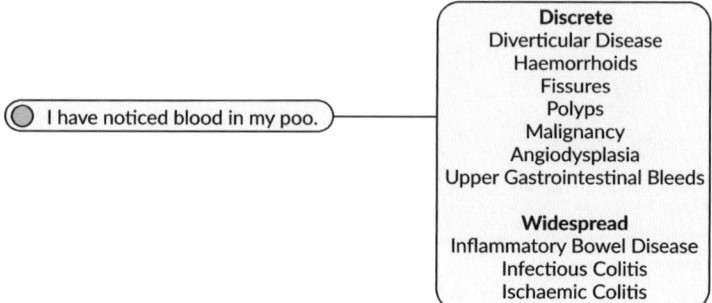

The differentials can be broadly categorised into **discrete** structural abnormalities and more **widespread** conditions that affect a greater portion of the gastrointestinal tract.

Examples of discrete insults that can cause rectal bleeding include varices (oesophageal and rectal), bleeding diverticula, haemorrhoids, anal fissures, polyps, angiodysplasia and colorectal cancer.

Diseases that affect a more widespread area of the gastrointestinal tract include inflammatory bowel disease (Crohn's disease and ulcerative colitis), ischaemic colitis (primarily in older patients) and infectious colitis (e.g. *Clostridium difficile* colitis).

Read through the classical presentations table in the following section to develop an understanding of how the main differentials are classically present.

# Classical Presentations

| Differential | Classical Presentation |
|---|---|
| **Diverticular Disease** | **Diverticulitis**: Gradual onset left iliac fossa pain which may be associated with diarrhoea and rectal bleeding. Patients may also have a fever. **Diverticular Bleed**: May be identified after anaemia is incidentally noted on a full blood count. Patients may present with a change in bowel habit or may present acutely with severe rectal bleeding. |

| | |
|---|---|
| **Haemorrhoids** | Painless rectal bleeding that is usually described as being bright red and dripping into the pan after defecation. Prolapsed haemorrhoids may be visible when sitting on the commode and may be palpable. Patients often have a preceding history of constipation. |
| **Anal Fissure** | Tearing pain around the anal opening when attempting to pass a bowel motion. Stools may be streaked in blood or fresh blood may be evident upon wiping with toilet paper. |
| **Colorectal Cancer** | Gradual onset of worsening constipation that may be associated with rectal bleeding and unintentional weight loss. May sometimes present with bowel obstruction secondary to a malignant stricture. May be identified after incidentally noting iron deficiency anaemia on a routine blood test. **Polyps** are outgrowths of the wall of the bowel that may be benign and can bleed. |
| **Gastrointestinal Angiodysplasia** | Painless blood noticed in the stools (relationship between blood and stool will depend on the site of angiodysplasia). May present with a large episode of bleeding. |
| **Upper Gastrointestinal Bleed** | Presents with melaena that usually occurs in the context of persistent epigastric pain (peptic ulcer disease) or a background of alcohol excess (oesophageal varices). May present more dramatically with haematemesis and haemodynamic compromise. |
| **Inflammatory Bowel Disease** | Crohn's disease tends to present with subacute onset RIF pain associated with diarrhoea (due to terminal ileitis). There may be a background of episodic diarrhoea and systemic upset. Ulcerative colitis is more commonly associated with rectal bleeding. |

| | |
|---|---|
| **Infectious Colitis** | Explosive watery diarrhoea that often occurs in elderly hospital inpatients who have recently received a course of antibiotics (in particular, clindamycin, ciprofloxacin, co-amoxiclav and cephalosporins). |
| **Ischaemic Colitis** | Acute onset abdominal pain and rectal bleeding that usually occurs in elderly patients. More common in patients with atrial fibrillation (embolic source). |

## Red Flags

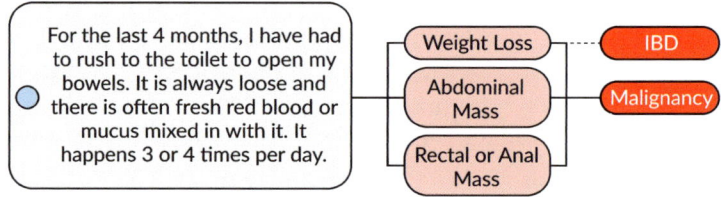

Most cases of rectal bleeding are caused by simple structural defects such as haemorrhoids and anal fissures and can be safely managed in a primary care setting. It is important, however, to be able to identify the dangerous causes of rectal bleeding that require more intensive investigation and management.

If patients are presenting with rectal bleeding on a background of systemic upset and **weight loss**, it may be suggestive of an underlying colorectal malignancy or of inflammatory bowel disease.

A **palpable mass within the abdomen or upon digital rectal examination** may be suggestive of colorectal cancer which should, subsequently, be visualised using rigid sigmoidoscopy, flexible sigmoidoscopy or colonoscopy.

# Relationship with Stool

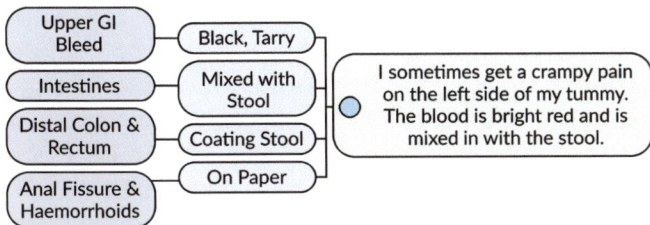

As food passes along the gastrointestinal tract, its material properties change and, hence, the relationship between the blood and the stools will provide useful information about where the bleed is likely to be. Though it may seem like an awkward line of enquiry, it is essential that you ask the patient to provide a detailed description of the appearance of their stools.

Upper gastrointestinal bleeds (i.e. from the oesophagus, stomach and proximal small intestine) will manifest with melaena which is classically described as **black, tarry stools** that are especially **foul-smelling**.

If the bleeding is arising from a point along much of the small bowel and proximal large bowel, the blood will appear **mixed with the stools**, and if arising from the distal colon and rectum, the blood may be described as **coating the stools**. Finally, bleeding arising from haemorrhoids or fissures within the anal canal may only be apparent **on the paper** when wiping.

# Assessment

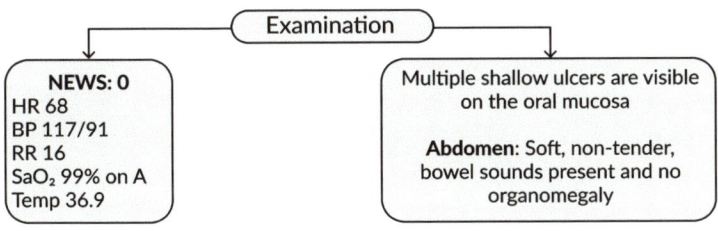

## *Observations*

Much of the time, patients presenting with rectal bleeding will complain of a small amount of bleeding that has been noted over a prolonged period. In such cases, the volume of blood loss is usually relatively small and unlikely to cause any changes in their vital signs. In some cases, however, such as a severe flare of inflammatory bowel disease or ischaemic colitis, significant blood loss can cause **hypovolaemic shock** (hypotension and tachycardia with associated end organ hypoperfusion).

## *Examination*

The assessment of a patient with rectal bleeding will likely involve performing an abdominal examination and a digital rectal examination.

- **Abdominal Examination**: In more widespread disease states such as inflammatory bowel disease, infectious colitis and ischaemic colitis, the abdomen may be **tender**. In severe cases, the abdomen will be **rigid** with **rebound tenderness** and **involuntary guarding** — suggestive of peritonitis. In peptic ulcer disease, the patient may be tender in the epigastrium.
- **Digital Rectal Examination**: Anal **fissures** and external **haemorrhoids** may be visualised; however, some fissures and internal haemorrhoids may be impalpable and difficult to visualise. **Low-lying rectal tumours** may also be palpable as an irregular mass within the rectum. It is also important to **inspect the colour of the blood** upon withdrawal of the finger during a digital rectal examination.

# Inflammatory Bowel Disease

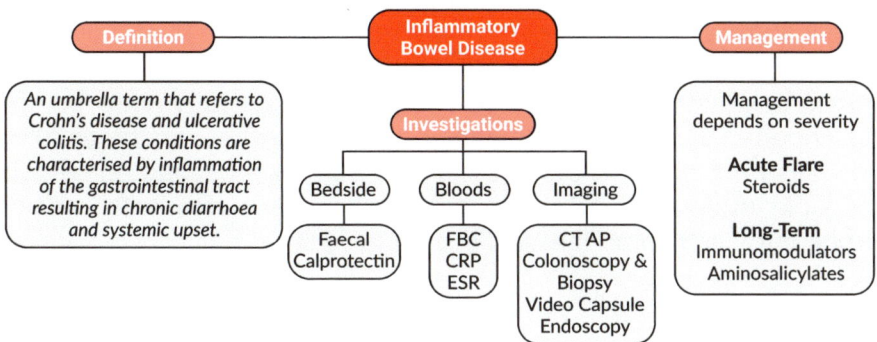

## *Definition*

Inflammatory bowel disease (IBD) is an umbrella term that encompasses Crohn's disease and ulcerative colitis. They are characterised by inflammation of the gastrointestinal tract resulting in chronic diarrhoea and systemic upset.

## *Investigations*

There are several causes of chronic diarrhoea in young people which can be difficult to distinguish (namely IBD, coeliac disease and irritable bowel syndrome). **Faecal calprotectin** is a convenient, non-invasive stool test that can be used to detect evidence of inflammation within the gastrointestinal tract which would point you towards a diagnosis of IBD.

Patients with suspected IBD should have an **FBC** to check whether the disease has caused a drop in their haemoglobin (which can occur both due to bleeding and due to anaemia of chronic disease) and to assess their **inflammatory markers** (white cell and neutrophil count). An **ESR** is another useful investigation which, if raised, is suggestive of an ongoing chronic inflammatory process.

Ultimately, diagnosis will involve performing an **endoscopy and biopsy** of the affected section of the gastrointestinal tract. In ulcerative colitis, this can be achieved with a colonoscopy as the disease will begin distally and progress proximally in a continuous manner. Histology will reveal mucosal and submucosal inflammation with crypt abscesses.

In Crohn's disease, the affected tissue may lie at any point along the gastrointestinal tract. Therefore, visualisation may be difficult depending on the area affected. Methods that may be used to visualise the affected areas include OGD, colonoscopy and video capsule endoscopy. Crohn's disease is associated with patchy transmural inflammation and histology will reveal non-caseating granulomas.

## Management

The management of IBD depends very much on the severity of the condition, the extent of bowel involved and the presence of complications (e.g. fistulae). Generally, acute flares are managed with **steroids**. Once remission has been induced, it can be maintained using **aminosalicylates** (mainstay in ulcerative colitis) and **immunomodulating agents** (mainstay in Crohn's disease).

# Bridge Box

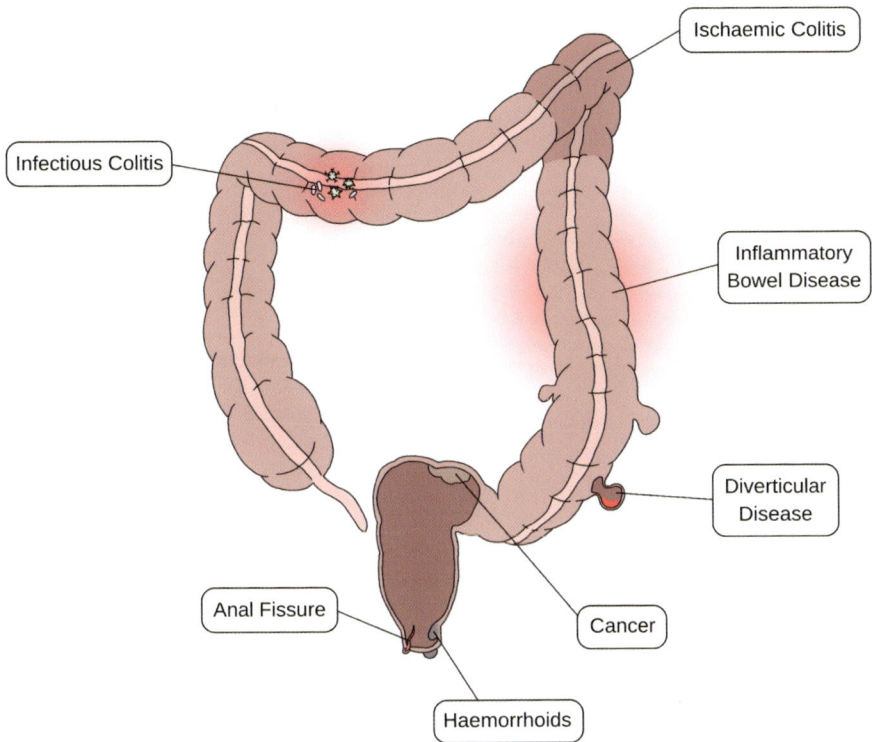

Ischaemic Colitis

Infectious Colitis

Inflammatory Bowel Disease

Diverticular Disease

Anal Fissure

Cancer

Haemorrhoids

Differentials for rectal bleeding.

# Chapter 19

# Scrotal Mass

Scrotal masses can arise due to both testicular and non-testicular causes. A thorough examination helps identify potentially dangerous causes of scrotal swelling.

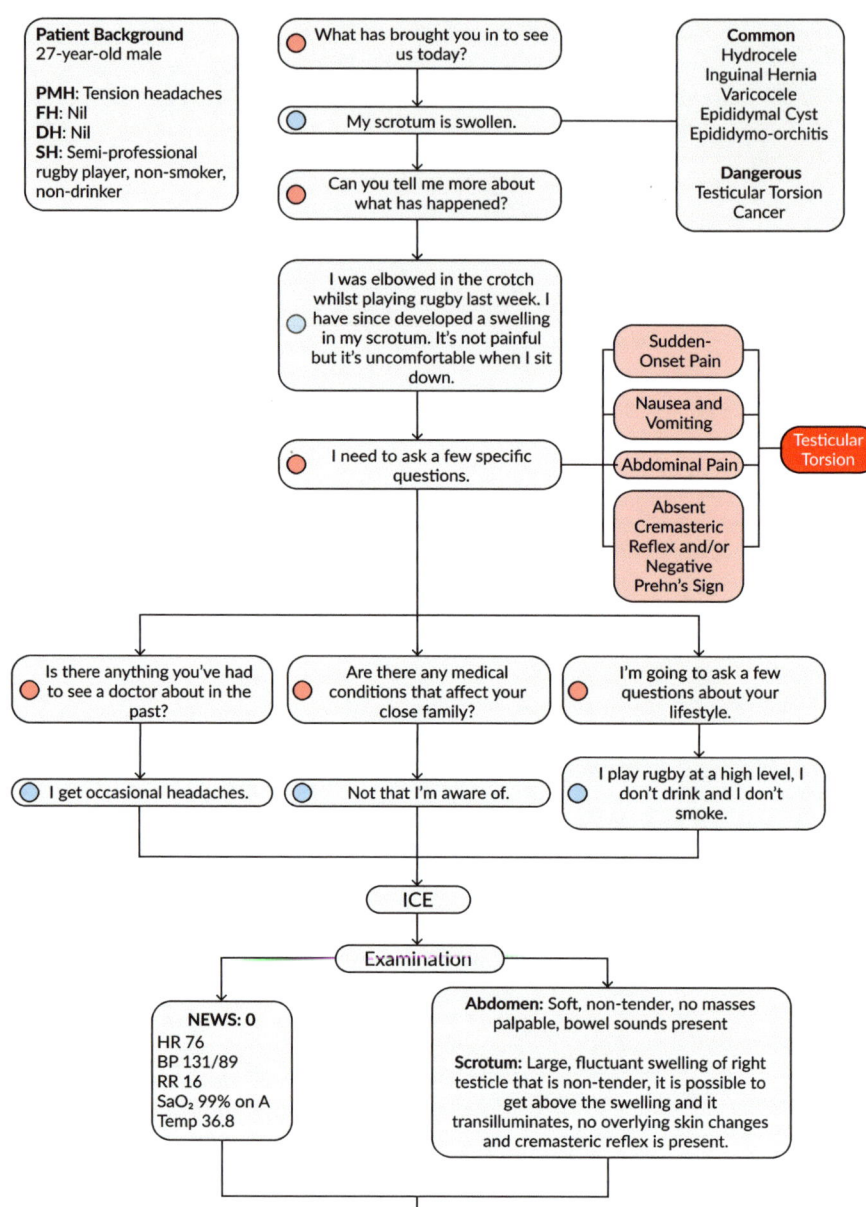

**Patient Background**
27-year-old male

**PMH:** Tension headaches
**FH:** Nil
**DH:** Nil
**SH:** Semi-professional rugby player, non-smoker, non-drinker

What has brought you in to see us today?

My scrotum is swollen.

Can you tell me more about what has happened?

I was elbowed in the crotch whilst playing rugby last week. I have since developed a swelling in my scrotum. It's not painful but it's uncomfortable when I sit down.

I need to ask a few specific questions.

**Common**
Hydrocele
Inguinal Hernia
Varicocele
Epididymal Cyst
Epididymo-orchitis

**Dangerous**
Testicular Torsion
Cancer

Sudden-Onset Pain

Nausea and Vomiting

Abdominal Pain

Absent Cremasteric Reflex and/or Negative Prehn's Sign

**Testicular Torsion**

Is there anything you've had to see a doctor about in the past?

Are there any medical conditions that affect your close family?

I'm going to ask a few questions about your lifestyle.

I get occasional headaches.

Not that I'm aware of.

I play rugby at a high level, I don't drink and I don't smoke.

ICE

Examination

**NEWS: 0**
HR 76
BP 131/89
RR 16
$SaO_2$ 99% on A
Temp 36.8

**Abdomen:** Soft, non-tender, no masses palpable, bowel sounds present

**Scrotum:** Large, fluctuant swelling of right testicle that is non-tender, it is possible to get above the swelling and it transilluminates, no overlying skin changes and cremasteric reflex is present.

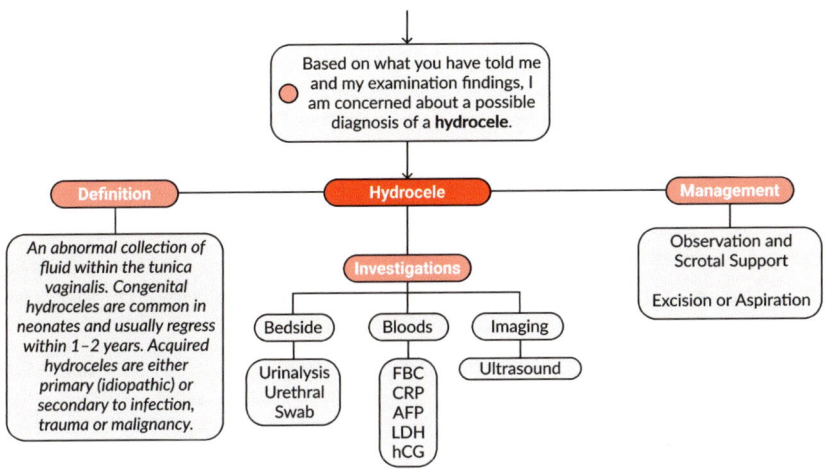

# Patient Background

| Patient Background |
|---|
| 27-year-old male |
| **PMH**: Tension headaches |
| **FH**: Nil |
| **DH**: Nil |
| **SH**: Semi-professional rugby player, non-smoker, non-drinker |

Unlike most other presentations, scrotal masses are most commonly present in **younger men and boys**. Both the acute causes of scrotal masses (testicular torsion and epididymo-orchitis) and chronic causes (inguinal hernia and testicular cancer) are more likely to present in younger men.

# Differential Diagnosis

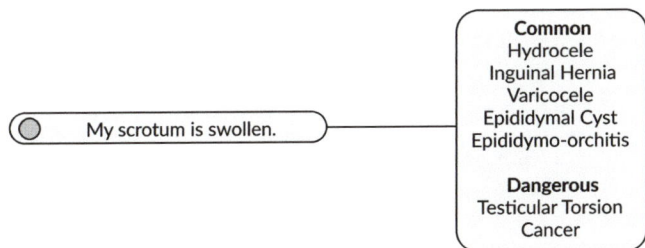

When any patient presents with acute scrotal pain, they should be examined by a suitably trained individual *immediately* to assess whether there is any clinical suspicion of **testicular torsion**. Patients with torsion will need exploratory surgery *within 4–6 hours* to stand a chance of saving the affected testicle.

The main causes of scrotal pain and tenderness are **epididymo-orchitis**, **testicular torsion** and **incarcerated or strangulated inguinal hernias**. In most other cases, patients may complain of discomfort but not significant pain. Painless masses in and around the testicle may be caused by **varicoceles** (dilation of the pampiniform plexus), **testicular tumours**, **hydroceles** and **epididymal cysts**.

Read through the classical presentations table in the following section to develop an understanding of how the main differentials are classically present.

## Classical Presentations

| Differential | Classical Presentation |
|---|---|
| **Hydrocele** | Gradual onset scrotal swelling that is usually soft, fluctuant and non-tender. Able to get above the swelling but it may not be possible to separate the testicle from the swelling. May transilluminate. |
| **Inguinal Hernia** | May present to primary care as a painless mass noted in the groin or scrotum. The swelling is separate from the testicle, and it is not possible to get above the swelling. The swelling may be reducible and bowel sounds may be heard upon auscultation of the swelling. May present acutely with severe pain and vomiting if the hernia has become incarcerated or obstructed. |
| **Varicocele** | Gradual onset scrotal swelling and discomfort that feels like a "bag of worms" above the scrotum. The swelling may reduce when the patient is lying down. More common on the left. |
| **Epididymal Cyst** | Gradual onset swelling located posterior to the testicle. Usually not particularly painful and may transilluminate. The swelling is separate from the testicle. |

| Epididymo-Orchitis | Subacute onset scrotal pain and tenderness that may be associated with dysuria and penile discharge. May occur secondary to a UTI or an STI. |
| --- | --- |
| Testicular Torsion | Sudden onset severe scrotal pain associated with nausea and vomiting. Absent cremasteric reflex and negative Prehn's sign. |
| Testicular Cancer | Gradual onset scrotal heaviness and discomfort associated with a palpable mass within the testicle. May be associated with a secondary hydrocele. |

# Red Flags

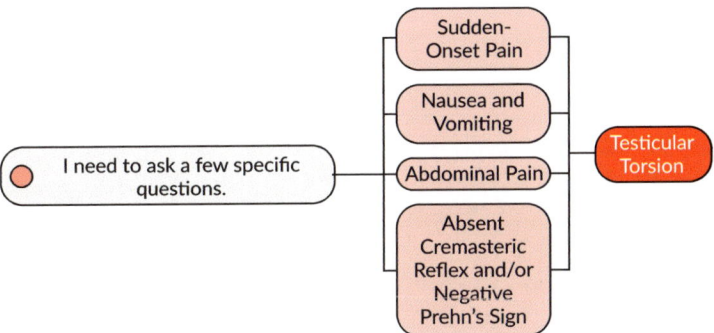

In the acute setting, the most important step in management is to determine the likelihood of the patient having testicular torsion. **Sudden onset intense scrotal pain** associated with **nausea and vomiting** is suggestive of a diagnosis of testicular torsion. Furthermore, upon examination, an **absent cremasteric reflex** and **negative Prehn's sign** are also in keeping with a diagnosis of testicular torsion (though these tests are not very specific). Patients with testicular torsion may also mention that they experienced some **recent trauma** to the region (e.g. during a rugby match). If clinically suspected, the on-call urology team should be contacted immediately.

# Assessment

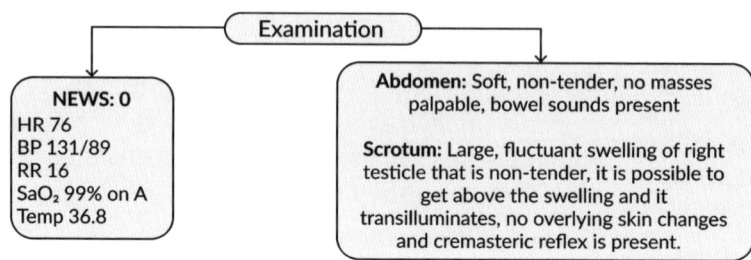

**NEWS: 0**
HR 76
BP 131/89
RR 16
SaO₂ 99% on A
Temp 36.8

**Abdomen:** Soft, non-tender, no masses palpable, bowel sounds present

**Scrotum:** Large, fluctuant swelling of right testicle that is non-tender, it is possible to get above the swelling and it transilluminates, no overlying skin changes and cremasteric reflex is present.

## *Observations*

In most patients presenting with a scrotal mass, their observations will be stable. If presenting with epididymo-orchitis, some patients may be febrile because of the infection.

## *Examination*

When approaching a patient with a scrotal mass or pain, it is important to examine the abdomen as well as the scrotum.

- **Scrotal Examination**
  - **Testicular Torsion**: Swollen and tender hemiscrotum with an absent cremasteric reflex and negative Prehn's sign.
  - **Epididymo-Orchitis**: Swollen and tender hemiscrotum that can be difficult to clinically distinguish from testicular torsion. Patients may mention that they had noted some penile discharge or dysuria and the history is usually less acute than in testicular torsion.
  - **Varicocele**: Palpable soft mass that feels like a '*bag of worms*' that is separate from the testicle and may disappear when lying flat. It is possible to get above the swelling.
  - **Hydrocele**: Enlarged, non-tender hemiscrotum where the testicle cannot be palpated beneath the mass. It is possible to get above the swelling and the swelling may transilluminate.
  - **Epididymal Cyst**: Soft, fluctuant mass that is palpable behind or just superior to the testicle. It may transilluminate and it is possible to get above the swelling.

- ○ **Inguinal Hernia**: It is not possible to get above the mass and the mass can be tracked back to the superficial inguinal ring. Bowel sounds may be heard on auscultation of the lump, and it may be reducible.
- **Abdominal Examination**
  - ○ **Epididymo-Orchitis**: Some patients may complain of suprapubic tenderness due to a urinary tract infection that has led to epididymo-orchitis.
  - ○ **Inguinal Hernia**: An incarcerated or strangulated inguinal hernia could cause bowel obstruction, so it is important to assess the abdomen for evidence of bowel obstruction (distension and absent or tinkling bowel sounds).
  - ○ **Varicocele**: A left-sided varicocele may be the first presentation of an underlying renal malignancy. Though it may be difficult to do so depending on the patient's body habitus, an attempt should be made to ballot the kidneys to feel for masses.

# Hydrocele

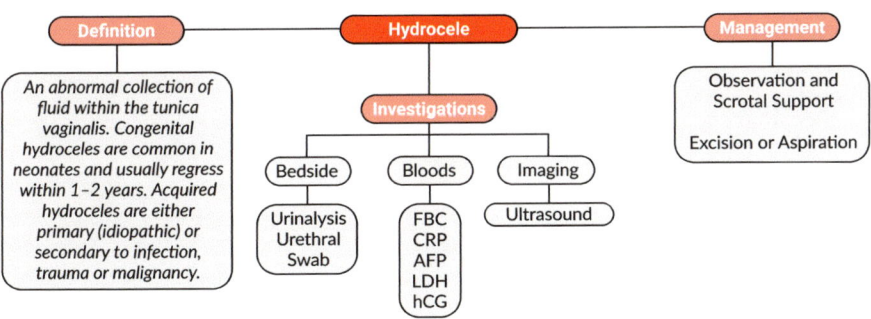

## *Definition*

A hydrocele is an abnormal collection of fluid within the tunica vaginalis that can be congenital (present at birth) or acquired (idiopathic or secondary to infection, trauma or malignancy).

## Investigations

At the bedside, **urinalysis** and **urethral swab** can help determine the underlying cause of a hydrocele that has arisen secondary to infection (i.e. UTI vs STI). Patients may also have raised inflammatory markers (**FBC** and **CRP**). Furthermore, hydroceles may occur secondary to malignancy, so the **tumour markers (alpha-fetoprotein, hCG and lactate dehydrogenase)** should be requested.

An **ultrasound** scan will help determine if there is an underlying disease process (e.g. malignancy) that has precipitated the formation of the hydrocele.

## Management

If the hydrocele is asymptomatic or minimally symptomatic and sinister underlying causes have been excluded, patients can be managed conservatively with **observation and scrotal support**. If the hydrocele is particularly large or causing trouble for the patient, **excision or aspiration** should be offered.

# Bridge Box

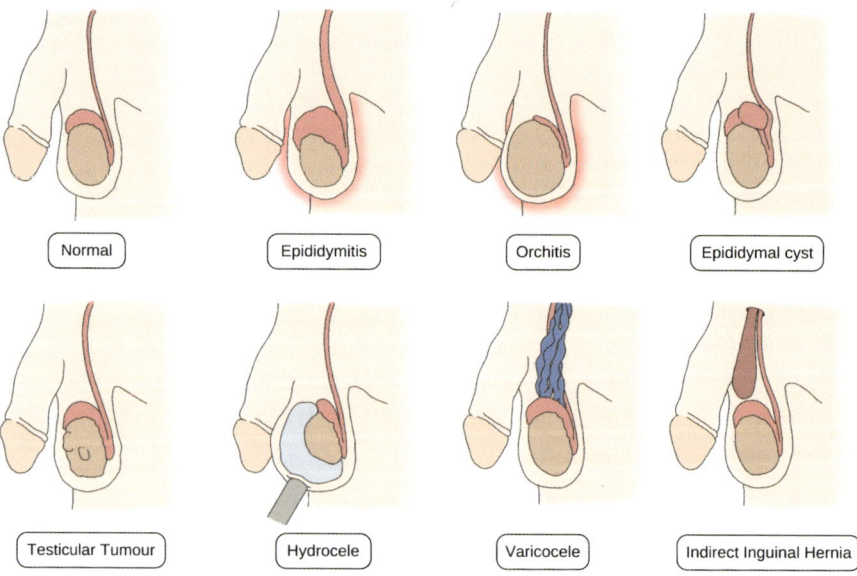

Differentials for scrotal mass.

# Chapter 20

# Back Pain

Back pain is an extremely common presentation in primary and secondary care. Though, much of the time, the cause is benign, there are a few sinister causes that must be excluded through a clear history and comprehensive examination.

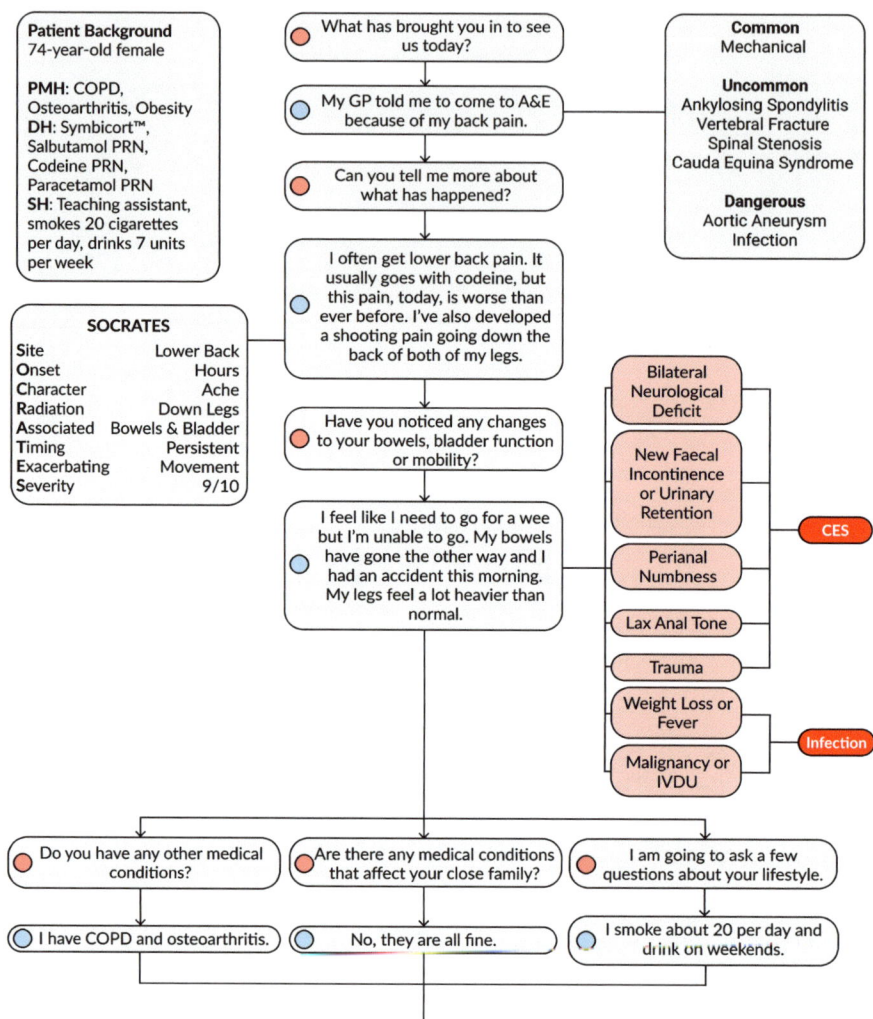

**Patient Background**
74-year-old female

**PMH**: COPD,
Osteoarthritis, Obesity
**DH**: Symbicort™,
Salbutamol PRN,
Codeine PRN,
Paracetamol PRN
**SH**: Teaching assistant,
smokes 20 cigarettes
per day, drinks 7 units
per week

**SOCRATES**

| | |
|---|---|
| Site | Lower Back |
| Onset | Hours |
| Character | Ache |
| Radiation | Down Legs |
| Associated | Bowels & Bladder |
| Timing | Persistent |
| Exacerbating | Movement |
| Severity | 9/10 |

What has brought you in to see us today?

My GP told me to come to A&E because of my back pain.

Can you tell me more about what has happened?

I often get lower back pain. It usually goes with codeine, but this pain, today, is worse than ever before. I've also developed a shooting pain going down the back of both of my legs.

Have you noticed any changes to your bowels, bladder function or mobility?

I feel like I need to go for a wee but I'm unable to. My bowels have gone the other way and I had an accident this morning. My legs feel a lot heavier than normal.

**Common**
Mechanical

**Uncommon**
Ankylosing Spondylitis
Vertebral Fracture
Spinal Stenosis
Cauda Equina Syndrome

**Dangerous**
Aortic Aneurysm
Infection

Bilateral Neurological Deficit

New Faecal Incontinence or Urinary Retention

Perianal Numbness

Lax Anal Tone

Trauma

Weight Loss or Fever

Malignancy or IVDU

**CES**

**Infection**

Do you have any other medical conditions?

I have COPD and osteoarthritis.

Are there any medical conditions that affect your close family?

No, they are all fine.

I am going to ask a few questions about your lifestyle.

I smoke about 20 per day and drink on weekends.

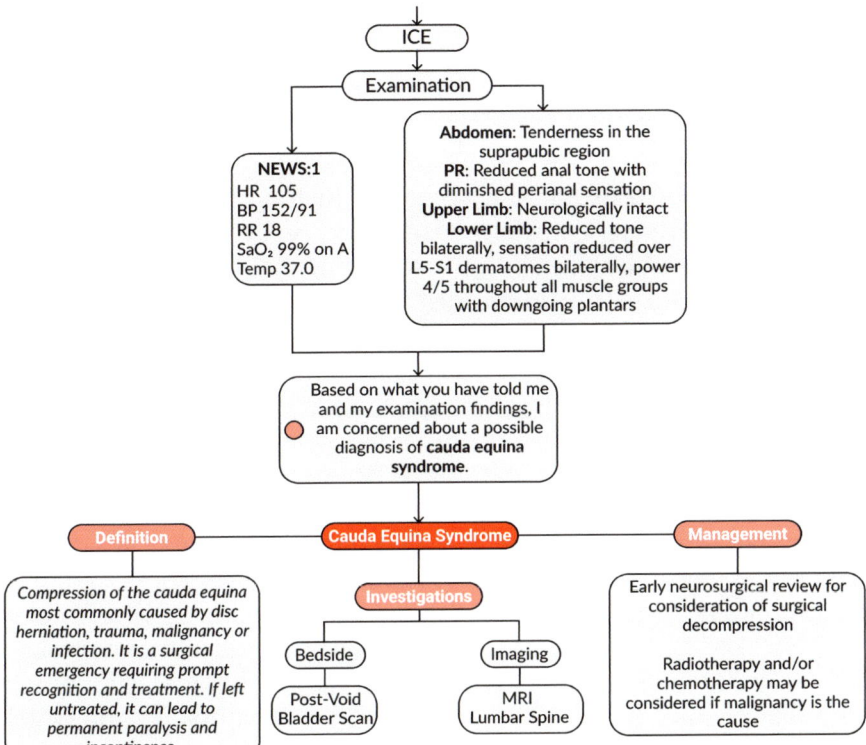

ICE

Examination

**NEWS:1**
HR 105
BP 152/91
RR 18
SaO₂ 99% on A
Temp 37.0

**Abdomen**: Tenderness in the
suprapubic region
**PR**: Reduced anal tone with
diminshed perianal sensation
**Upper Limb**: Neurologically intact
**Lower Limb**: Reduced tone
bilaterally, sensation reduced over
L5-S1 dermatomes bilaterally, power
4/5 throughout all muscle groups
with downgoing plantars

Based on what you have told me
and my examination findings, I
am concerned about a possible
diagnosis of **cauda equina
syndrome**.

**Definition** — **Cauda Equina Syndrome** — **Management**

Compression of the cauda equina
most commonly caused by disc
herniation, trauma, malignancy or
infection. It is a surgical
emergency requiring prompt
recognition and treatment. If left
untreated, it can lead to
permanent paralysis and
incontinence.

**Investigations**

Bedside

Post-Void
Bladder Scan

Imaging

MRI
Lumbar Spine

Early neurosurgical review for
consideration of surgical
decompression

Radiotherapy and/or
chemotherapy may be
considered if malignancy is the
cause

# Patient Background

**Patient Background**
74-year-old female

**PMH**: COPD,
Osteoarthritis, Obesity
**DH**: Symbicort™,
Salbutamol PRN,
Codeine PRN,
Paracetamol PRN
**SH**: Teaching assistant,
smokes 20 cigarettes
per day, drinks 7 units
per week

The background details of a patient with back pain can help you assess their risk of developing a dangerous cause of back pain (e.g. cauda equina syndrome).

## *Dangerous Causes*

The main concern in a patient presenting to A&E with a sudden worsening in their back pain is cauda equina syndrome. **Older patients** are at greater risk of developing osteoporotic fractures of the vertebral column and they are also at greater risk of developing malignancies (e.g. prostate and breast cancer) that can give rise to bone metastases which, in turn, can lead to pathological fractures of the vertebrae.

### Benign Causes

Several clues in the patient's medical history, social history and general appearance can help assess the risk of them developing benign causes of back pain (i.e. musculoskeletal back pain).

Patients who are **overweight or obese** will be placing their lumbar spine under greater strain thereby increasing the risk of developing musculoskeletal back pain. The patient's **occupation** and **levels of activity** can also significantly influence the likelihood of them developing musculoskeletal back pain. In particular, those who have sedentary jobs (e.g. office workers) and get relatively little exercise are at greater risk.

Some patients will develop **osteoarthritis** because their cartilage is too weak to bear the stresses that they are placed under. If patients have osteoarthritic changes in their knees or hands, they are also likely to have some osteoarthritic changes in their vertebral column that can give rise to back pain. Finally, patients with chronic lung diseases (e.g. COPD) may suffer from a chronic cough which can strain the muscles of the lower back, causing pain.

## Differential Diagnosis

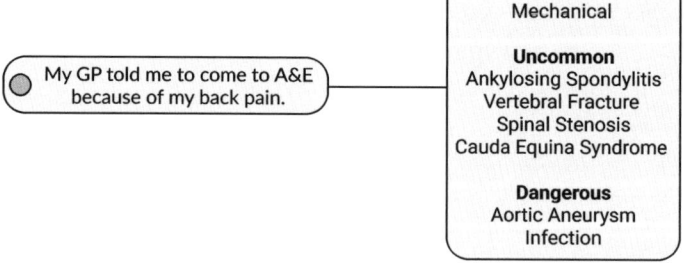

## *Common*

Most cases of back pain that present to primary care or A&E will be mechanical back pain. This can include muscle sprains and disc prolapses, and they are generally managed conservatively with a combination of simple analgesia and physiotherapy.

## *Uncommon and Dangerous*

Differentials for back pain are considered dangerous if they place the spinal cord or the cauda equina at risk. This can lead to irreversible nerve damage and significant morbidity if not attended to urgently.

Furthermore, it is imperative to consider non-skeletal causes of lower back pain. **Abdominal aortic aneurysms** can present for the first time with back pain. This is particularly important to consider in **older male patients**. **Discitis** and **epidural abscesses** are other rare but important differentials to consider, especially in febrile patients and those with risk factors for serious infections (e.g. immunodeficiency and intravenous drug use).

# SOCRATES

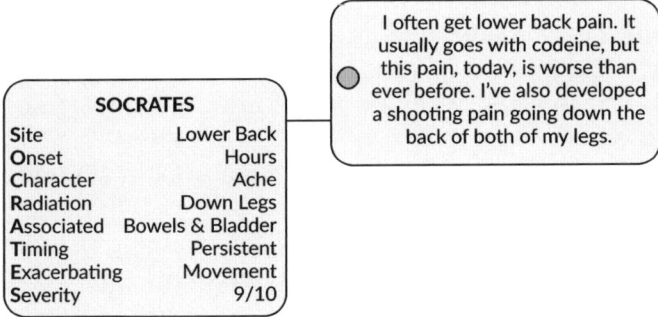

I often get lower back pain. It usually goes with codeine, but this pain, today, is worse than ever before. I've also developed a shooting pain going down the back of both of my legs.

| SOCRATES | |
| --- | --- |
| Site | Lower Back |
| Onset | Hours |
| Character | Ache |
| Radiation | Down Legs |
| Associated | Bowels & Bladder |
| Timing | Persistent |
| Exacerbating | Movement |
| Severity | 9/10 |

There are a few patterns of symptoms that are worth keeping at the back of your mind while you explore SOCRATES in a patient presenting with back pain.

- **Site**
  - ○ **Lower Back**: Most causes of back pain.
  - ○ **Thoracic Back Pain**: Red flag feature that may be suggestive of dangerous underlying diagnosis (e.g. unstable fracture).
- **Onset**
  - ○ **Sudden**: Vertebral fracture and cauda equina syndrome
  - ○ **Over Days**: Discitis and epidural abscesses
  - ○ **Over Weeks or Months**: Mechanical, ankylosing spondylitis, spinal stenosis and aortic aneurysm
    - It is worth noting that mechanical back pain can come on suddenly after an abnormal strain is placed on the back (e.g. lifting a heavy object). In addition, aortic aneurysms may be asymptomatic until they leak or rupture causing sudden back/abdominal pain.
- **Character**
  - ○ **Aching**: Mechanical, ankylosing spondylitis and spinal stenosis
  - ○ **Intense**: Vertebral fracture and cauda equina syndrome
- **Radiation**
  - ○ **Down Legs**: Cauda equina syndrome and spinal stenosis
- **Associated Symptoms**
  - ○ **Bilateral Lower Limb Weakness**: Cauda equina syndrome
  - ○ **Bilateral Lower Limb Pain**: Spinal stenosis (often occurs on exertion and is worse when walking uphill)
  - ○ **Fever**: Discitis and epidural abscesses
  - ○ **Other Evidence of Trauma**: Fracture
  - ○ **Anterior uveitis, Achilles tendinitis**: Ankylosing spondylitis
- **Timing**
  - ○ **Persistent**: Vertebral fracture, cauda equina syndrome, aortic aneurysm and infection
  - ○ **Intermittent**: Ankylosing spondylitis (mornings), spinal stenosis (exertion) and mechanical (movement)
- **Exacerbating**
  - ○ **Movement**: Most causes of back pain tend to be worse with movement, except for ankylosing spondylitis and some cases of mechanical back pain.

- **Severity**: The causes of back pain can vary in severity, and it is difficult to categorise a cause as being more or less severe than another cause.

Read through the classical presentations table in the following section to develop an understanding of how the main differentials are classically present.

# Classical Presentations

| Differential | Classical Presentation |
|---|---|
| **Mechanical Back Pain** | Chronic history of lower back pain that is worse with activity in a patient whose back is excessively loaded because of their constitution (e.g. obesity) or activity (e.g. heavy lifting). |
| **Ankylosing Spondylitis** | Chronic lower back pain and reduced range of spinal mobility in a young patient. The pain is worse in the morning and improves with activity. May be associated with extra-articular manifestations, such as anterior uveitis, Achilles tendinitis, apical lung fibrosis, amyloidosis and aortic regurgitation. |
| **Vertebral Fracture** | **Traumatic**: Sudden onset lower back pain following a fall. May be associated with downstream neurological sequelae if fracture fragments are impinging on the spinal cord. **Compression**: Common in elderly patients and are usually asymptomatic. |
| **Spinal Stenosis** | Chronic history of exertional lower limb pain that is better when walking uphill/sitting and worse when walking downhill. |
| **Cauda Equina Syndrome** | Acute onset severe lower back pain associated with bilateral leg weakness and numbness, urinary retention and faecal incontinence. Examination will reveal saddle anaesthesia and lax anal tone. |

| | |
|---|---|
| **Abdominal Aortic Aneurysm** | May present with an insidious history of back-ache, classically in men over the age of 60 years. If the aneurysm is **leaking** or **ruptured**, patients may present with acute onset central abdominal pain with evidence of hypovolaemic shock (low blood pressure and tachycardia). |
| **Discitis or Epidural Abscess** | Acute onset back pain associated with a fever. It is more common in intravenous drug users. Epidural abscesses can lead to rapidly progressing neurology that relates to the spinal level at which it is found. |

## Red Flags

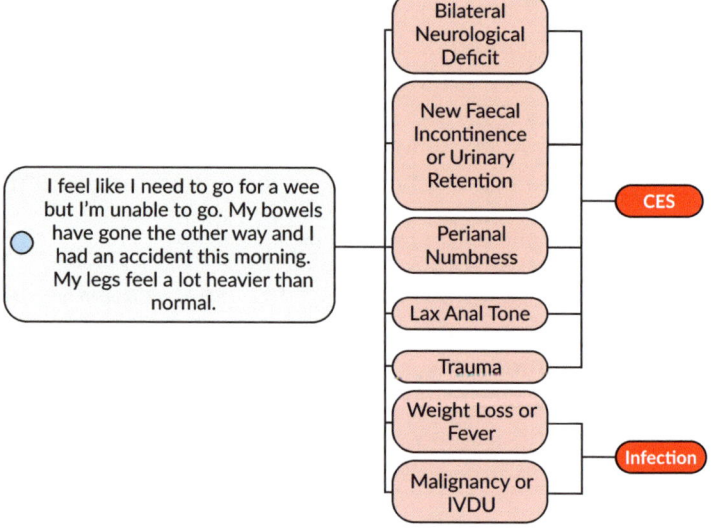

A detailed history that enquires specifically about associated symptoms can help you confidently rule out some of the dangerous causes of back pain.

Compression of the cauda equina leads to disruption of the fibres that make up the sciatic nerve. Therefore, patients will present with **bilateral** sciatica-type features (pain and weakness).

Furthermore, as the fibres of the cauda equina contribute to the pelvic splanchnic nerves that are responsible for the maintenance of urinary and faecal continence, damage to these structures can manifest with **saddle anaesthesia (perianal numbness), lax anal tone, urinary retention** and **faecal incontinence**. It is also important to ask about **trauma** to the area, as a fracture of the vertebra could lead to compression of the cauda equina.

Spinal infections and abscesses should be considered in patients presenting with new back pain and features of infection (e.g. **fever**). Furthermore, **intravenous drug users** are at particularly increased risk of developing discitis as they will frequently introduce *Staphylococcus aureus* into their bloodstreams when injecting.

Acuity alone cannot be used to rule out infectious causes of back pain. **Tuberculosis**, for example, can cause a chronic infection of the vertebrae resulting in bone destruction and paraplegia (known as **Pott's disease**). It is, therefore, important to ask about associated features suggestive of systemic upset (e.g. night sweats and unintentional weight loss).

# Assessment

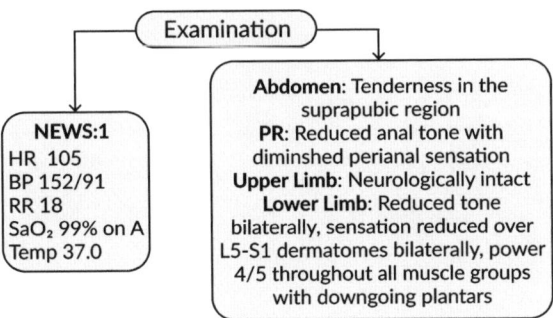

**Examination**

**NEWS:1**
HR 105
BP 152/91
RR 18
SaO₂ 99% on A
Temp 37.0

**Abdomen:** Tenderness in the suprapubic region
**PR:** Reduced anal tone with diminshed perianal sensation
**Upper Limb:** Neurologically intact
**Lower Limb:** Reduced tone bilaterally, sensation reduced over L5-S1 dermatomes bilaterally, power 4/5 throughout all muscle groups with downgoing plantars

## *Observations*

Most patients with back pain will be systemically well. If patients are showing features of infection (e.g. **fever**, tachycardia and hypotension), discitis and epidural abscess should be considered.

## *Examination*

A thorough examination can help prevent unnecessary further investigations (e.g. MRI) by providing you with sufficient clinical information to safely rule out dangerous causes of lower back pain.

The following examinations should be performed to assess for evidence of cauda equina syndrome:

- **Lower Limb Neurology**: In cauda equina syndrome, patients will demonstrate weakness in all muscle groups and impaired sensation over the L5-S1 dermatomes. Most importantly, the symptoms are *bilateral*. A straight leg raise will be difficult to perform and will likely elicit significant pain.
- **Abdominal Examination**: Patients with cauda equina syndrome are at risk of developing urinary retention, so the **bladder may be palpable** and tender. Furthermore, given that an aortic aneurysm is a plausible, if rare, cause of lower back pain, the abdomen should be palpated for a central and expansile mass.
- **Digital Rectal Examination**: Assess the patient's **perianal and perineal sensation** and the **laxity of their anal tone**.

# Cauda Equina Syndrome

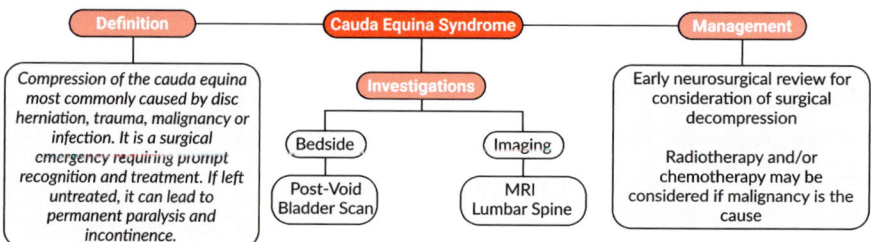

## *Definition*

Cauda equina syndrome refers to the constellation of symptoms that arise due to compression of the cauda equina. This usually involves sudden onset lower back pain, bilateral leg weakness and sensory impairment, urinary retention, faecal incontinence, perianal numbness and lax anal tone.

## Investigations

During the initial assessment, a few simple bedside tests can be used to aid your diagnosis. A **post-void bladder scan** will provide an objective measure of whether the patient is in urinary retention. Furthermore, **urinalysis** can help identify other causes of urinary retention (e.g. UTI).

Ultimately, if cauda equina syndrome is suspected, the patient should undergo an urgent **MRI scan** of their lumbar spine.

## Management

If confirmed by an MRI scan, patients will require urgent neuro-surgical review for consideration of **surgical decompression**. In some cases, especially if malignant causes are suspected, **high-dose steroids** may be administered to reduce oedema. Furthermore, radiotherapy and/or chemotherapy may also be considered for malignant causes of cauda equina syndrome.

# Bridge Box

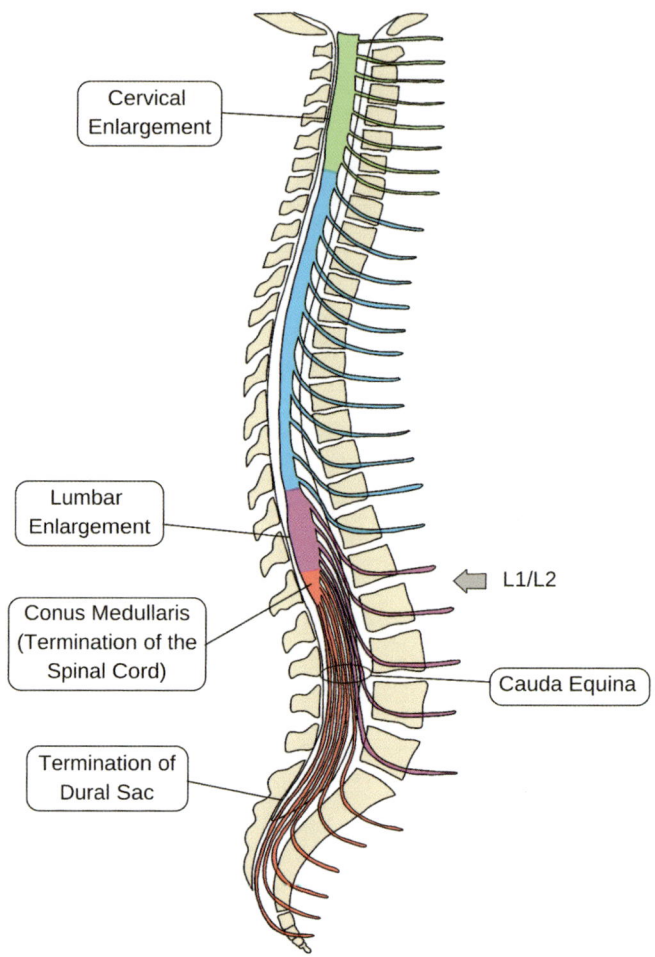

Anatomy of the cauda equina.

# Chapter 21

# Joint Pain

Joint pain is a common complaint among patients presenting to both primary and secondary care services. Establishing the site, onset and precipitating factors can help identify the likely cause.

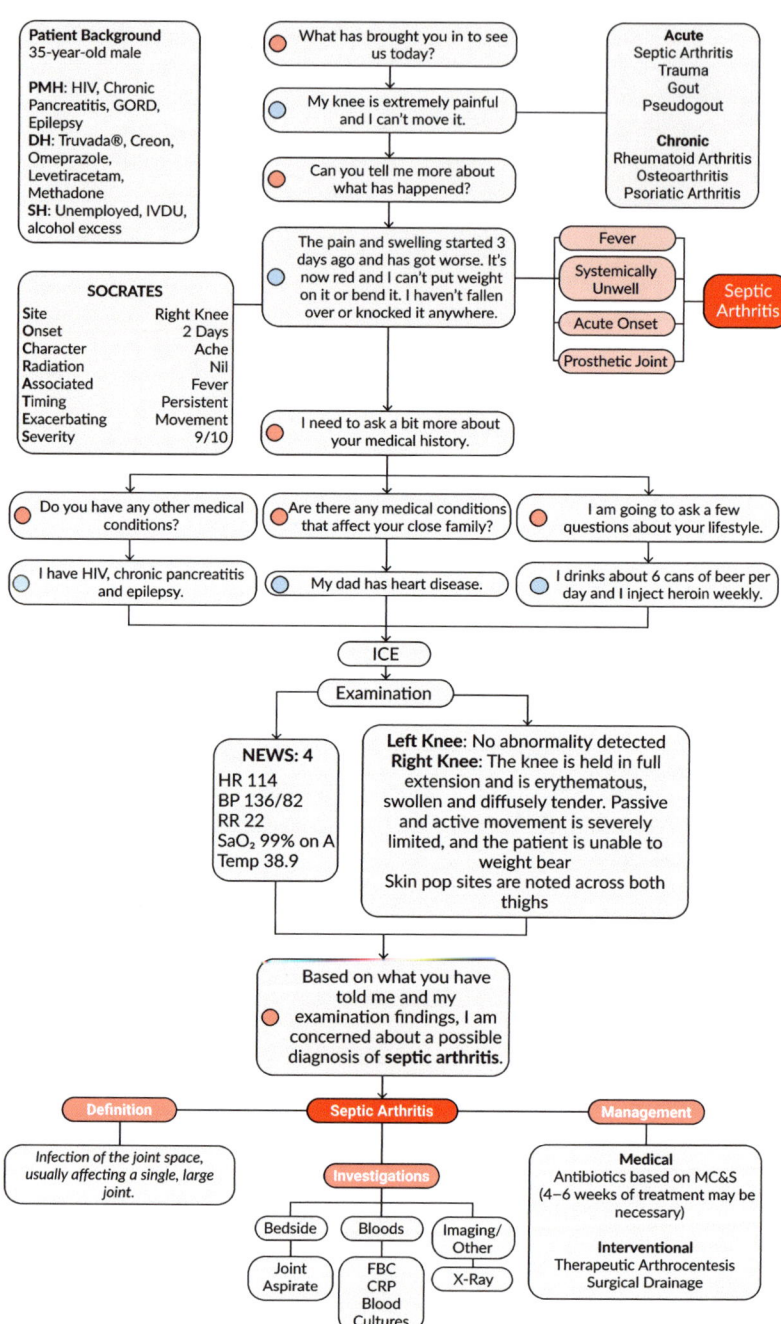

**Patient Background**
35-year-old male

**PMH:** HIV, Chronic Pancreatitis, GORD, Epilepsy
**DH:** Truvada®, Creon, Omeprazole, Levetiracetam, Methadone
**SH:** Unemployed, IVDU, alcohol excess

What has brought you in to see us today?

My knee is extremely painful and I can't move it.

Can you tell me more about what has happened?

The pain and swelling started 3 days ago and has got worse. It's now red and I can't put weight on it or bend it. I haven't fallen over or knocked it anywhere.

**Acute**
Septic Arthritis
Trauma
Gout
Pseudogout

**Chronic**
Rheumatoid Arthritis
Osteoarthritis
Psoriatic Arthritis

Fever

Systemically Unwell

Acute Onset

Prosthetic Joint

**Septic Arthritis**

**SOCRATES**

| | |
|---|---|
| Site | Right Knee |
| Onset | 2 Days |
| Character | Ache |
| Radiation | Nil |
| Associated | Fever |
| Timing | Persistent |
| Exacerbating | Movement |
| Severity | 9/10 |

I need to ask a bit more about your medical history.

Do you have any other medical conditions?

Are there any medical conditions that affect your close family?

I am going to ask a few questions about your lifestyle.

I have HIV, chronic pancreatitis and epilepsy.

My dad has heart disease.

I drinks about 6 cans of beer per day and I inject heroin weekly.

ICE

Examination

**NEWS: 4**

HR 114
BP 136/82
RR 22
SaO$_2$ 99% on A
Temp 38.9

**Left Knee:** No abnormality detected
**Right Knee:** The knee is held in full extension and is erythematous, swollen and diffusely tender. Passive and active movement is severely limited, and the patient is unable to weight bear
Skin pop sites are noted across both thighs

Based on what you have told me and my examination findings, I am concerned about a possible diagnosis of **septic arthritis**.

**Definition**

**Septic Arthritis**

**Management**

Infection of the joint space, usually affecting a single, large joint.

**Medical**
Antibiotics based on MC&S (4–6 weeks of treatment may be necessary)

**Interventional**
Therapeutic Arthrocentesis
Surgical Drainage

**Investigations**

Bedside

Bloods

Imaging/Other

Joint Aspirate

FBC
CRP
Blood Cultures

X-Ray

# Patient Background

The **age** and **sex** of a patient with joint pain can often be helpful in determining the probability of the various differentials. For example, **men** more commonly develop gout, whereas **women** more commonly develop rheumatoid arthritis. Furthermore, septic arthritis can happen at any age, however, younger patients are more likely to develop septic arthritis secondary to sexually transmitted infections, whereas in older patients it is more likely to be caused by enteric bacteria.

In addition, factors that increase the risk of developing serious infection (e.g. **immunodeficiency**) and introducing dangerous bacteria into the bloodstream (e.g. **intravenous drug use**) can lead to a greater risk of developing septic arthritis.

# Differential Diagnosis

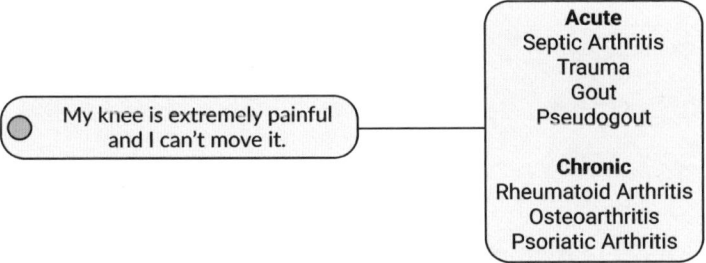

The causes of joint pain can be broadly divided into acute and chronic. The main acute causes that are seen in A&E and primary care are trauma, septic arthritis and crystal arthropathies (gout and pseudogout). Chronic causes of joint pain are more likely to present to a primary care provider and include rheumatoid arthritis, osteoarthritis and psoriatic arthritis.

The diagnoses can also be further delineated based on the pattern of joints affected.

- **Septic Arthritis, Gout and Pseudogout**: Mono- or oligoarthritis. Septic arthritis and pseudogout usually affect larger joints (e.g. knees), whereas gout has a tendency to affect the first metacarpophalangeal joint.
- **Rheumatoid Arthritis**: Symmetrical polyarthritis primarily affecting the small joints of the hands.
- **Osteoarthritis**: Symmetrical oligo- or polyarthritis that mainly affects large weight-bearing joints (e.g. hips and knees) and the small joints of the hands.
- **Psoriatic Arthritis**: Can follow any of the five patterns — symmetrical polyarthritis, asymmetrical oligoarthritis, distal interphalangeal joint involvement, arthritis mutilans and psoriatic spondylitis.

## SOCRATES

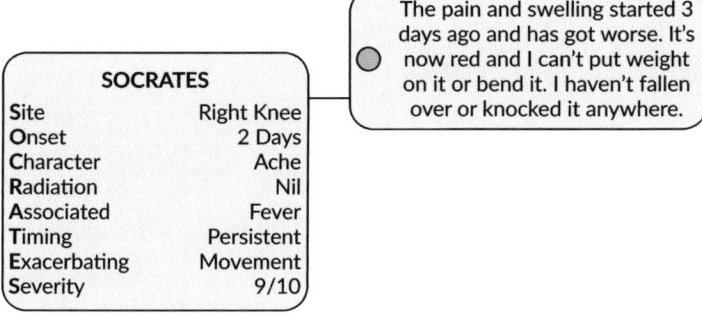

The pain and swelling started 3 days ago and has got worse. It's now red and I can't put weight on it or bend it. I haven't fallen over or knocked it anywhere.

| SOCRATES | |
|---|---|
| Site | Right Knee |
| Onset | 2 Days |
| Character | Ache |
| Radiation | Nil |
| Associated | Fever |
| Timing | Persistent |
| Exacerbating | Movement |
| Severity | 9/10 |

There are a few patterns of symptoms that are worth keeping at the back of your mind while you explore SOCRATES in a patient presenting with joint pain.

- **Site**
  - **Small Joints**: Osteoarthritis, rheumatoid arthritis and psoriatic arthritis
  - **Large Joints**: Gout, pseudogout, septic arthritis and osteoarthritis
- **Onset**
  - **Acute**: Trauma, septic arthritis, gout and pseudogout

- ○ **Chronic**: Osteoarthritis, rheumatoid arthritis and psoriatic arthritis
- **Character**
  - ○ **Stiffness and Ache**: Osteoarthritis, rheumatoid arthritis and psoriatic arthritis
  - ○ **Intense**: Gout, pseudogout and septic arthritis
- **Radiation**: Most causes of joint pain are confined to one or a group of joints.
- **Associated Symptoms**
  - ○ **Fever**: Septic arthritis
  - ○ **Psoriasis and Nail Changes**: Psoriatic arthritis
  - ○ **Fatigue and Weakness**: Rheumatoid arthritis
- **Timing**
  - ○ **Worse in the morning**: Rheumatoid arthritis
  - ○ **Worse after activity**: Osteoarthritis
  - ○ **Persistent**: Gout, pseudogout and septic arthritis
- **Exacerbating**: Most causes of joint pain are worse when moving the affected joint except for rheumatoid arthritis.
- **Severity**: Generally speaking, the acute causes of joint pain are particularly severe (e.g. septic arthritis and gout), whereas the chronic causes may be better tolerated.

Read through the classical presentations table in the following section to develop an understanding of how the main differentials are classically present.

## Classical Presentations

| Differential | Classical Presentation |
|---|---|
| **Septic Arthritis** | Acute onset severe joint pain associated with swelling, redness, tenderness and marked limitation in the range of motion. The patient may be systemically unwell with a fever. |
| **Trauma** | Joint pain that occurs after sustaining trauma to the area. The pain may be immediate in the case of a fracture, or it may be delayed in the case of ligamentous injury. |

| | |
|---|---|
| **Gout and Pseudogout** | Acute onset severe joint pain associated with swelling, tenderness and limited range of motion. It is not commonly associated with systemic upset but can mimic septic arthritis. Gout most commonly affects the first metatarsophalangeal joint and pseudogout usually affects large joints (e.g. knee). |
| **Rheumatoid Arthritis** | Chronic history of pain and stiffness in the small joints of the hands (sparing the distal interphalangeal joints) and feet that progress over time. The pain is worse in the morning and improves with the use of the affected joints. Classically present in middle-aged women. |
| **Osteoarthritis** | Chronic history of pain that is worse when using the affected joints and improves with rest. Can affect large weight-bearing joints and the small joints of the hands and feet. |
| **Psoriatic Arthritis** | Chronic history of joint pain in patients with a background of psoriasis. Patients may also have nail changes, such as pitting, onycholysis and subungual hyperkeratosis. The arthritis usually follows five possible patterns: symmetrical polyarthritis, asymmetrical oligoarthritis, distal interphalangeal joint involvement, arthritis mutilans and psoriatic spondylitis. |

# Red Flags

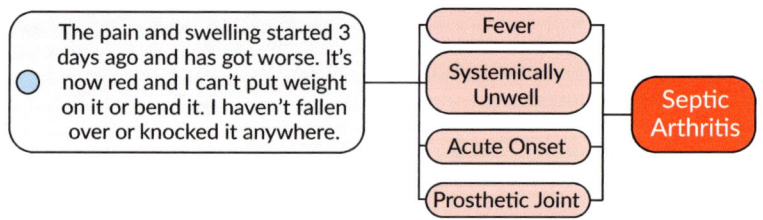

Septic arthritis is the most concerning form of monoarthritis as it can progress rapidly and cause extensive joint destruction.

Classically, the joint in septic arthritis will appear **red, hot, swollen and extremely tender** with a marked **limitation in the range of motion**. These changes would have arisen over a period of hours or days. Though this description may also be in keeping with a diagnosis of gout or pseudogout, if there is any concern about a possible diagnosis of septic arthritis, the patient should be commenced on antibiotics and the joint should be aspirated urgently. In some cases, patients with septic arthritis may also have a **fever** and be **systemically unwell**.

# Assessment

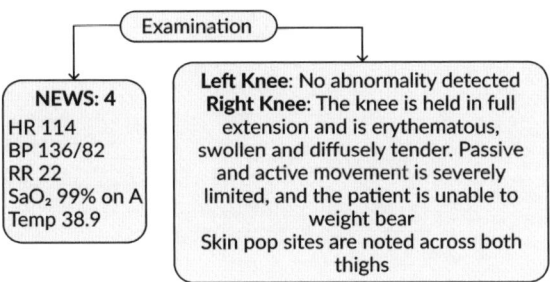

## Observations

In most cases of acute joint pain, patients will have normal observations. An important exception, however, is septic arthritis — in such cases, the patients may have developed a **fever** and be showing signs of sepsis (**tachycardia and hypotension**).

## Examination

Comparing symmetrical joints is useful to more accurately assess the changes that have taken place within the affected joint. In acute monoarthritides (septic arthritis, gout and pseudogout), the joint will be **red, hot, swollen and extremely tender** with a **limited range of active and passive motion**.

Though this will likely be apparent from the history, the presence of **surgical scars** in the skin surrounding the joint may allude to the presence of prosthetic material within the joint. Furthermore, the skin should be checked for any **penetrating injuries** that may have introduced bacteria into the region.

Patients presenting with chronic arthritis may have some evidence of deformity if they present relatively late in the course of the disease. This includes **Heberden's** and **Bouchard's nodes** which are bony swellings in the hands seen in osteoarthritis. Patients with rheumatoid arthritis, on the other hand, may develop **Swan neck** and **Boutonniere deformity**.

# Septic Arthritis

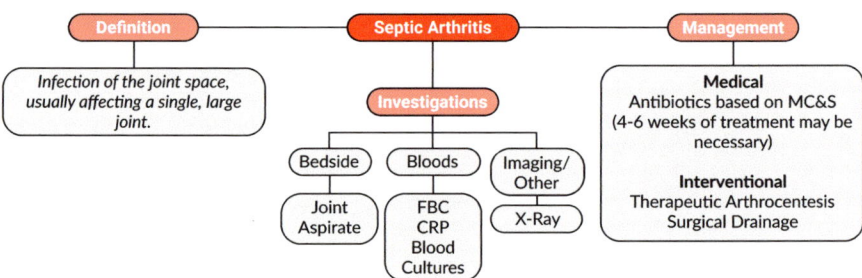

## *Definition*

Septic arthritis refers to an infection of the joint space that can cause rapidly progressive joint destruction.

## *Investigations*

A **joint aspirate** is a crucial investigation that can help confirm the diagnosis in patients presenting with an acute monoarthritis. It can be sent for microscopy and culture to confirm the diagnosis of septic arthritis and identify the causative organism. Microscopy will also help diagnose gout (negatively birefringent, needle-shaped crystals) and pseudogout (positively birefringent, rhomboid-shaped crystals).

The patient's inflammatory markers are likely to be raised (**FBC** and **CRP**) and **blood cultures** should be taken, ideally before starting treatment, to identify the causative organism. An **X-Ray** should also be requested to check for any evidence of trauma.

## Management

Patients with septic arthritis should have the **joint aspirated** and they will also need a prolonged course of **antibiotics** based on the culture and sensitivity results. If septic arthritis has developed in a prosthetic joint, the prosthesis may need to be revised.

# Bridge Box

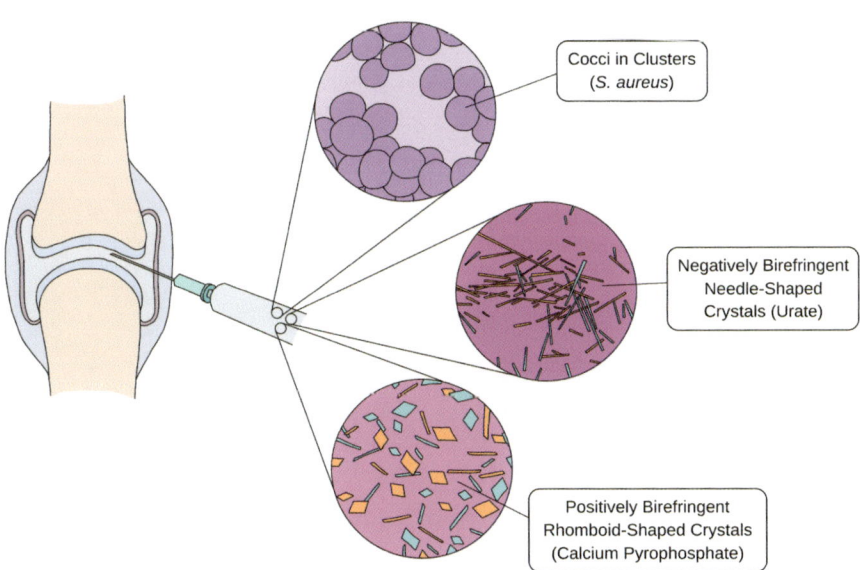

Differentials for joint pain.

# Chapter 22

# Leg Pain

Leg pain is a relatively straightforward presentation to assess due to the narrow differential. Important differentials that should not be missed include DVT and acute limb ischaemia.

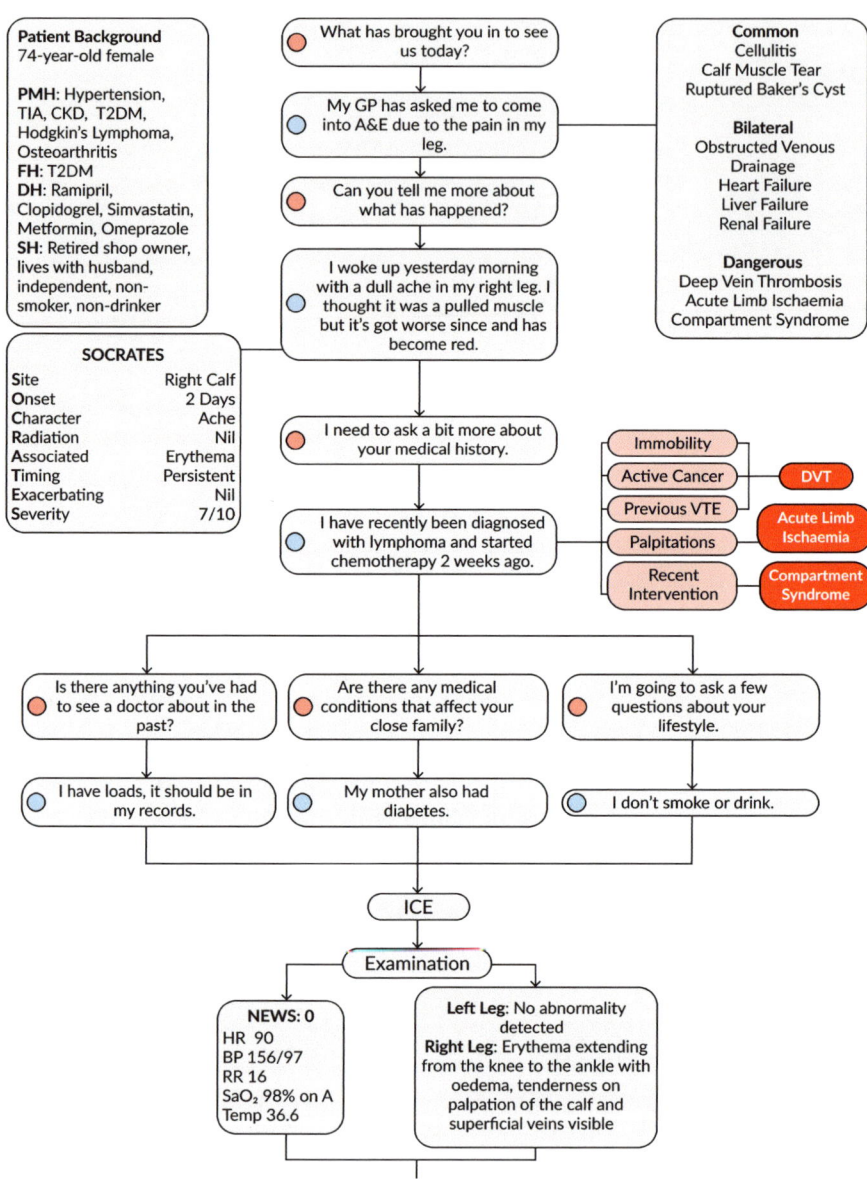

**Patient Background**
74-year-old female

**PMH:** Hypertension, TIA, CKD, T2DM, Hodgkin's Lymphoma, Osteoarthritis
**FH:** T2DM
**DH:** Ramipril, Clopidogrel, Simvastatin, Metformin, Omeprazole
**SH:** Retired shop owner, lives with husband, independent, non-smoker, non-drinker

**SOCRATES**

| | |
|---|---|
| Site | Right Calf |
| Onset | 2 Days |
| Character | Ache |
| Radiation | Nil |
| Associated | Erythema |
| Timing | Persistent |
| Exacerbating | Nil |
| Severity | 7/10 |

What has brought you in to see us today?

My GP has asked me to come into A&E due to the pain in my leg.

Can you tell me more about what has happened?

I woke up yesterday morning with a dull ache in my right leg. I thought it was a pulled muscle but it's got worse since and has become red.

I need to ask a bit more about your medical history.

I have recently been diagnosed with lymphoma and started chemotherapy 2 weeks ago.

Is there anything you've had to see a doctor about in the past?

I have loads, it should be in my records.

Are there any medical conditions that affect your close family?

My mother also had diabetes.

I'm going to ask a few questions about your lifestyle.

I don't smoke or drink.

**Common**
Cellulitis
Calf Muscle Tear
Ruptured Baker's Cyst

**Bilateral**
Obstructed Venous Drainage
Heart Failure
Liver Failure
Renal Failure

**Dangerous**
Deep Vein Thrombosis
Acute Limb Ischaemia
Compartment Syndrome

Immobility
Active Cancer
Previous VTE
Palpitations
Recent Intervention

DVT
Acute Limb Ischaemia
Compartment Syndrome

ICE

Examination

**NEWS: 0**
HR 90
BP 156/97
RR 16
SaO₂ 98% on A
Temp 36.6

**Left Leg:** No abnormality detected
**Right Leg:** Erythema extending from the knee to the ankle with oedema, tenderness on palpation of the calf and superficial veins visible

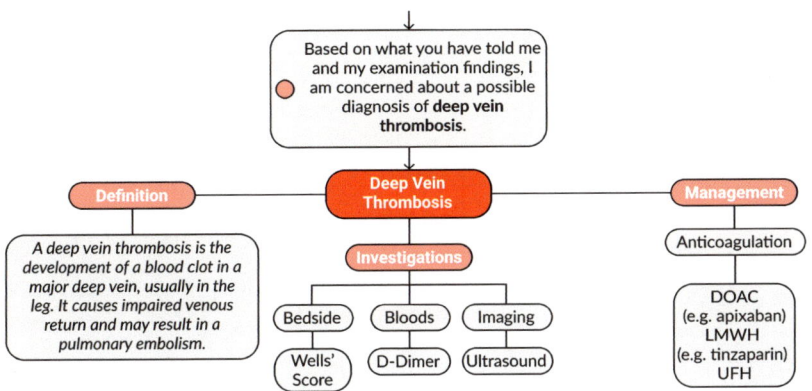

# Patient Background

**Patient Background**
74-year-old female

**PMH:** Hypertension, TIA, CKD, T2DM, Hodgkin's Lymphoma, Osteoarthritis
**FH:** T2DM
**DH:** Ramipril, Clopidogrel, Simvastatin, Metformin, Omeprazole
**SH:** Retired shop owner, lives with husband, independent, non-smoker, non-drinker

Deep vein thrombosis (DVT) is a concerning cause of leg pain and usually arises in the context of multiple risk factors. Several of these can be elicited from the patient background. For example, patients who are **pregnant**, have **active cancer** or have **recent surgery** are at significantly increased risk of developing a DVT. It should be noted if patients have a **family history of venous thromboembolism** as it may be suggestive of an inherited defect resulting in hypercoagulability (e.g. Factor V Leiden). Common medications that can increase the risk of VTE include the **combined oral contraceptive pill**, **hormone replacement therapy** and **tamoxifen**.

Acute limb ischaemia is another serious cause of acute limb pain and **atrial fibrillation** is a significant risk factor as it leads to the formation of clots within the left atrium which can then embolise to a peripheral artery causing limb ischaemia. The same risk factors for ischaemic heart disease apply to peripheral vascular disease (e.g. hypertension, smoking and obesity).

**Diabetes mellitus** can predispose patients to develop infections (e.g. cellulitis), as can the presence of known defects in the skin (e.g. ulcers).

## Differential Diagnosis

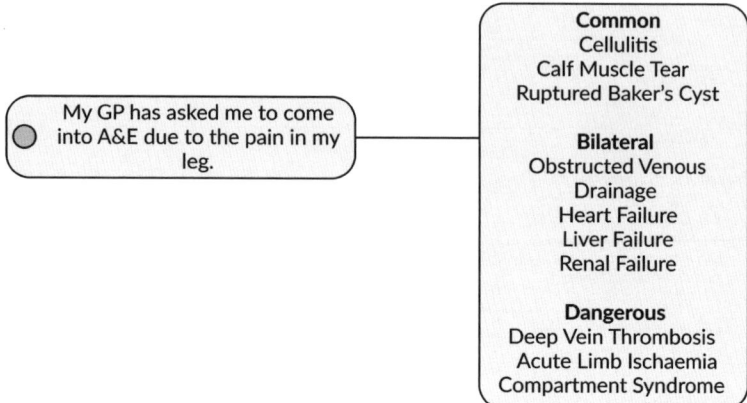

Most cases of leg pain will arise due to muscular injuries (e.g. calf muscle strain) which typically have a **preceding history of exercise** or **abnormal exertion**. A Baker's cyst is a collection of fluid within the popliteal fossa which may cause some discomfort in the area and, if it bursts, can cause acute onset calf pain. It typically happens in patients with a background of knee problems (e.g. osteoarthritis and rheumatoid arthritis).

Subacute onset lower limb pain associated with a **red, tender swelling** may be suggestive of cellulitis. Often such infections are mild, however, if severe, they can cause systemic upset requiring admission for inpatient antibiotics. It is good practice to mark the area of cellulitis upon initial assessment to monitor the response to treatment. If the pain in a limb is out of proportion with the clinical appearance, **necrotising fasciitis** is a crucial differential to consider as it can spread rapidly across the fascial planes and cause widespread soft tissue destruction. Similarly, **compartment syndrome** should be considered in a patient who has recently undergone an intervention on the leg (e.g. embolectomy and fracture repair) presenting with sudden onset pain that is out of proportion with the clinical findings.

Acute limb ischaemia classically presents with sudden onset severe pain in one of the lower limbs. Upon assessment, the limb may demonstrate the **5 Ps**: **p**ale, **p**ulseless, **p**ainful, **p**erishingly cold and **p**aralysis/**p**araesthesia. It is worth noting that patients with a known background of peripheral vascular disease are less likely to present so acutely, as they would have had time to develop collateral blood vessels which reduces the risk of acute ischaemia. Most cases of acute limb ischaemia will be embolic (usually due to emboli arising from the heart).

In patients with **progressive, bilateral oedema** without any other obvious cause (e.g. heart, liver or renal failure), obstructed venous or lymphatic drainage should be considered as a possible cause. Certain abdominal and pelvic malignancies, such as ovarian cancer, often present insidiously and leg swelling may be the first sign that is noticed by the patient.

## SOCRATES

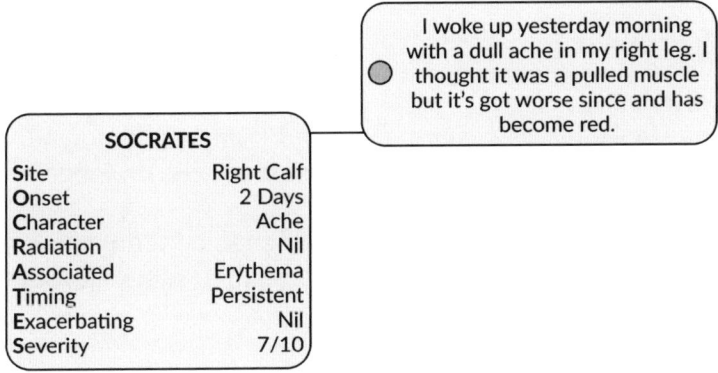

| SOCRATES | |
|---|---|
| Site | Right Calf |
| Onset | 2 Days |
| Character | Ache |
| Radiation | Nil |
| Associated | Erythema |
| Timing | Persistent |
| Exacerbating | Nil |
| Severity | 7/10 |

I woke up yesterday morning with a dull ache in my right leg. I thought it was a pulled muscle but it's got worse since and has become red.

There are a few patterns of symptoms that are worth keeping at the back of your mind while you explore SOCRATES in a patient presenting with leg pain.

- **Site**
  - **Unilateral**: Ruptured Baker's cyst, calf muscle tear, DVT, cellulitis, acute limb ischaemia and compartment syndrome
  - **Bilateral**: Obstructed venous drainage and organ failure
- **Onset**
  - **Sudden**: Ruptured Baker's cyst, acute limb ischaemia and compartment syndrome
  - **Gradual**: DVT, cellulitis, obstructed venous drainage and organ failure

- **Character**
  - **Ache**: DVT and cellulitis
  - **Intense**: Acute limb ischaemia and compartment syndrome
- **Radiation**: Most cases of leg pain will be confined to the affected leg.
- **Associated Symptoms**
  - **Fever**: Cellulitis
  - **Erythema**: Cellulitis and DVT
  - **Pale**: Acute limb ischaemia
  - **Pulseless, Paraesthesia, Paralysis**: Acute limb ischaemia and compartment syndrome
- **Timing**
  - **After Exercise/Exertion**: Calf muscle tear
  - **After Intervention (e.g. fracture repair)**: Compartment syndrome
- **Exacerbating**: Most causes of leg pain will be worse when moving the leg.
- **Severity**
  - **Severe**: Acute limb ischaemia and compartment syndrome
  - **Discomfort**: Organ failure, obstructed venous drainage and DVT

Read through the classical presentations table in the following section to develop an understanding of how the main differentials are classically present.

## Classical Presentations

| Differential | Classical Presentation |
|---|---|
| **Cellulitis** | Superficial, spreading area of erythematous, swollen and tender skin. There may be a clear puncture site or another breach in the skin (e.g. ulcer). Patients may also be systemically unwell with a fever. |
| **Pulled or Torn Calf Muscle** | Sudden onset pain in the calf that usually occurs soon after exercise or abnormal exertion. |

| | |
|---|---|
| **Ruptured Baker's Cyst** | Sudden pain along the posterior aspect of the lower leg with a preceding history of a swelling around the popliteal fossa. |
| **Obstructed Venous Drainage** | Gradual onset bilateral leg swelling with evidence of chronic venous insufficiency (e.g. venous ulcers and varicose veins). Patients may have other symptoms related to the cause of the compression (e.g. abdominal bloating in ovarian cancer). |
| **Organ Failure** | **Heart Failure**: Chronic history of worsening exercise tolerance and bilateral leg swelling in a patient with cardiovascular risk factors. Other features include orthopnoea and paroxysmal nocturnal dyspnoea.<br>**Liver Failure**: History of jaundice, abdominal distension, easy bruising and bilateral leg swelling in a patient with a background of liver disease (e.g. alcoholic liver disease).<br>**Renal Failure**: Progressive breathlessness and bilateral leg swelling in a patient with known renal impairment. Other features include low urine output, fatigue and itching. |
| **Deep Vein Thrombosis** | Subacute onset unilateral leg swelling, pain and redness. May have evidence of risk factors in recent history (e.g. cancer, immobility and surgery). |
| **Acute Limb Ischaemia** | Sudden onset unilateral leg pain. The leg will look pale and feel cold with impalpable pulses and, sometimes, patients may complain of paralysis or paraesthesia. Patients may have a background of cardiovascular risk factors, in particular, atrial fibrillation. |
| **Compartment Syndrome** | Unilateral pain, swelling and tenderness in a limb that is out of proportion with the visible signs. Usually occurs in the context of a fracture, recent surgery or revascularisation of ischaemic limbs. |

# Red Flags

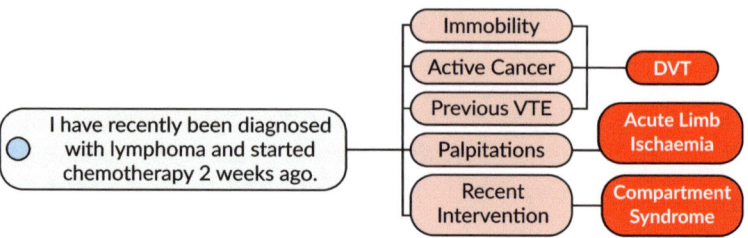

As mentioned earlier, DVT and acute limb ischaemia are the main concerning causes of acute onset limb pain in a patient presenting to the emergency department or primary care. The precipitants of DVT can be remembered by considering **Virchow's triad**: hyper-coagulability, vessel wall injury and stasis. Venous clots, in general, arise due to stasis, and causes of stasis include **prolonged immobility** (e.g. due to a recent illness) and **obesity**. Some patients may be hypercoagulable due to a **genetic predisposition** (e.g. Factor V Leiden) or it may be acquired (e.g. **pregnancy, cancer and inflammatory diseases**).

Many cases of embolic acute limb ischaemia arise in patients with **atrial fibrillation**. If it has not previously been diagnosed, patients should be asked whether they tend to experience **palpitations** and an ECG should be performed.

# Assessment

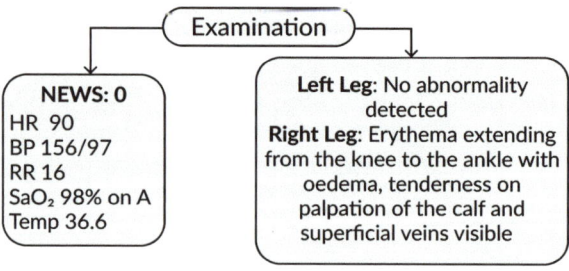

## *Observations*

Some patients with cellulitis may develop features of **sepsis** (fever, tachycardia and hypotension). Tachycardia, tachypnoea and desaturation in a patient with acute lower limb pain should also alert you about the possibility of a **pulmonary embolism** arising from a DVT. An **irregular tachycardia** may be suggestive of atrial fibrillation which is a major risk factor for acute limb ischaemia.

## *Examination*

It is useful to compare both legs to assess whether the changes are bilateral and to gauge how significant the described changes are. **Swelling, erythema, warmth and tenderness** of an area of the lower limb could be suggestive of cellulitis or DVT. The erythema is likely to be more pronounced in cellulitis and, in some cases, patients may develop a **palpable subcutaneous collection**. It is worth noting the presence of **ulcers** as this would significantly increase the risk of a patient developing cellulitis. Thready or absent pulses in a cold, painful foot are suggestive of limb ischaemia.

# Deep Vein Thrombosis

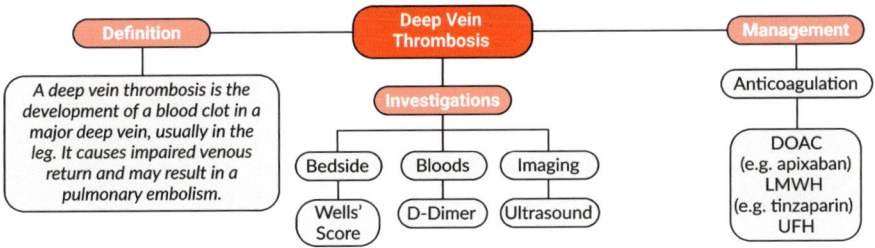

## *Definition*

A DVT is a blood clot within a major deep vein, usually in a leg. It is a medical emergency as it could give rise to a pulmonary embolism.

## Investigations

The initial assessment of a suspected DVT involves calculating the **Wells' score**. This is a risk assessment tool that determines whether a patient should have a **D-Dimer** or be referred directly for an urgent **ultrasound** of the affected limb. As cellulitis can be difficult to distinguish from a DVT, an **FBC** and a **CRP** should be requested as raised inflammatory markers are in keeping with an infectious process.

## Management

The first-line treatment for DVT is a **direct acting oral anticoagulant** (e.g. apixaban). In some cases, if DOACs are contraindicated, **low molecular weight heparins** (e.g. tinzaparin) may be used. **Unfractionated heparin** tends to be used primarily in patients with renal failure and in those that may require rapid reversal of anticoagulation (usually due to high bleeding risk). If the DVT is considered provoked (i.e. there is a clear precipitant such as recent surgery), anticoagulation should be continued for at least 3 months. If it is unprovoked, anticoagulation should be continued for 6 months, and **thrombophilia screening** should be arranged. This normally involves assessing for occult malignancy and inherited defects in clotting factors.

# Bridge Box

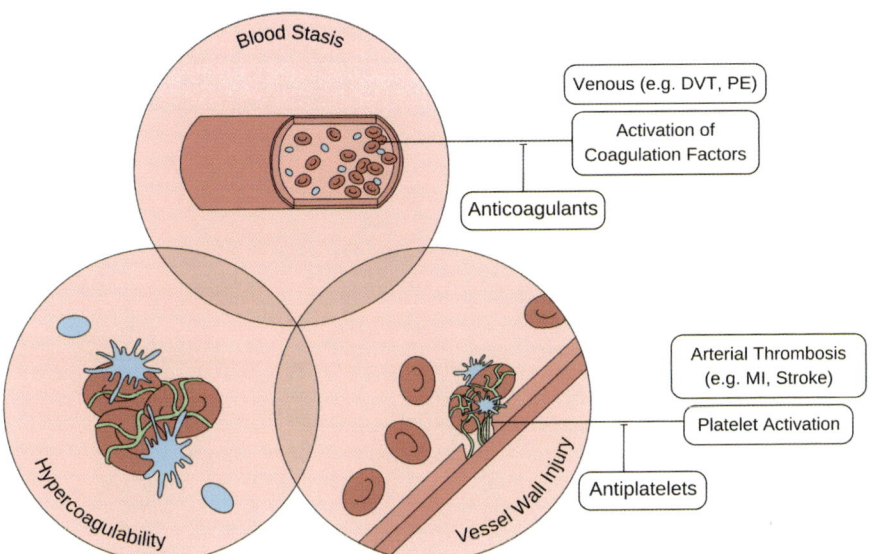

Factors contributing to intravascular thrombus formation.

# Chapter 23

# Weight Loss

Weight loss can often be attributed to lifestyle factors (e.g. changes in diet and exercise levels), however, it may also be suggestive of underlying catabolic processes that require further investigation and management.

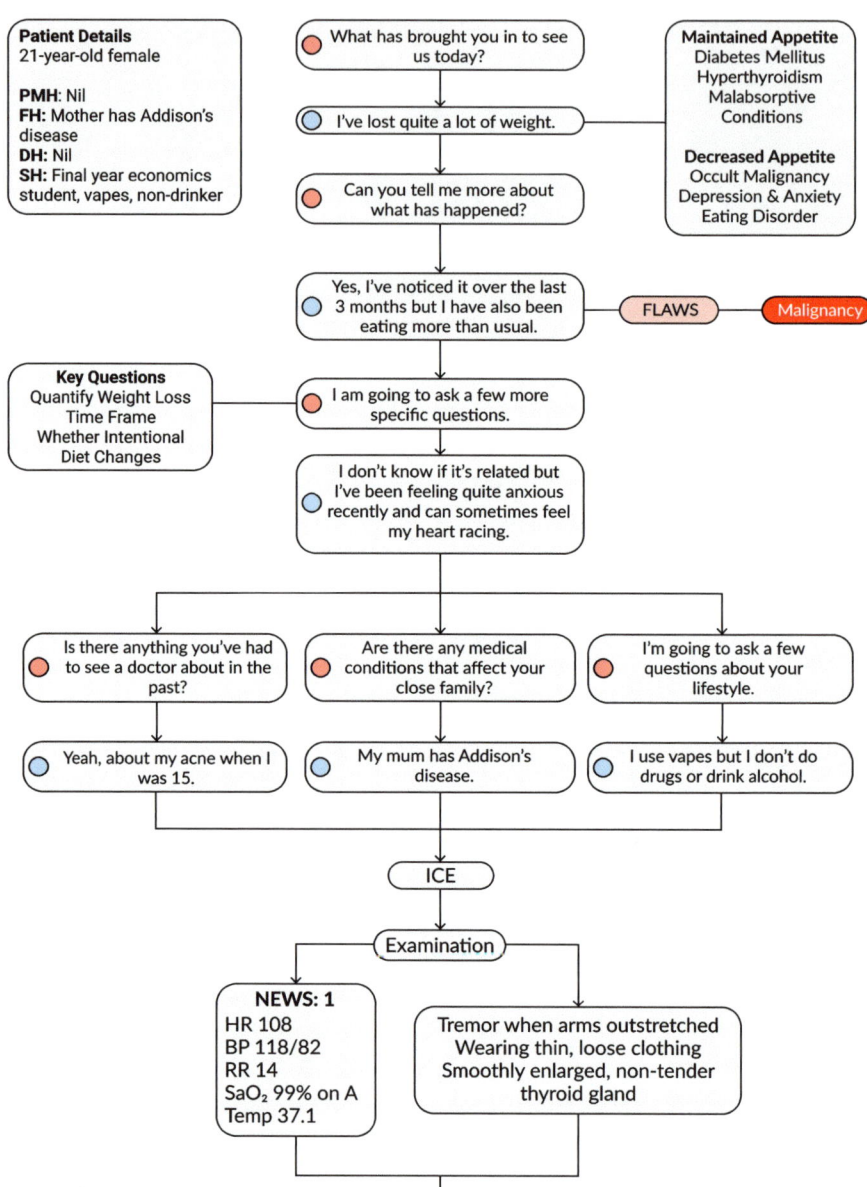

**Patient Details**
21-year-old female

**PMH:** Nil
**FH:** Mother has Addison's disease
**DH:** Nil
**SH:** Final year economics student, vapes, non-drinker

What has brought you in to see us today?

I've lost quite a lot of weight.

**Maintained Appetite**
Diabetes Mellitus
Hyperthyroidism
Malabsorptive Conditions

**Decreased Appetite**
Occult Malignancy
Depression & Anxiety
Eating Disorder

Can you tell me more about what has happened?

Yes, I've noticed it over the last 3 months but I have also been eating more than usual.

FLAWS    Malignancy

**Key Questions**
Quantify Weight Loss
Time Frame
Whether Intentional
Diet Changes

I am going to ask a few more specific questions.

I don't know if it's related but I've been feeling quite anxious recently and can sometimes feel my heart racing.

Is there anything you've had to see a doctor about in the past?

Are there any medical conditions that affect your close family?

I'm going to ask a few questions about your lifestyle.

Yeah, about my acne when I was 15.

My mum has Addison's disease.

I use vapes but I don't do drugs or drink alcohol.

ICE

Examination

**NEWS: 1**
HR 108
BP 118/82
RR 14
$SaO_2$ 99% on A
Temp 37.1

Tremor when arms outstretched
Wearing thin, loose clothing
Smoothly enlarged, non-tender thyroid gland

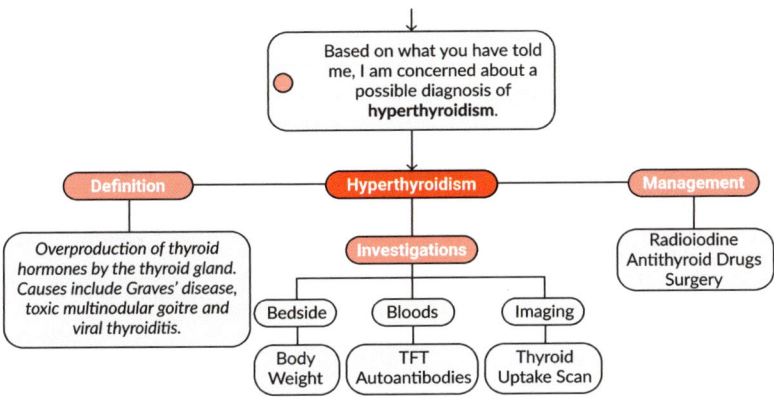

## Patient Background

**Patient Details**
21-year-old female

**PMH**: Nil
**FH**: Mother has Addison's disease
**DH**: Nil
**SH**: Final year economics student, vapes, non-drinker

Causes of weight loss that are generally more common in **younger patients** include eating disorders, depression, anxiety disorder, inflammatory bowel disease and coeliac disease. In **older patients**, there should be a low threshold for considering underlying malignancy as a potential cause for unintentional weight loss. It is important to ask detailed questions about the patient's lifestyle and their current mental state and stress levels. A common cause of unintentional weight loss is depression and anxiety that may be precipitated by lifestyle factors, such as work or relationships. It is appropriate to enquire in detail about their **dietary habits**, **sleep hygiene** and **activity levels** to determine which simple adjustments may help resolve the symptoms.

## Differential Diagnosis

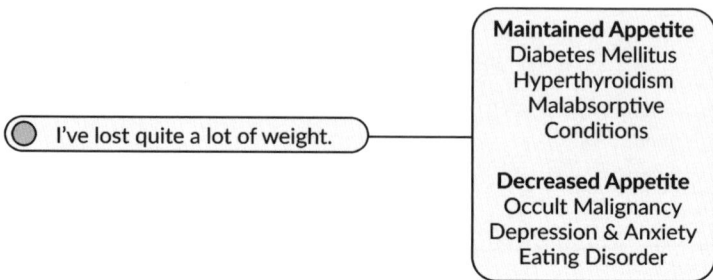

Broadly speaking, the causes of weight loss can be categorised into those associated with maintained appetite and decreased appetite. The causes that are associated with a maintained appetite are generally **metabolic conditions** (e.g. diabetes mellitus and hyperthyroidism) and **malabsorptive conditions** (e.g. inflammatory bowel disease and coeliac disease).

Causes that are associated with decreased appetite are generally **catabolic conditions** that increase the body's energy requirements (e.g. malignancy) and **mental health conditions** (e.g. depression, anxiety disorder and eating disorders).

## Key Questions

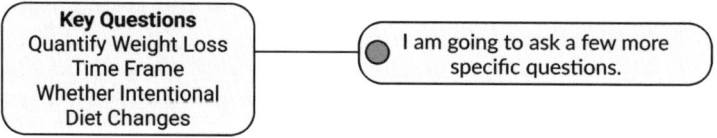

Unintentional weight loss occurs when energy consumption exceeds energy intake. Therefore, it is important to ask detailed questions about the **quantity** of weight lost (the patient should be weighed during the consultation to have some objective measurement on record), the **time frame** over which they believe this happened and whether they had any **intention** of losing weight. Furthermore, a detailed **dietary history** should be taken to determine whether undernourishment due to poor dietary habits has precipitated the weight loss. If a patient's diet is deemed insufficient to meet their calorie requirements, you should enquire about why they maintain such a diet. This may expose contributing factors, such as being unable to cook, losing their appetite and lacking energy to make or source food.

Read through the classical presentations table in the following section to develop an understanding of how the main differentials are classically present.

## Classical Presentations

| Differential | Classical Presentation |
|---|---|
| Diabetes Mellitus | **Type 1 Diabetes Mellitus**: Presenting in young people with a history of polyuria and nocturia. They may describe some weight loss and trouble gaining weight. They may present acutely with diabetic ketoacidosis. **Type 2 Diabetes Mellitus**: Presenting in adults with polyuria and nocturia. Patients are often overweight and there may be a family history. |
| Hyperthyroidism | Chronic history of anxiety, excessive sweating, palpitations, tremor, heat intolerance and diarrhoea. Some patients may even notice a midline enlargement in their neck. |
| Malabsorptive Conditions | Chronic history of diarrhoea that may be pale and difficult to flush away (in coeliac disease) or may be associated with rectal bleeding (inflammatory bowel disease). |
| Occult Malignancy | Chronic history of fatigue and weight loss that may be associated with loss of appetite and night sweats. There may be localising symptoms (e.g. lymphadenopathy in lymphoma, cough in lung cancer or rectal bleeding in colorectal cancer). |

| | |
|---|---|
| **Depression and Anxiety Disorder** | **Depression**: Chronic history of low mood, low energy and little interest doing activities that they previously enjoyed. Often associated with sleep and appetite disturbance, and impaired concentration and memory. **Anxiety Disorder**: Characterised by excessive anxiety that may be free-floating (generalised) or related to a more specific trigger or circumstance (e.g. social phobia). |
| **Eating Disorders** | **Anorexia Nervosa**: Chronic history of poor oral intake, morbid preoccupation with body weight and appearance and significant weight loss. May be associated with purging behaviours. **Bulimia Nervosa**: Chronic history of bingeing (eating large amounts of food) followed by purging (e.g. forced vomiting and laxative abuse). Patients may maintain a normal body weight. |

## Red Flags

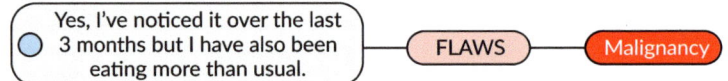

Though all organic causes of unintentional weight loss require a thorough assessment, an underlying malignancy is the most urgent cause that must be identified and treated. Manifestations of constitutional upset that are classically associated with malignancy can be remembered using the mnemonic **FLAWS**, which stands for **F**ever, **L**ethargy, **A**ppetite loss, **W**eight loss and night **S**weats. There may, in some cases, be localising symptoms of the malignancy, for example, an altered bowel habit may be suggestive of underlying colorectal cancer.

# Assessment

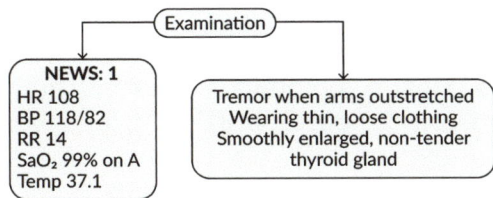

## Observations

In most cases, patients with unintentional weight loss will present to primary care with a chronic history and they are unlikely to have any significant abnormalities in their observations. Patients with hyperthyroidism may be noted to be **tachycardic**.

## Examination

The appearance of the patient can help gauge the extent of their weight loss, for example, by looking at how their clothes fit. Examination findings that are in keeping with hyperthyroidism include **exophthalmos**, **tremor**, **goitre** and **pretibial myxoedema**. The patient's abdomen should also be examined to feel for any potential masses. The patient should be **formally weighed** during the consultation and the weight should be recorded for monitoring purposes.

# Hyperthyroidism

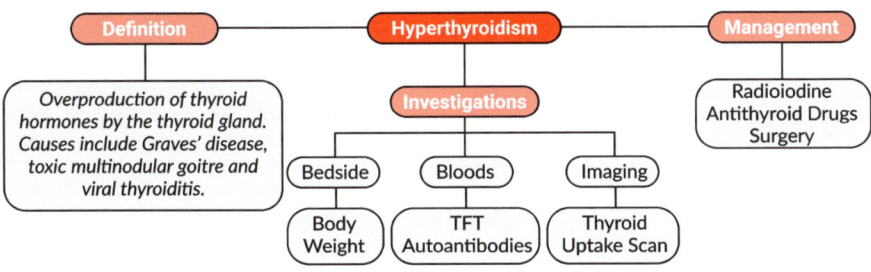

## Definition

Hyperthyroidism refers to the excess production and activity of thyroid hormones and it can be caused by several conditions including Graves' disease (most common), toxic multinodular goitre and viral thyroiditis (also known as de Quervain's thyroiditis).

## Investigations

As mentioned earlier, the patient's **body weight** should be recorded. A **TFT** should be sent which will likely show a suppressed TSH level and raised $T_4$ level. There is a panel of **autoantibodies** that are also sent in patients with suspected thyroid disease: TSH receptor-stimulating antibodies (most sensitive and specific), anti-thyroid peroxidase antibodies and anti-thyroglobulin antibodies. A **thyroid uptake scan** may also be performed as the scintigraphy pattern will allow you to distinguish between the various causes of hyperthyroidism.

## Management

The management depends on the cause, for example, viral thyroiditis is often managed conservatively as it is self-limiting. Graves' disease and toxic multinodular goitre may be treated with **radioiodine**, **antithyroid drugs** (e.g. carbimazole) and **surgery** (e.g. thyroidectomy).

# Bridge Box

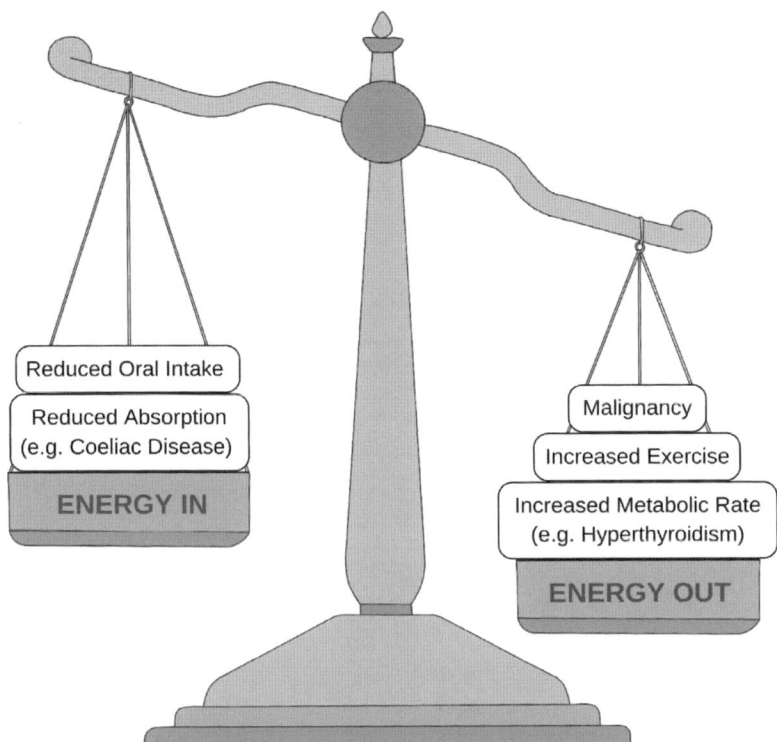

Factors contributing to weight loss.

# Chapter 24

# Fatigue

Fatigue is one of the most frequent presenting complaints in primary care. It can be daunting to encounter due to the extensive range of differentials.

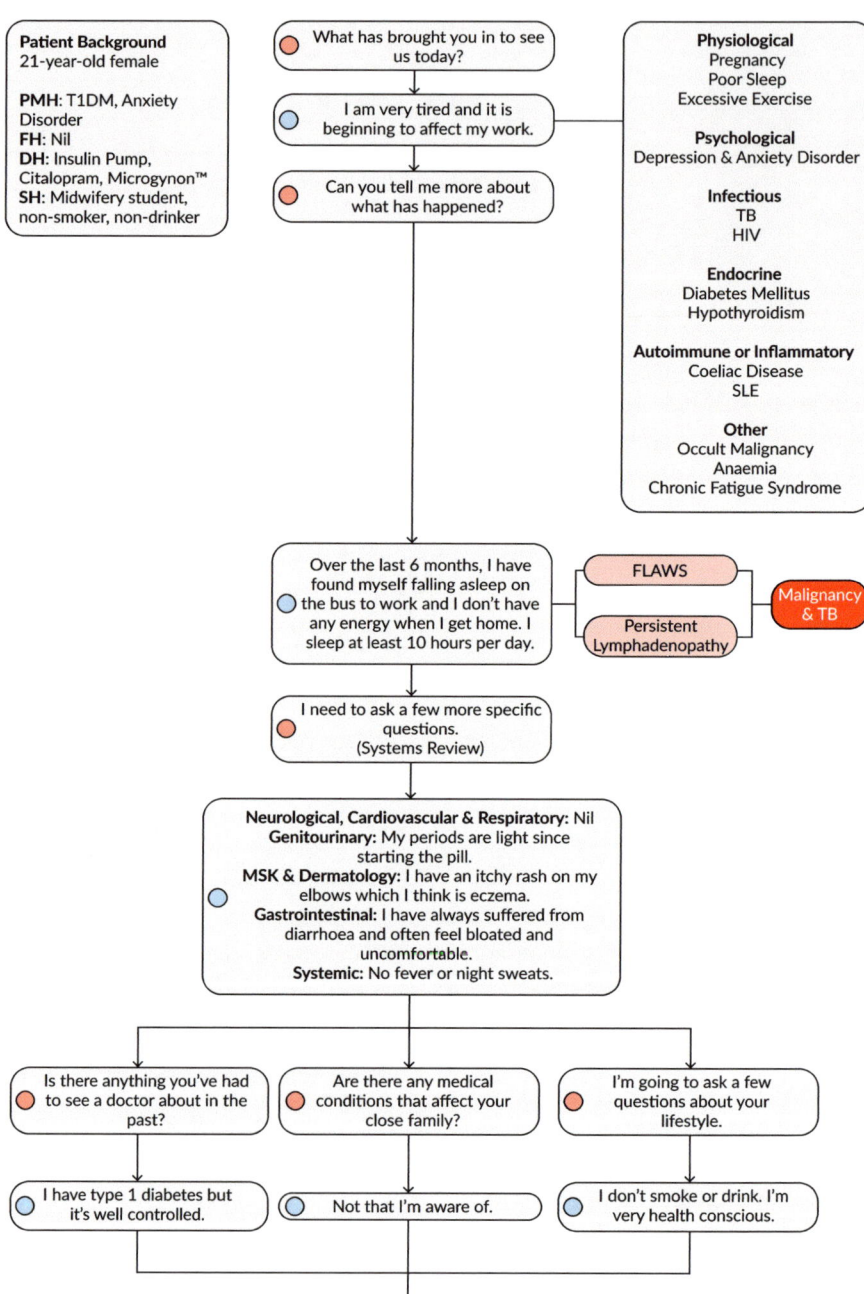

**Patient Background**
21-year-old female

**PMH**: T1DM, Anxiety Disorder
**FH**: Nil
**DH**: Insulin Pump, Citalopram, Microgynon™
**SH**: Midwifery student, non-smoker, non-drinker

What has brought you in to see us today?

I am very tired and it is beginning to affect my work.

Can you tell me more about what has happened?

**Physiological**
Pregnancy
Poor Sleep
Excessive Exercise

**Psychological**
Depression & Anxiety Disorder

**Infectious**
TB
HIV

**Endocrine**
Diabetes Mellitus
Hypothyroidism

**Autoimmune or Inflammatory**
Coeliac Disease
SLE

**Other**
Occult Malignancy
Anaemia
Chronic Fatigue Syndrome

Over the last 6 months, I have found myself falling asleep on the bus to work and I don't have any energy when I get home. I sleep at least 10 hours per day.

FLAWS

Persistent Lymphadenopathy

Malignancy & TB

I need to ask a few more specific questions.
(Systems Review)

**Neurological, Cardiovascular & Respiratory:** Nil
**Genitourinary:** My periods are light since starting the pill.
**MSK & Dermatology:** I have an itchy rash on my elbows which I think is eczema.
**Gastrointestinal:** I have always suffered from diarrhoea and often feel bloated and uncomfortable.
**Systemic:** No fever or night sweats.

Is there anything you've had to see a doctor about in the past?

Are there any medical conditions that affect your close family?

I'm going to ask a few questions about your lifestyle.

I have type 1 diabetes but it's well controlled.

Not that I'm aware of.

I don't smoke or drink. I'm very health conscious.

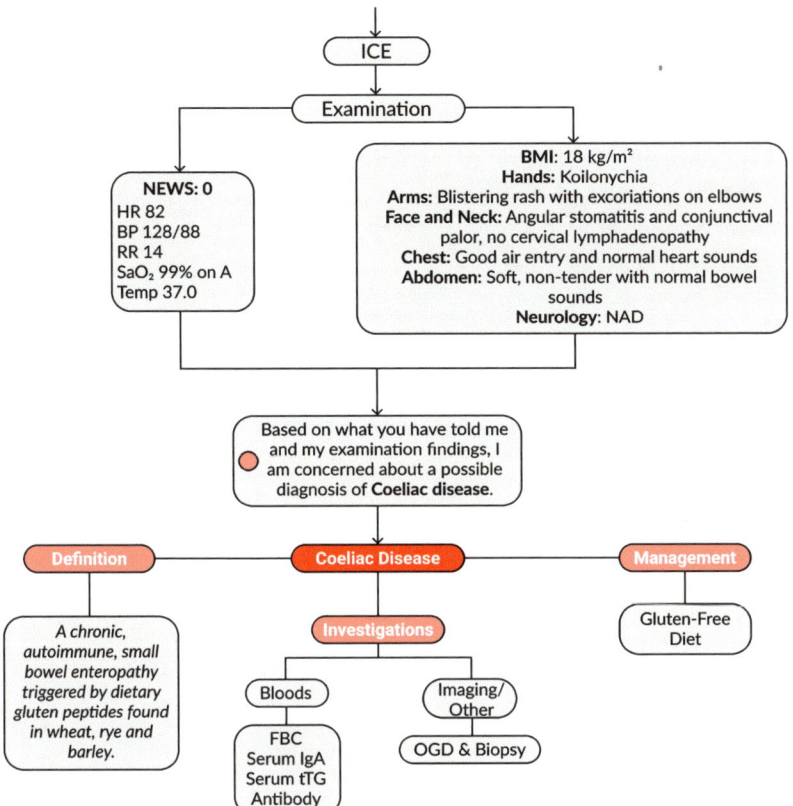

## Patient Background

**Patient Background**
21-year-old female

**PMH:** T1DM, Anxiety Disorder
**FH:** Nil
**DH:** Insulin Pump, Citalopram, Microgynon™
**SH:** Midwifery student, non-smoker, non-drinker

Fatigue is a vague yet common presentation in primary care and it can be challenging to tease apart functional fatigue (e.g. as a result of lifestyle factors) from fatigue associated with underlying organic disease processes.

Most cases of fatigue are likely to be related to **lifestyle and psychiatric factors**, such as stress, low mood, anxiety and poor sleep hygiene. It is, therefore, important to establish a clear understanding of the patient's lifestyle and potential stressors. This includes enquiring about their daily routines, relationships and work stressors and anything else that may be causing psychological strain. Other factors such as **caffeine intake** and **shift work** should be explored to see how their lifestyle is contributing to their sense of fatigue and how this can be mitigated.

A background history of **autoimmune disease** and **risk factors for anaemia** (e.g. heavy menstrual bleeding) may point you towards an organic cause of fatigue, such as hypothyroidism or iron deficiency anaemia.

# Differential Diagnosis

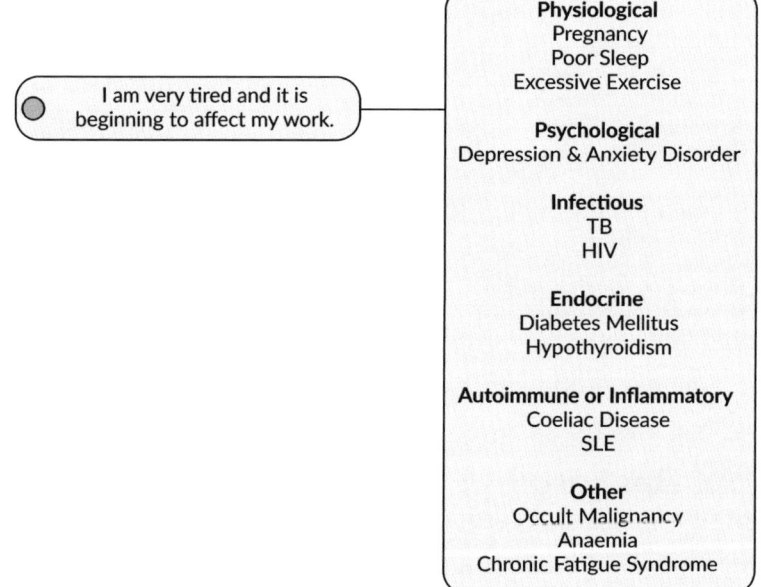

Fatigue has a broad range of differential diagnoses. Though it will most commonly be caused by a lifestyle that is not conducive to adequate rest and recuperation, a systems review is required to screen for potential organic causes. Examples of psychological or physiological causes of fatigue include pregnancy, poor sleep, depression and anxiety.

Fatigue is also a very common symptom associated with chronic disease including several **autoimmune diseases** (e.g. hypothyroidism and SLE). **Anaemia** is one of the most common organic causes of fatigue, particularly in young women of reproductive age who suffer from heavy periods. More rarely, fatigue may be an aspect of the presentation in patients with chronic infections, such as TB and HIV.

Read through the classical presentations table in the following section to develop an understanding of how the main differentials are classically present.

## Classical Presentations

| Differential | Classical Presentation |
|---|---|
| Lifestyle Factors | Often arising from a combination of poor sleep hygiene, excessive caffeine intake, poor diet, stress and limited exercise. |
| Depression and Anxiety Disorder | **Depression**: Chronic history of low mood, low energy and little interest doing activities that they previously enjoyed. Often associated with sleep and appetite disturbance, and impaired concentration and memory. **Anxiety Disorder**: Characterised by excessive anxiety that may be free-floating (generalised) or related to a more specific trigger or circumstance (e.g. social phobia). |
| Tuberculosis | Chronic history of a productive cough, shortness of breath, fatigue, night sweats and weight loss. Usually occurs in patients who have spent time in a tuberculosis endemic region. |
| HIV | May present acutely with a seroconversion illness (rash and flu-like symptoms) or chronically with a history of recurrent infections and weight loss. |

| | |
|---|---|
| **Diabetes Mellitus** | **Type 1 Diabetes Mellitus**: Presenting in young people with a history of polyuria and nocturia. They may describe some weight loss and trouble gaining weight. They may present acutely with diabetic ketoacidosis. **Type 2 Diabetes Mellitus**: Presenting in adults with polyuria and nocturia. Patients are often overweight and there may be a family history. |
| **Hypothyroidism** | Chronic history of fatigue, weight gain, cold intolerance, constipation and low mood. |
| **Coeliac Disease** | Chronic history of diarrhoea that may be pale and difficult to flush away (steatorrhoea), and weight loss. May be associated with a vesicular rash on the extensor surfaces (dermatitis herpetiformis) and some patients may have a family history. |
| **Systemic Lupus Erythematosus** | Chronic history of a constellation of symptoms including a rash, photosensitivity, arthralgia and fatigue. May be incidentally noted to have low cell counts on a routine blood test. |
| **Occult Malignancy** | Chronic history of fatigue and weight loss that may be associated with loss of appetite and night sweats. There may be localising symptoms (e.g. lymphadenopathy in lymphoma, cough in lung cancer and rectal bleeding in colorectal cancer). |
| **Anaemia** | Chronic history of shortness of breath, reduced exercise tolerance and fatigue. Patients may have an obvious source of excess bleeding (e.g. heavy menstrual bleeding) or it may be occult (e.g. colorectal malignancy). |

| | |
|---|---|
| **Chronic Fatigue Syndrome** | Chronic history of generalised fatigue often associated with pain and weakness in various parts of the body. Usually a diagnosis of exclusion. |

# Red Flags

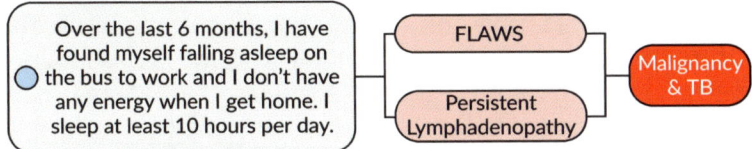

Though, much of the time, fatigue has clear lifestyle precipitants, it may occasionally be the first presentation of an underlying catabolic process such as malignancy or infection that is depleting the patient's physiological reserve. Associated symptoms that are classically associated with malignancy (e.g. lymphoma) and tuberculosis include **fever**, **night sweats**, **weight loss** and **non-tender lymphadenopathy**.

# Systems Review

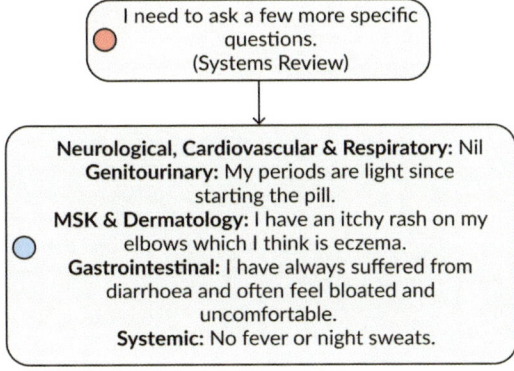

Given the broad range of differentials, a systems review should be performed to identify any associated symptoms that could help localise any organic disease processes that are driving the patient's fatigue.

- **Neuropsychiatric**: An exploration of the patient's mood and stress can help identify factors that are contributing to their fatigue.
- **Genitourinary**: In women of childbearing age, it is important to enquire about their periods. Patients with particularly heavy periods may become anaemic which contributes to their fatigue. Furthermore, menstrual irregularities may be suggestive of an underlying autoimmune disease (e.g. hypothyroidism).
- **Skin and Musculoskeletal**: Rashes and joint pains are symptoms that are commonly associated with autoimmune conditions, such as SLE and rheumatoid arthritis.
- **Gastrointestinal**: In young people with chronic diarrhoea, organic causes like inflammatory bowel disease and coeliac disease should be considered before making a diagnosis of exclusion, such as irritable bowel syndrome. Conditions like coeliac disease and Crohn's disease, in particular, can cause malabsorption resulting in sequelae that further worsen the patient's fatigue (e.g. anaemia due to iron and vitamin B12 malabsorption).

# Assessment

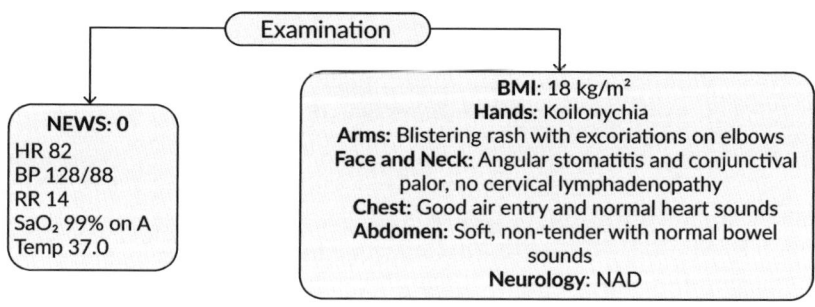

Examination

NEWS: 0
HR 82
BP 128/88
RR 14
SaO$_2$ 99% on A
Temp 37.0

BMI: 18 kg/m$^2$
**Hands:** Koilonychia
**Arms:** Blistering rash with excoriations on elbows
**Face and Neck:** Angular stomatitis and conjunctival palor, no cervical lymphadenopathy
**Chest:** Good air entry and normal heart sounds
**Abdomen:** Soft, non-tender with normal bowel sounds
**Neurology:** NAD

## Observations

Much of the time, patients presenting with fatigue will be physiologically well, in which case the observations will not provide much useful information. Patients who are dehydrated, anxious or anaemic may sometimes be noted to be tachycardic at rest.

## Examination

The examination findings in a patient with fatigue may be subtle but can help significantly narrow your differential diagnosis.

Patients with anaemia may appear **pale** and, if severe, may have fingernail changes such as **koilonychia**. The patient's body habitus may also provide useful clues. Patients with chronic gastrointestinal conditions and some autoimmune conditions (e.g. SLE and diabetes mellitus) may appear **underweight** with **loose-fitting clothing**. On the other hand, patients with hypothyroidism may have gained weight.

# Coeliac Disease

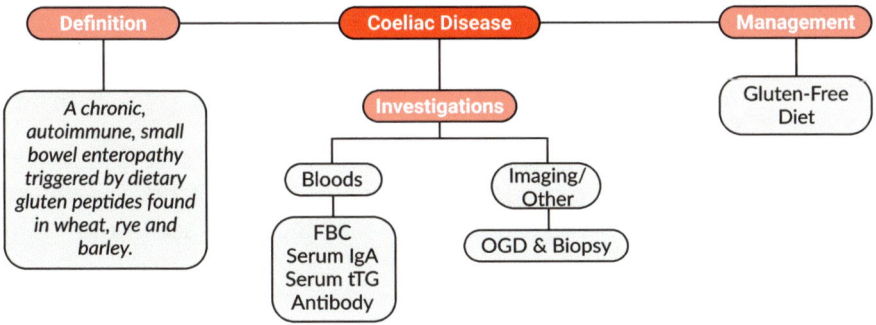

## Definition

Coeliac disease is an autoimmune disease that is characterised by subtotal villous atrophy, crypt hyperplasia and an increase in intraepithelial lymphocytes in response to exposure to gliadin (protein component of gluten). It is often diagnosed when children present with failure to thrive. It can, sometimes, present much later as it may be misdiagnosed as irritable bowel syndrome or patients may find ways of coping with the symptoms without seeking health-care attention.

## Investigations

A **faecal calprotectin** is a non-invasive stool test that acts as a marker of gastrointestinal inflammation. It is particularly useful when trying to distinguish inflammatory causes of chronic diar-rhoea (e.g. Crohn's disease) from irritable bowel syndrome.

   The first step in investigating a possible diagnosis of coeliac disease involves sending a blood sample to check for the presence of **anti-tissue transglutaminase** (anti-tTG) antibodies. This should be paired with a test for **total serum IgA** titres as selective IgA deficiency is relatively common in patients with coeliac disease and, so, it can give rise to a false negative anti-tTG result. An **FBC** and **vitamin B12** and **folate** levels should also be requested as patients with coeliac disease are prone to developing a mixed anaemia due to nutrient deficiencies.

   The gold standard diagnostic test for coeliac disease is an **oesophagogastroduodenoscopy (OGD) and biopsy**. The biopsy is usually taken from the duodenum or jejunum and will demon-strate subtotal villous atrophy with crypt hyperplasia and an increase in the proportion of intraepithelial lymphocytes. This test should be performed while the patient maintains a diet containing gluten as avoiding gluten can resolve the microarchitectural changes associated with coeliac disease, thereby leading to diag-nostic uncertainty.

## Management

Patients with coeliac disease can manage their condition effectively by omitting gluten-containing foods from their diet.

# Bridge Box

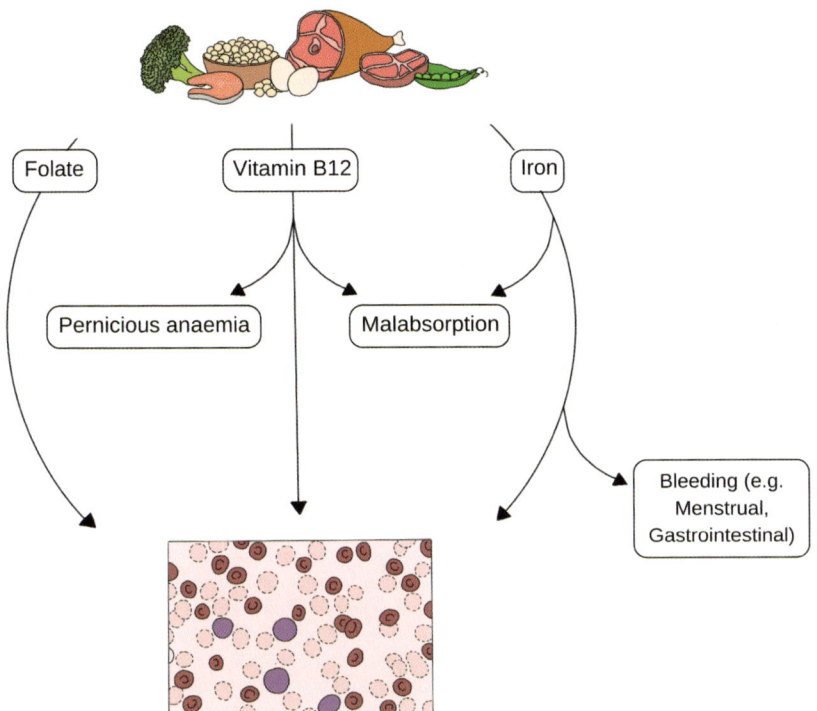

Nutrient-related causes of anaemia.

# Chapter 25

# Differentials in Detail

# Abdominal Aortic Aneurysm

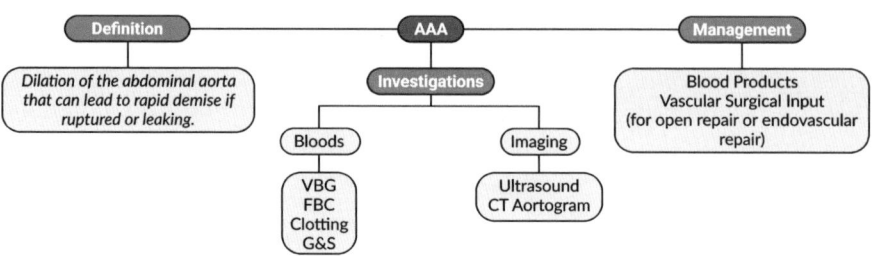

**Presentations**: Epigastric Pain, Back Pain

## *Definition*

An abdominal aortic aneurysm (AAA) is a dilation of the abdominal aorta which is often asymptomatic but can rupture or leak resulting in a rapid blood loss and often death if not identified and treated promptly.

## *Investigations*

AAAs may be identified upon routine screening (ultrasound scan) offered to men in the UK once they turn 65 years old. In a patient presenting acutely with a suspected leaking or ruptured AAA, a **VBG** will provide a useful early indication of the patient's haemoglobin and lactate. An **FBC**, a **clotting screen** and a **G&S** are all important as the patient will likely need multiple blood products and emergency surgery under the vascular surgical team. A point-of-care **ultrasound scan** should be performed on older men presenting with acute abdominal pain to check for the presence of an AAA, though a **CT aortogram** would be required to better describe the anatomy and determine whether it has ruptured.

## *Management*

Acute management involves multiple blood products and urgent vascular surgical input.

# Achalasia

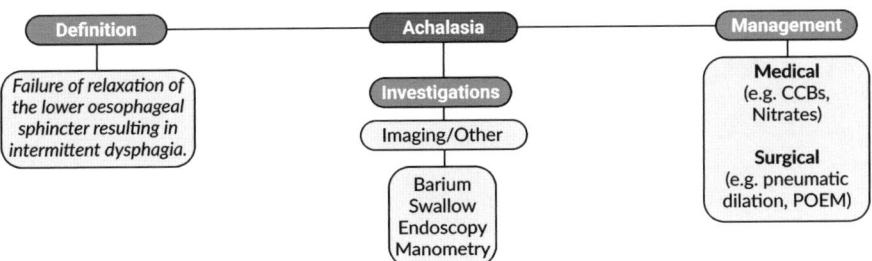

**Presentation**: Dysphagia

## *Definition*

Achalasia is characterised by a failure of relaxation of the lower oesophageal sphincter resulting in intermittent dysphagia to both solids and liquids.

## *Investigations*

The history of intermittent dysphagia is classical of achalasia, however, the diagnosis can be confirmed by performing **oesophageal manometry** to demonstrate raised pressures at the lower oesophageal sphincter. Furthermore, a **barium swallow** may reveal a '*bird's beak*' appearance. **Endoscopy** is often performed as the clinical presentation may be difficult to distinguish from oesophageal cancer.

## *Management*

Certain medications, such as **calcium channel blockers** and **nitrates**, may be used to relax the lower oesophageal sphincter. Interventions that could be performed include **pneumatic dilation** and **peroral endoscopic myotomy (POEM)**.

# Acute Abdomen

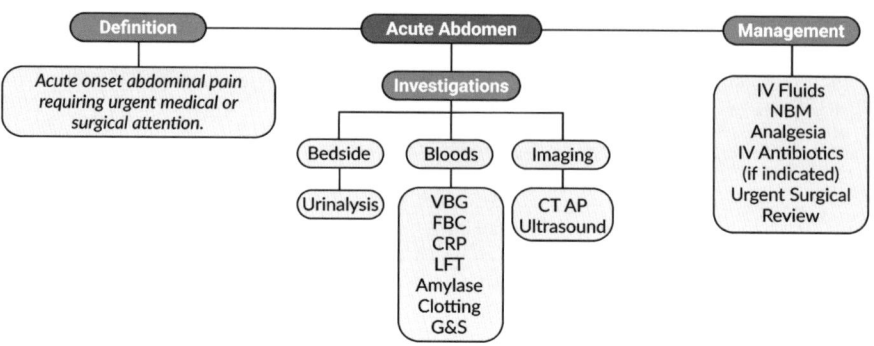

**Presentations**: Nausea and Vomiting, All Abdominal Pain

## Definition

Acute abdomen is a generic term that is used to refer to acute abdominal pain that is likely to require urgent surgical intervention (e.g. cholecystitis and appendicitis).

## Investigations

**Urinalysis** and, in people of child-bearing potential, a **urine pregnancy test** should be requested to check for urinary or early pregnancy-related causes of the pain. A **VBG** allows lactate and haemoglobin to be checked early. **FBC** and **CRP** may demonstrate raised inflammatory markers and **LFT** will likely be deranged in hepatobiliary causes of acute abdomen (e.g. cholecystitis). **Amylase** is often raised in most cases of acute abdomen, but it will be particularly raised in acute pancreatitis (3 times the upper limit of normal is sometimes used as a benchmark for pancreatitis). As many patients are likely to require surgical intervention, a **clotting screen** and **G&S** should be requested. Once stabilised, the patient will likely require a **CT abdomen and pelvis with contrast** to identify the cause of acute abdomen. In younger patients, **ultrasound** may be a preferred option.

## Management

The initial management of undifferentiated acute abdomen involves keeping the patient **nil-by-mouth**, administering **IV fluids**, providing **analgesia**, starting **antibiotics** if indicated and arranging **urgent surgical review**.

# Acute Coronary Syndrome

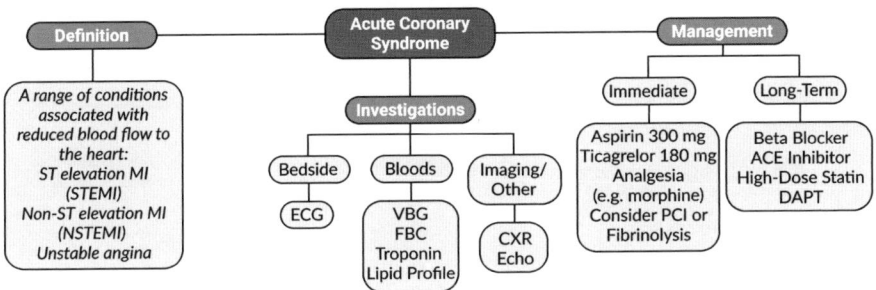

**Presentations**: Collapse, Chest Pain, Epigastric Pain

## Definition

Acute coronary syndrome (ACS) is an umbrella term referring to a constellation of symptoms that arise due to sudden, reduced blood flow to the myocardium. It encompasses ST-elevation myocardial infarction (STEMI), non-ST-elevation myocardial infarction (NSTEMI) and unstable angina pectoris (UAP).

## Investigations

At the bedside, an **ECG** may demonstrate changes associated with myocardial ischaemia or infarction (e.g. ST elevation or depression and T wave inversion). A raised serum **troponin** concentration would be suggestive of a myocardial infarction (cell death) as opposed to just ischaemia (impaired oxygen delivery to cells). A **chest X-ray** is often performed to rule out other potential causes of acute chest pain (e.g. pneumothorax). An **echocardiogram** can identify regional wall motion abnormalities and allows visualisation of valvular defects and estimation of systolic function.

## Management

Initial management involves loading the patient with **two antiplatelet agents** (e.g. aspirin and ticagrelor) and managing the patient's pain with **opioid analgesia**. Patients may also find that a GTN spray or infusion improves their pain. Depending on whether the patient has a STEMI, an NSTEMI or unstable angina, and on the facilities available at the time, patients will either undergo percutaneous coronary intervention (inserting a stent to re-establish myocardial perfusion), thrombolysis or medical management.

# Acute Limb Ischaemia

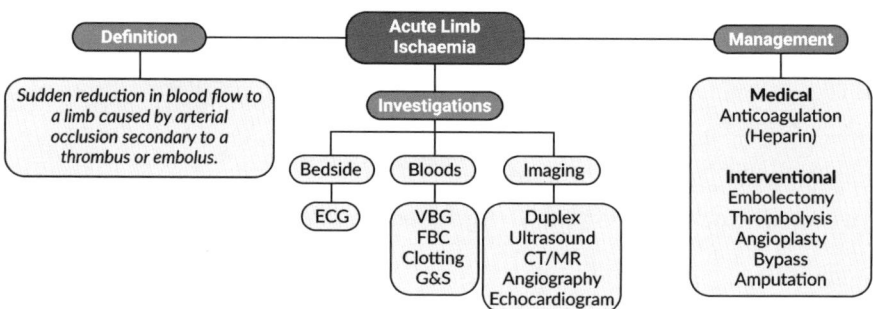

**Presentation**: Leg Pain

## Definition

Acute limb ischaemia arises when a thrombus or embolus causes a sudden occlusion in the arterial supply to the affected limb.

## Investigations

Atrial fibrillation is a major risk factor for the development of acute limb ischaemia — stasis within the heart leads to the formation of a clot which can then embolise to a peripheral artery causing acute limb ischaemia. This can be captured on an **ECG**. The tissue ischaemia can lead to a raised lactate that would be demonstrated by a **VBG**. Patients will likely need an intervention to re-establish perfusion to the affected leg so an **FBC**, a **clotting**

**screen** and a **G&S** should be requested. A lack of flow can be observed using a **duplex ultrasound** and **CT/MR angiography**. An **echocardiogram** may be performed at a later stage to check for a mural thrombus or valvular abnormalities that could have given rise to the clot that caused acute limb ischaemia.

## Management

Initially, the patient should be established on **anticoagulation**, usually with IV heparin. The case should then be discussed with the on-call vascular surgeons and interventional radiologists who may consider a variety of different interventions (e.g. embolectomy) to relieve the blocked vessel and re-perfuse the ischaemic leg.

# Adrenal Insufficiency

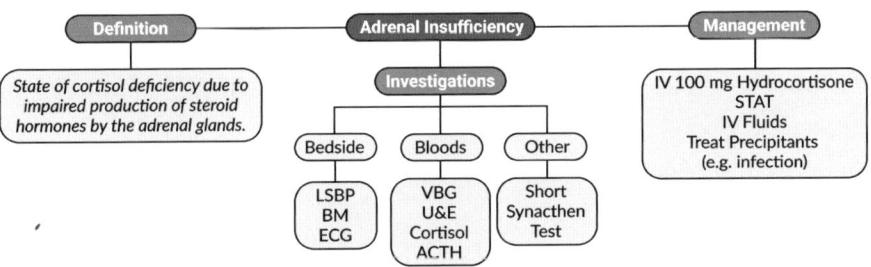

**Presentations**: Nausea and Vomiting

## Definition

Adrenal insufficiency refers to an impairment in the functioning of the adrenal gland resulting in insufficient output of cortisol and aldosterone. It may occur due to autoimmune attack (Addison's disease) and tuberculosis is the most common cause worldwide.

## Investigations

Patients with adrenal insufficiency often present with vague symptoms, such as fatigue and dizziness. Their lack of cortisol can impair their ability to maintain their blood pressure during postural changes, so a **lying-standing blood pressure** is a simple investigation that can be performed at the bedside. As cortisol is one of the hormonal mechanisms involved in regulating blood glucose concentration, its deficiency can result in hypoglycaemia so the patient's **BM** should be tested upon assessment. A deficiency of cortisol and aldosterone can lead to electrolyte derangement (hyponatraemia and hyperkalaemia) which would be detected on a **VBG** and **U&E**. Hyperkalaemia can lead to **ECG** changes. In primary adrenocortical failure, the patient will have a low **cortisol** level and a raised **ACTH** level. A **short synacthen test** involves administering a synthetic form of ACTH and measuring the cortisol level to see whether the patient's adrenal glands are able to respond to stimulation — the cortisol will fail to rise in patients with primary adrenocortical failure.

## Management

If presenting acutely with an adrenal crisis, patients should be managed with **IV hydrocortisone**, **IV fluids** and **glucose** if hypoglycaemic. It is also important to identify and treat any precipitants for their crisis.

# Anaemia

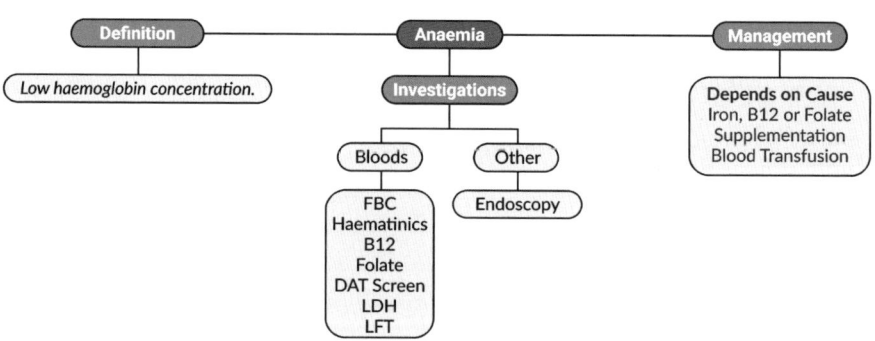

**Presentations**: Shortness of Breath, Fatigue

## Definition

Anaemia refers to a low haemoglobin concentration.

## Investigations

An **FBC** will allow the haemoglobin to be quantified and will provide the mean cell volume which allows the anaemia to be categorised (microcytic, normocytic or macrocytic). Microcytic anaemia often occurs due to iron deficiency (identified using **haematinics**) and thalassemia (identified using **haemoglobin electrophoresis**). Macrocytic anaemia often occurs due to **vitamin B12** and **folate** deficiency, so assays for these nutrients should be requested. Haemolytic anaemia results in a raised bilirubin (demonstrated by **LFT**) and an increase in **LDH**. If autoimmune haemolytic anaemia is suspected, a **direct antiglobulin test (DAT)** should be requested. In cases of unexplained iron deficiency anaemia, patients should be considered for **endoscopy** (an OGD and colonoscopy) to check for an occult malignancy.

## Management

The management depends very much on the case of the anaemia. It often involves optimising the levels of nutrients that contribute to red cell development while also attending to any underlying causes of deficiency (e.g. poor dietary intake and malabsorption). In severe, symptomatic anaemia, **blood transfusions** should be considered.

# Anal Fissure

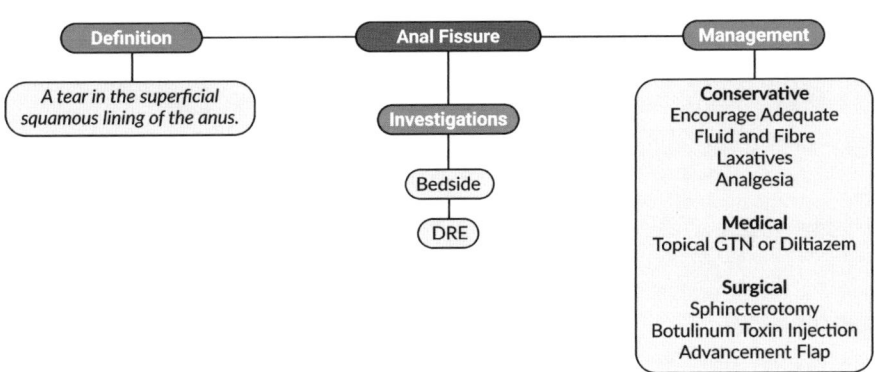

**Presentations**: Constipation, Rectal Bleeding

## Definition

An anal fissure is a tear in the lining of the anus that usually presents with intense pain upon defecation and mild rectal bleeding (mainly upon wiping).

## Investigations

It is largely a clinical diagnosis based on the symptoms described. When inspecting the anal opening during a **DRE**, the anal fissure may be visualised. Often, patients do not tolerate a DRE well because of the pain.

## Management

**Conservative measures** that can loosen the stools should be advised. **Topical GTN** and **diltiazem** can relax the anal sphincter and improve the blood flow to the fissure to help it heal. If conservative and medical measures fail, surgical interventions may be considered.

# Ankylosing Spondylitis

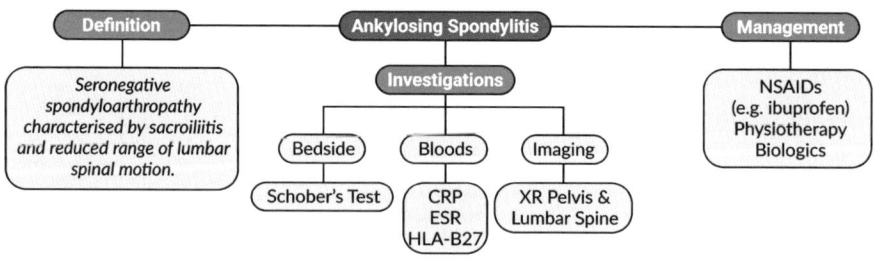

**Presentation**: Back Pain

## Definition

Ankylosing spondylitis is a seronegative spondyloarthropathy, which means that it is not associated with any particular autoantibodies (seronegative) and it primarily affects the axial skeleton (spondyloarthropathy). It classically presents in young patients with a chronic history of lower back pain and a limited range of motion.

## *Investigations*

At the bedside, **Schober's test** is a clinical examination that demonstrates a limited range of lumbar spinal flexion. Blood may reveal a raised **CRP** and **ESR**, in keeping with chronic inflammation, and initial **X-rays** of the lumbar spine and pelvis may reveal sacroiliitis. Patients may also undergo an **HLA-B27** test which looks for the presence of the HLA-B27 antigen in their blood cells — this is strongly associated with ankylosing spondylitis.

## *Management*

The pain often responds well to **NSAIDs** and **physiotherapy**. If these measures are ineffective, **biologics** may be considered.

# Aortic Dissection

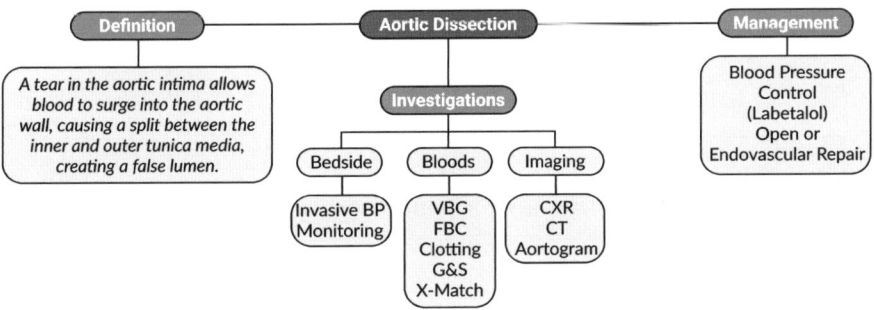

**Presentation**: Chest Pain

## *Definition*

Aortic dissection refers to a tear in the lining of the aorta that classically occurs in patients with uncontrolled hypertension. It usually presents with sudden onset tearing chest pain that radiates through to the back between the scapulae.

### Investigations

To prevent further propagation of the tear in the aorta, **invasive blood pressure monitoring** (arterial line insertion) and control are required. The patient may require urgent vascular intervention so **FBC**, **clotting screen**, **G&S** and **X-match** should be requested. Furthermore, propagation of the dissection can lead to tissue ischaemia which would lead to a raised lactate on the **VBG**. A **chest X-ray** may reveal a widened mediastinum (though this is not very sensitive or specific). A **CT aortogram** is the gold-standard investigation.

### Management

Intravenous agents (e.g. labetalol) should be used to maintain the patient's **blood pressure** within an acceptable range. Urgent discussion with the on-call **vascular surgery** team is required to plan ongoing management.

# Appendicitis

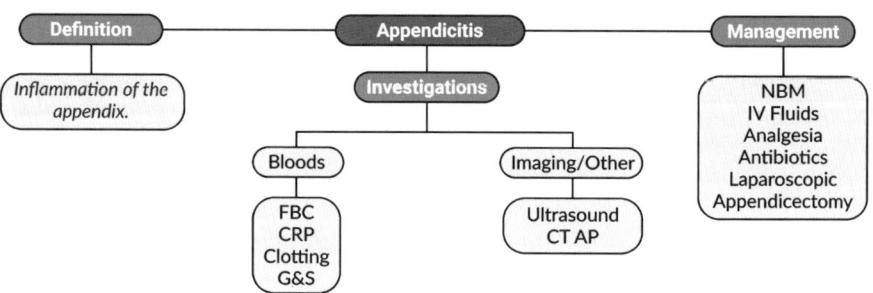

**Presentation**: Iliac Fossa Pain

## Definition

Appendicitis refers to inflammation of the appendix that usually presents with acute right iliac fossa pain in children and young adults.

## Investigations

An **FBC** and a **CRP** will reveal raised inflammatory markers and, as the patient will likely be undergoing an emergency operation, a **clotting screen** and **G&S** should be requested. An **ultrasound** scan will be an appropriate imaging modality in younger patients to avoid exposure to ionising radiation. In older patients where the diagnosis may be uncertain or in obese patients in whom an ultrasound scan is technically difficult, a **CT abdomen and pelvis with contrast** should be considered.

## Management

The initial management involves keeping the patient **nil-by-mouth**, administering **IV fluids** and **antibiotics**, and managing the patient's pain with strong **analgesia**. It can be definitively managed with a **laparoscopic appendicectomy**.

# Arrhythmia

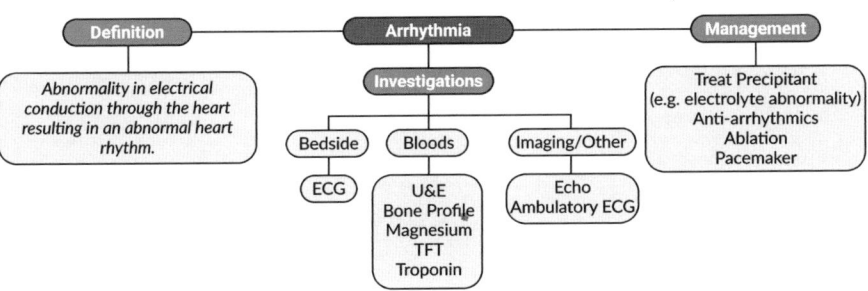

**Presentation**: Collapse

## Definition

An arrhythmia is an abnormal rhythm that arises due to aberrant electrical activity within the heart. It can present with palpitations or can cause a brief reduction in cardiac output resulting in syncope.

## Investigations

An **ECG** may capture the arrhythmia, however, patients may require **ambulatory ECG monitoring** if the arrhythmia is intermittent (e.g. paroxysmal atrial fibrillation). Arrhythmias can be precipitated by electrolyte derangements (**U&E**, **bone profile** and **magnesium**), thyroid abnormalities (**TFT**) or ischaemic events (**troponin**). An **echocardiogram** may reveal structural abnormalities (e.g. valve defects) that are strongly associated with arrhythmias.

## Management

Initial management involves treating any reversible precipitants (e.g. hypomagnesaemia). Depending on the arrhythmia, various antiarrhythmics (e.g. beta-blockers) may be used. Interventions that may be considered for certain arrhythmias include **ablation** and **pacemaker** insertion.

# Asthma

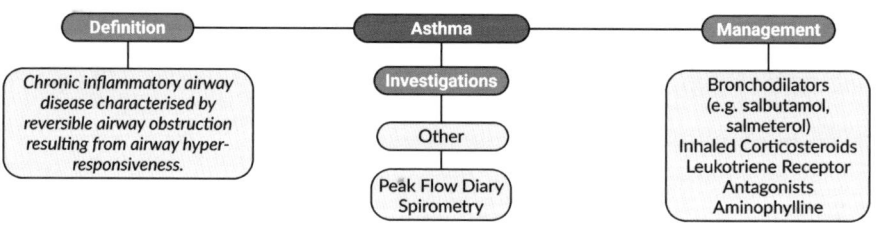

**Presentations**: Cough, Shortness of Breath

## *Definition*

Asthma is a common condition that is characterised by episodes of reversible bronchoconstriction and airway hyper-responsiveness. It is often associated with other atopic conditions (allergic rhinitis, eczema and food allergies).

## *Investigations*

Asthma is often diagnosed clinically in primary care, however, patients can be asked to keep a **peak flow diary** which may demonstrate a diurnal variation that is in keeping with a diagnosis of asthma. Some patients may undergo **spirometry** that will reveal a reversible obstructive pattern (FEV1/FVC < 0.7).

## *Management*

Asthma follows a stepwise management plan that includes the use of short-acting (e.g. salbutamol) and long-acting beta agonists (e.g. salmeterol) and muscarinic antagonists (e.g. tiotropium bromide), leukotriene receptor antagonists (e.g. montelukast), inhaled steroids (e.g. beclomethasone) and aminophylline.

# Benign Prostatic Hyperplasia

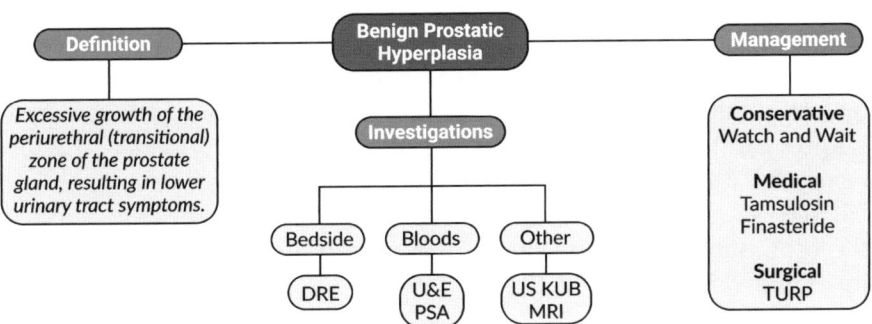

**Presentations**: Dysuria, Polyuria

## Definition

Benign prostatic hyperplasia (BPH) is a common condition that mostly affects older men and is characterised by excessive growth of the periurethral transitional zone of the prostate gland. This can cause a partial or complete urinary outflow obstruction.

## Investigations

A **DRE** will likely reveal a smoothly enlarged prostate gland with a palpable central sulcus. If a patient presents with urinary retention, their **U&E** should be checked as the obstruction could cause hydronephrosis (detected on an **ultrasound KUB**), resulting in a post-renal AKI. Furthermore, once the obstruction has been relieved, patients can develop postobstructive diuresis that leads to derangement of their renal function. If there is any concern about a possible diagnosis of prostate cancer, the **PSA level** should be checked (though care must be taken to ensure that the sample is taken at a time when confounding variables will not affect the result, such as recent DRE or urinary infections). If there is any uncertainty about a possible alternative diagnosis of prostate cancer, a **multiparametric MRI scan** may be requested.

## Management

If the symptoms are mild, a **watch and wait** approach may be employed. **Tamsulosin** is an alpha-blocker that can relax the smooth muscle encircling the prostatic urethra and **finasteride** is a $5\alpha$-reductase inhibitor that can reduce the volume of the prostate gland. Both medications can facilitate improved urinary outflow from the bladder. A **transurethral resection of the prostate (TURP)** is a common urological procedure that removes some of the prostatic tissue that is impinging on the urethra thereby allowing for better flow to be achieved.

# Biliary Colic

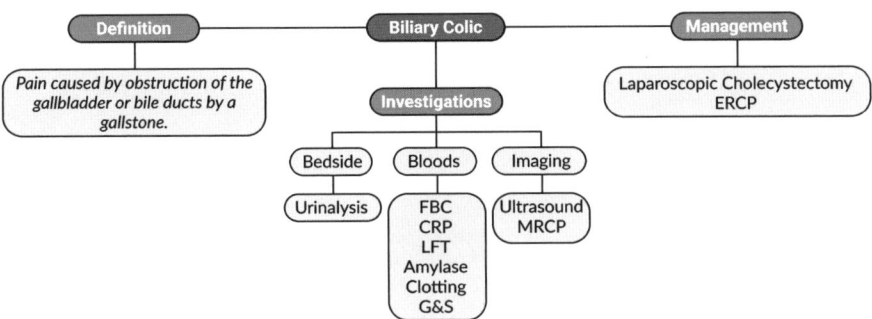

**Presentation**: RUQ Pain

## *Definition*

Biliary colic refers to intermittent right upper quadrant pain that occurs due to temporary obstruction of the biliary tree by a gallstone.

## *Investigations*

If a gallstone gets stuck within the common bile duct (CBD), it will block the flow of bile into the small bowel. This, in turn, will lead to a lack of urobilinogen in the urine (which can be detected by performing **urinalysis**). Biliary colic can be clinically difficult to distinguish from cholecystitis — an **FBC** and a **CRP** should be requested as significantly raised inflammatory markers would be in keeping with an infectious process. Biliary colic may also cause some derangement in the **LFTs** (in particular, a raised ALP and GGT). If a gallstone gets impacted near the pancreatic duct, it can cause gallstone pancreatitis which would cause a significantly raised **amylase**. As the patient may need urgent surgery, a **clotting screen** and **G&S** should be requested. The gallstone can be visualised using **ultrasound** and **MRCP**.

## Management

Patients with symptomatic gallstones should undergo an elective **laparoscopic cholecystectomy**. If a CBD stone is causing a biliary outflow obstruction, it will need to be relieved using **ERCP**.

# Brain Tumour

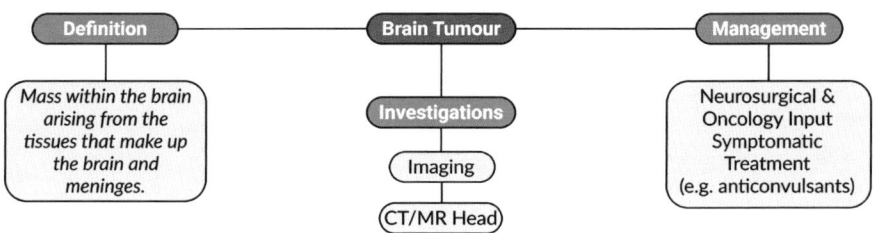

**Presentations**: Headache, Confusion, Nausea and Vomiting

## Definition

A brain tumour is an abnormal growth of brain tissue that can have serious consequences given the space-sensitive nature of the cranium and the impact of the tumour on normal brain activity (i.e. manifesting with seizures and confusion).

## Investigations

Cross-sectional imaging in the form of **CT** and **MRI head** scans is the mainstay of identifying brain tumours.

## Management

The management of brain tumours is complex and will involve input from both neurosurgery and oncology.

# Bronchiectasis

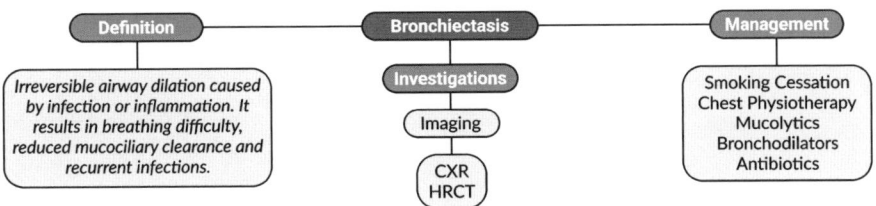

**Presentation**: Cough

## *Definition*

Bronchiectasis refers to the permanent dilation of the airways due to a chronic infective or inflammatory process. Patients often complain of suffering from a chronic, productive cough, frequent respiratory tract infections and shortness of breath.

## *Investigations*

Some subtle changes suggestive of bronchiectasis may be noted on a **chest X-ray**, such as tram-track opacities, however, the gold-standard imaging modality is a **high-resolution CT (HRCT) scan**. Patients who have presented with an infective exacerbation of bronchiectasis should be asked to provide a sputum sample as they are at risk of becoming colonised by resistant organisms, such as *Pseudomonas aeruginosa*.

## *Management*

The management of bronchiectasis focuses on risk factor modification (e.g. **smoking cessation**) and assisting the clearance of mucous with **chest physiotherapy** and **mucolytics**. **Bronchodilators** may be helpful in patients presenting with an exacerbation and some patients may be considered for long-term **antibiotics**.

# Calf Muscle Tear

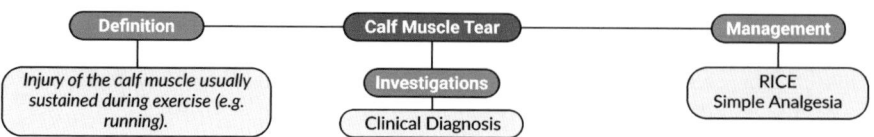

**Presentation**: Leg Pain

## *Definition*

A calf muscle tear is a common injury that usually affects athletes. It refers to a tear of the gastrocnemius or soleus muscles which, together, make up triceps surae.

## *Investigations*

It is a clinical diagnosis.

## *Management*

As with most mild sporting injuries, **simple analgesia** and **RICE** (**R**est, **I**ce, **C**ompress, **E**levate) should be recommended.

# Cellulitis

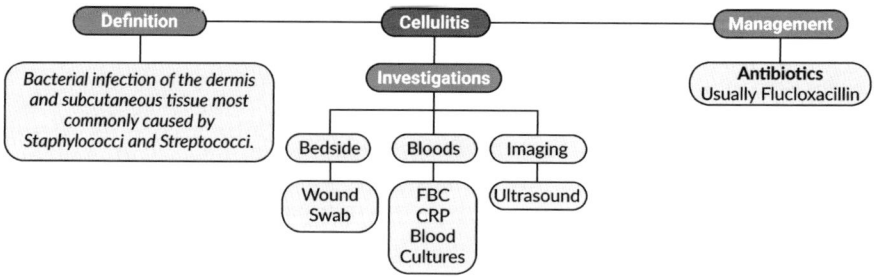

**Presentation**: Leg Pain

## Definition

Cellulitis is a common infection of the superficial layers of the skin. It is most commonly caused by *Staphylococci* and *Streptococci*, and significant risk factors include diabetes mellitus, vascular disease and breaks in the skin (e.g. ulcers).

## Investigations

If a break in the skin is identified within the cellulitic area, a **wound swab** should be taken for microscopy, culture and sensitivities. Blood will likely reveal a raised **FBC** and **CRP**. Though it is usually mild, some patients may become septic due to cellulitis, in which case **blood cultures** should be taken as part of the sepsis 6 protocol. **Ultrasound** can be used to identify subcutaneous collections that develop in the context of cellulitis.

## Management

Cellulitis can usually be treated with oral or IV antibiotics that target *Staphylococci* and *Streptococci* (usually **flucloxacillin**).

# Cholecystitis

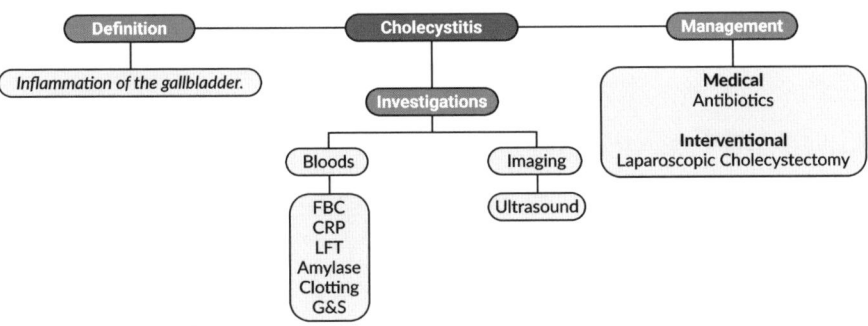

**Presentation**: RUQ Pain

## Definition

Cholecystitis is inflammation of the gallbladder that usually occurs secondary to an infection in a patient with gallstones. It usually manifests with persistent RUQ pain and a fever.

## Investigations

The patient's inflammatory markers (**FBC** and **CRP**) are likely to be raised and the **LFT** will show some abnormalities (most probably a raised ALP and GGT). **Amylase** is likely to be raised in any case of intra-abdominal inflammation, but it may be particularly raised if the patient has developed **gallstone pancreatitis**. As the patient is likely to need to undergo surgery, a **clotting screen** and **G&S** should also be requested. **Ultrasound** can be used to demonstrate an enlarged and thick-walled gallbladder. In some cases where there is some diagnostic uncertainty or where ultrasonography is not available, a **CT abdomen and pelvis with contrast** may be appropriate.

## Management

Patients are often managed initially with empirical **antibiotics** (ceftriaxone and metronidazole is a common combination) while awaiting intervention. The definitive treatment would be a **laparoscopic cholecystectomy**.

# Chronic Fatigue Syndrome

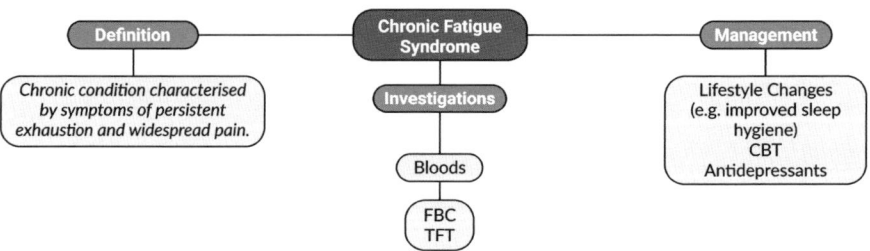

**Presentation**: Fatigue

## Definition

Chronic fatigue syndrome (also known as myalgic encephalomyelitis) refers to a constellation of symptoms characterised by persistent fatigue and widespread pain.

## Investigations

There is no test for chronic fatigue syndrome, and it remains largely a clinical diagnosis, however, an **FBC** and a **TFT** may be requested to rule out other causes of fatigue, such as anaemia and hypothyroidism.

## Management

Chronic fatigue syndrome is often complex to manage. **Lifestyle changes** that facilitate rest and recuperation can help optimise the patient, and they may also be recommended **antidepressants** and **CBT**.

# Cluster Headache

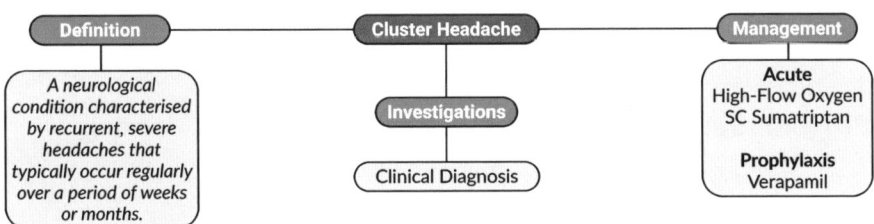

**Presentation**: Headache

## Definition

A cluster headache is a very debilitating type of headache that gains its name from the metronomic nature of the symptoms. Patients will often develop intense unilateral headaches associated with lacrimation and a red eye at around the same time, every day for weeks on end.

## Investigations

It is a clinical diagnosis.

## Management

Acute management of a cluster headache involves administering **high-flow oxygen** and **subcutaneous sumatriptan**. **Verapamil** (calcium channel blocker) can be used for long-term prevention.

# Central Nervous System (CNS) Inflammation

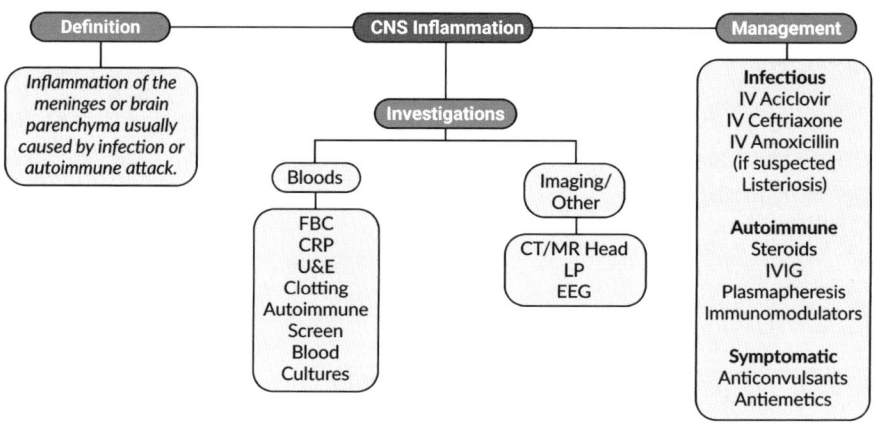

**Presentations**: Headache, Confusion, Nausea and Vomiting

## Definition

Inflammation of the brain (encephalitis) and meninges (meningitis) usually occurs due to infection but can also be caused by autoimmune attack.

## Investigations

As it is an inflammatory condition, the patient's inflammatory markers may be noted to be raised (**FBC** and **CRP**). In patients presenting with new confusion, electrolyte derangement (e.g. hyponatraemia) is a possible cause and would be detected on a **U&E**. Intracranial bleeds could also cause confusion, so a **clotting screen** should be requested. If the patient has new confusion with features of sepsis, **blood cultures** should be taken as the patient may have developed a bacterial meningoencephalitis. An **autoimmune screen** may identify certain antibodies that are associated with autoimmune encephalitis (e.g. NMDAR antibody). **CT/MR head** scans may be normal but may also reveal areas of enhancement (in particular, the temporal lobe) in encephalitis. A **lumbar puncture** will allow a CSF analysis to be performed which may demonstrate patterns that determine the likely cause of the condition (e.g. bacterial vs viral) and may even allow the causative organism to be identified. If there is any concern about the patient developing seizure activity, an **electroencephalogram (EEG)** may be requested.

### *Management*

As encephalitis can progress rapidly, patients are often treated empirically with **antibiotics** (e.g. ceftriaxone) and **antivirals** (e.g. aciclovir). The treatment of autoimmune encephalitis focuses on measures that reduce the level of causative antibodies (e.g. plasmapheresis). Symptom control measures include anticonvulsants and antiemetics.

## Colorectal Cancer

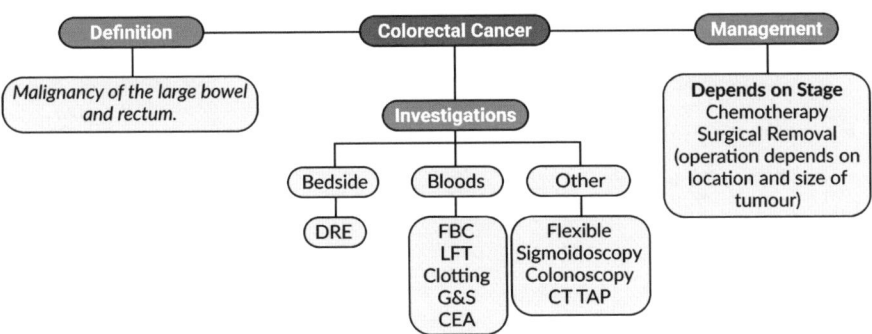

**Presentations**: Diarrhoea, Constipation, Rectal Bleeding

## Definition

Colorectal cancer is a common malignancy arising from the rectum and colon. It may present subtly with an unexplained change in bowel habit or unexplained iron deficiency anaemia.

## Investigations

A **DRE** may allow palpation of low-lying rectal tumours. An **FBC** may demonstrate a microcytic anaemia and a derangement in **LFT** may be suggestive of liver metastases. If the patient is having significant rectal bleeding or is being worked-up for surgery, a **clotting screen** and **G&S** should be requested. **Carcinoembryonic antigen (CEA)** is a tumour marker that is used in the diagnosis and monitoring of colorectal cancer. A **flexible sigmoidoscopy** or **colonoscopy** will enable the tumour to be visualised and a biopsy to be taken. A **CT thorax, abdomen and pelvis** will allow for staging.

## Management

The management depends largely on the location and stage of the tumour but will likely involve surgery, chemotherapy and radiotherapy.

# Compartment Syndrome

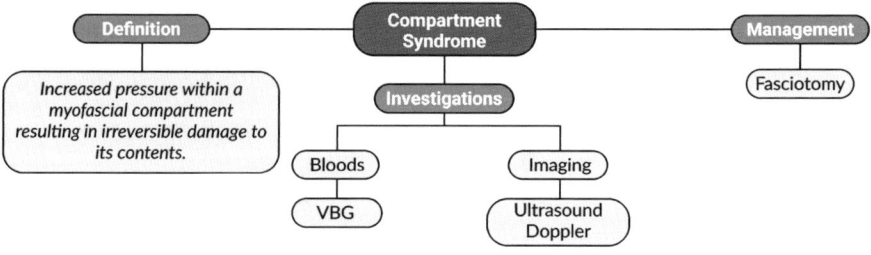

**Presentation**: Leg Pain

## Definition

Compartment syndrome is a surgical emergency in which the pressure within a myofascial compartment rises and can cause vascular compromise and irreversible tissue damage. It typically occurs after recent intervention on the affected leg (e.g. revascularisation or fracture repair).

## Investigations

Compartment syndrome is largely a clinical diagnosis but a **VBG** may reveal a raised lactate and an **ultrasound** can reveal muscle oedema.

## Management

Patient will require an emergency **fasciotomy** to decompress the compartment.

# Chronic Obstructive Pulmonary Disease (COPD)

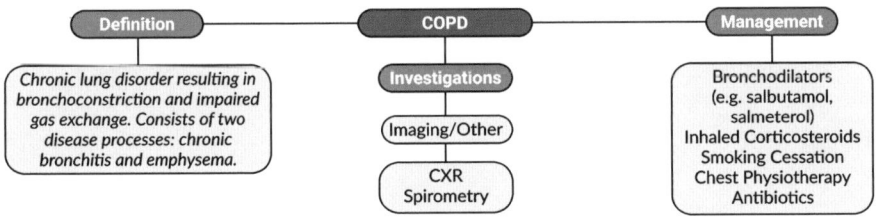

**Presentations**: Shortness of Breath, Cough

## Definition

COPD is a common, chronic lung disorder that consists of two disease processes: chronic bronchitis and emphysema. It is much more common in patients with a significant smoking history.

## Investigations

**Spirometry** will reveal an obstructive defect (FEV1/FVC $< 0.7$) and a **chest X-ray** may reveal hyperinflated lungs.

## Management

The long-term management of COPD involves using inhaled **bronchodilators** and **corticosteroids**. Patients should also be provided with **smoking cessation** advice and assistance. Patients may also benefit from **chest physiotherapy** to help clear mucus and, in some cases, long-term **antibiotics**. As they are at increased risk, patients with COPD should be offered the pneumococcal and influenza vaccine. For more information about the management of an *Exacerbation of COPD*, please refer to **page 93**.

# Costochondritis

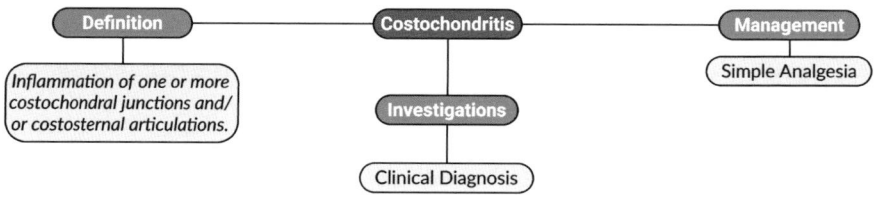

**Presentation**: Chest Pain

## Definition

Costochondritis is a common condition characterised by inflammation of the costochondral and costosternal junctions that presents with chest pain and reproducible chest wall tenderness.

## Investigations

It is largely a clinical diagnosis, however, patients may undergo some tests to rule out other causes of chest pain (e.g. ECG and troponin).

## Management

Costochondritis can usually be managed with simple analgesia (e.g. NSAIDs).

# Decompensated Chronic Liver Disease

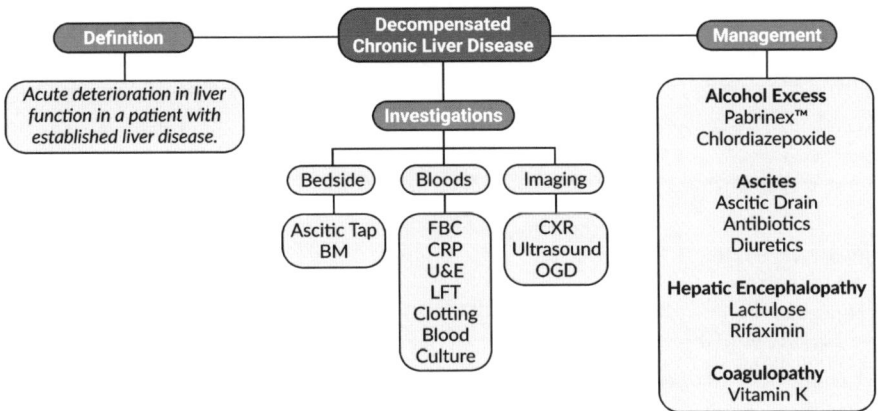

**Presentation**: Jaundice

## Definition

Decompensated chronic liver disease refers to a sudden worsening in liver function in a patient with established chronic liver disease. It may manifest with ascites, jaundice and encephalopathy.

## Investigations

At the bedside, an **ascitic tap** can be used to obtain a sample of ascitic fluid and send for microscopy and culture to diagnose spontaneous bacterial peritonitis (SBP). Patients with chronic liver disease are also at increased risk of hypoglycaemia due to dysfunctional hepatic glycogen stores, so their **BM** should be checked upon initial assessment. And **FBC** and **CRP** may reveal raised inflammatory markers suggestive of an infection that may have triggered their decompensation. Patients with chronic liver disease are also at risk of developing renal impairment (hepatorenal syndrome) so **U&E** should be requested. An **LFT** may demonstrate evidence of liver inflammation (transaminitis) or impairments in the liver's synthetic function (albumin and bilirubin). Impaired liver synthetic function will also lead to abnormalities on a **clotting screen**. If the patient is septic, **blood cultures** should be taken. A **chest X-ray** may reveal features of pulmonary oedema. An **ultrasound scan** is useful in visualising the nodularity seen in cirrhosis and identifying hepatocellular carcinoma which could precipitate decompensation. Patients with portal hypertension may have developed oesophageal varices which are prone to bleeding, so an **OGD** may be considered.

## Management

In patients with a known background of alcohol excess, **Pabrinex™** (vitamin B substances with ascorbic acid) should be started as they are at risk of Wernicke–Korsakoff syndrome due to thiamine deficiency. They should also have their CIWA score monitored and **chlordiazepoxide** administered to manage the symptoms of withdrawal.

Ascites should be managed by inserting a **drain**. If there is any concern about SBP, they should also be started on IV **antibiotics**. **Diuretics** such as spironolactone and furosemide are often used to reduce the reaccumulation of ascitic fluid. Hepatic encephalopathy can be managed by giving **lactulose** and aiming for at least 2 bowel motions per day. **Rifaximin** is an antibiotic that can modulate the gut microbiome and is also used in the treatment of hepatic encephalopathy. If the clotting screen reveals evidence of coagulopathy, the patient should receive **vitamin K**.

# Delirium

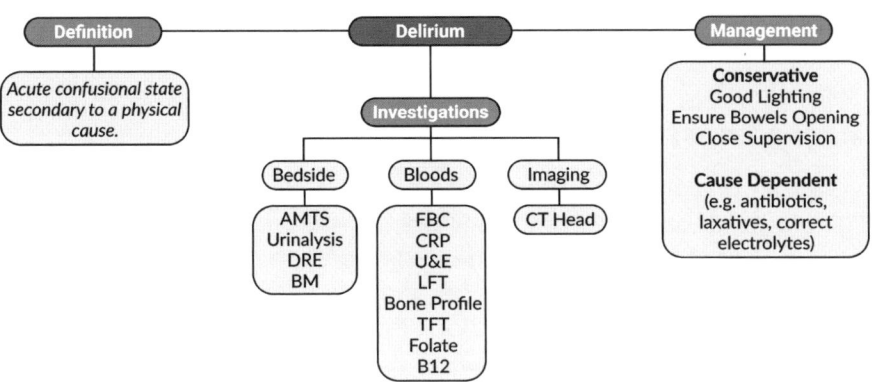

**Presentation**: Confusion

## *Definition*

Delirium refers to an acute confusional state that arises due to an underlying physical cause, such as constipation, pain and infections. It is a very common reason for hospital admission among elderly patients.

## *Investigations*

At the bedside, various scoring systems such as **AMTS**, 4AT and CAM may be used. The focus of investigating delirium is to identify reversible causes. **Urinalysis** should be performed to check for evidence of a UTI (though urinalysis may be unreliable in elderly patients, especially if they are incontinent). A bladder scan may be performed if urinary retention is suspected. Furthermore, both low and high **BM** can lead to delirium. A **DRE** may reveal impacted stool within the rectum.

FBC and **CRP** may reveal raised inflammatory markers suggestive of an underlying infection. Derangements in electrolytes (**U&E** and **bone profile**) and liver function (**LFT**) can also contribute to delirium. **TFT**, **vitamin B12** and **folate** often constitute a full '*Delirium Screen*'. If no obvious cause has been found for the delirium, a **CT head** scan should be considered as a subdural haemorrhage can present with a subacute history of confusion and there may not be a clear history of recent head injury.

## Management

Several **conservative measures** such as close supervision, good lighting and orientation tools (e.g. clocks) can help ameliorate patients' symptoms. Management is largely tailored towards identifying and **treating the cause**. In patients who are aggressive and pose a risk to themselves and/or others, sedatives such as haloperidol or lorazepam may be used.

# Dementia

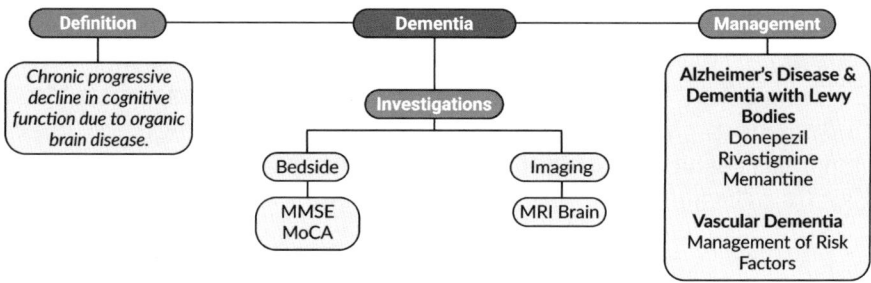

**Presentation**: Confusion

## Diagnosis

Dementia is an umbrella term referring to a chronic and progressive decline in cognitive function. Examples of types of dementia include Alzheimer's disease, vascular dementia and dementia with Lewy bodies.

## Investigations

By the bedside, assessments of cognitive function like a **Montreal Cognitive Assessment™ (MoCA)** and **Mini–Mental State Exam**

(**MMSE**) are useful for aiding a diagnosis and monitoring disease progression. An **MRI brain** scan can reveal features that are in keeping with causes of dementia, such as temporal lobe atrophy and small vessel disease.

### Management

The management of dementia depends on the type. Alzheimer's disease and dementia with Lewy bodies can be treated with acetyl-cholinesterase inhibitors (e.g. **donepezil** and **rivastigmine**). NMDA receptor antagonists such as **memantine** may also be used. The management of vascular dementia largely focuses on managing vascular risk factors, such as hypertension.

## Depression and Anxiety Disorder

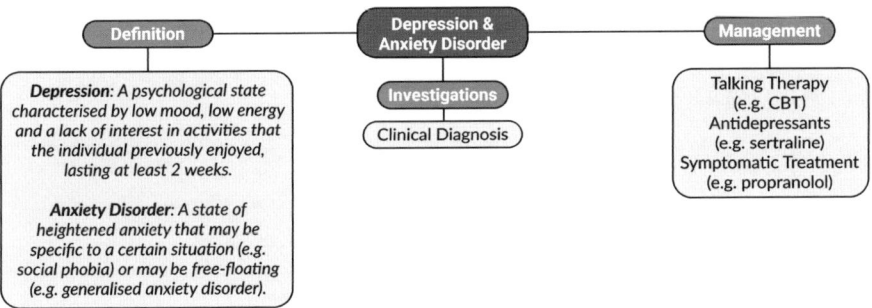

**Presentations**: Chest Pain, Weight Loss, Fatigue

### Definition

**Depression** is a common mental health condition that is characterised by core symptoms (low mood, anergia and anhedonia), biological symptoms (poor sleep, change in appetite and change in weight) and cognitive symptoms (changes in memory and focus). **Anxiety disorder** is an umbrella term that refers to a state of heightened anxiety that may be context-dependent (e.g. social phobia) or may be free-floating (generalised anxiety disorder).

## Investigations

These conditions are diagnosed by taking a detailed history, including a **mental state examination**. Assessment tools such as a **PHQ-9** and **GAD-7**.

## Management

The management of both depression and anxiety disorder usually involves a combination of **talking therapy** and **antidepressants**. Patients with physical manifestations of their anxiety disorder (e.g. palpitations and tremor) may benefit from **symptomatic treatment** with propranolol.

# Diabetes Insipidus

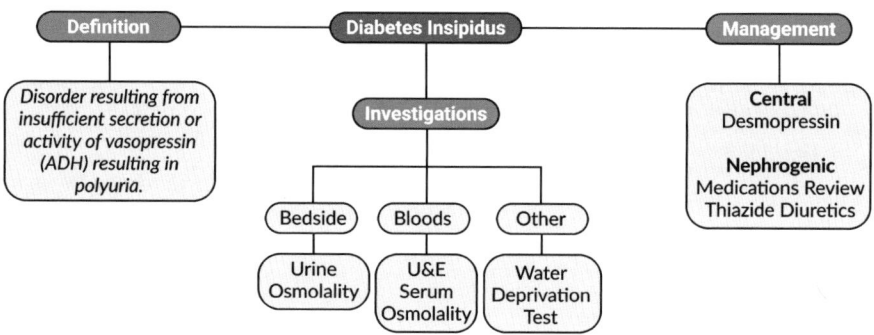

**Presentation**: Polyuria

## Definition

Diabetes insipidus is a condition in which insufficient production of antidiuretic hormone (ADH) or resistance to the action of ADH results in polyuria.

## Investigations

Diabetes insipidus is often initially investigated by comparing **urine and serum osmolality**. This can be assessed in the context of a **water deprivation test** where patients are prevented from drinking water and the urine and serum osmolality are measured on multiple occasions. As patients with diabetes insipidus are unable to concentrate their urine, they will continue to produce dilute urine even though their serum becomes increasingly concentrated. The subsequent administration of **desmopressin** (vasopressin analogue) can help distinguish between cranial and nephrogenic diabetes insipidus. In cranial diabetes insipidus, the kidneys will be able to respond to the exogenous vasopressin and start concentrating the urine. Patients with diabetes insipidus often become profoundly dehydrated and so may develop hypernatraemia and a pre-renal AKI (**U&E**).

## Management

Central diabetes insipidus is treated with **desmopressin**. Nephrogenic diabetes insipidus can be triggered by certain medications (e.g. lithium), so the patient's **drug history** should be reviewed. Some patients may also benefit from treatment with **thiazide diuretics**.

# Diabetes Mellitus

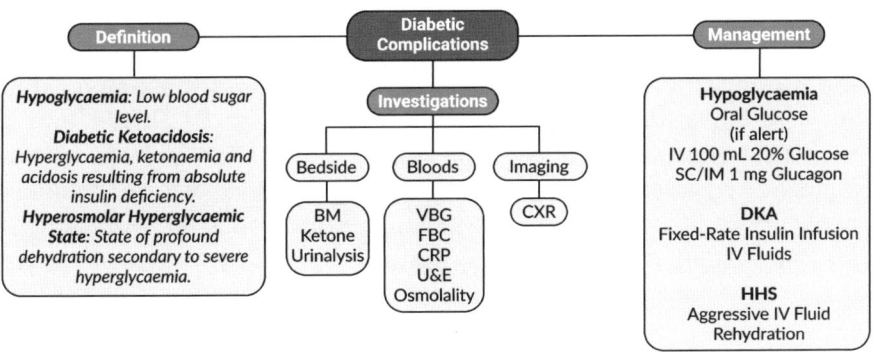

**Presentations**: Nausea and Vomiting

## Definition

Diabetes mellitus can be difficult to manage well and it can sometimes present to A&E with complications, such as diabetic ketoacidosis (DKA), hyperosmolar hyperglycaemic state (HHS) and hypoglycaemia.

## Investigations

At the bedside, a **BM** and **capillary ketones** should be checked. It should be noted that ketonaemia is usually accompanied by hyperglycaemia, however, patients who are on SGLT2 inhibitors (e.g. empagliflozin) are at risk of euglycaemic ketoacidosis. **Urinalysis** may also demonstrate ketones and glucose in the urine. A **VBG** provides an early value for the pH, bicarbonate and glucose which are important in the diagnosis of DKA. An **FBC** and a **CRP** may reveal raised inflammatory markers suggestive of an underlying infection that may have precipitated the complication. Dehydration resulting from DKA and HHS may lead to a pre-renal AKI (**U&E**). Furthermore, hyperglycaemia can cause a pseudohyponatraemia though profound dehydration can lead to hypernatraemia. The diagnosis of HHS involves measuring the **serum osmolality**. A **chest X-ray** may be performed as part of an infection screen.

## Management

The management of hypoglycaemia is guided by the conscious level of the patient. If alert, **oral glucose** can be used. If there are any concerns, **IV glucose** or **IM glucagon** can be administered. The management of DKA focuses on rehydrating the patient and suppressing ketone production by administering **IV fluids** and a **fixed-rate insulin infusion**. The main complication of HHS is profound dehydration, so patients require aggressive **IV fluid** resuscitation. If the fluids alone fail to lower the glucose at an appropriate rate, an insulin infusion may be started.

# Discitis and Epidural Abscess

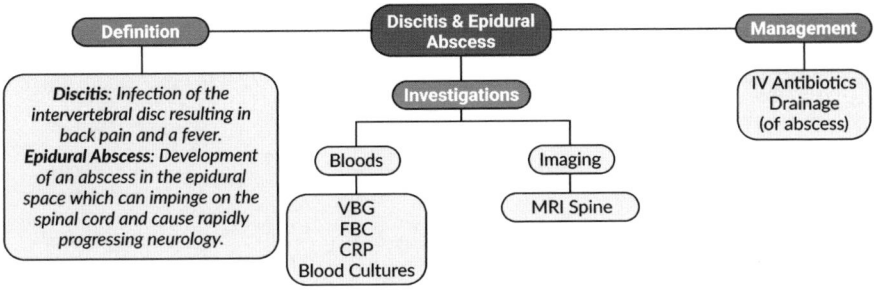

**Presentation**: Back Pain

## *Definition*

**Discitis** refers to an infection of the intervertebral disc, whereas an **epidural abscess** refers to the development of an abscess within the epidural space. Abscesses can enlarge causing rapidly progressing neurological impairments.

## *Investigations*

A **VBG** provides a measure of serum lactate concentration to help assess the severity of sepsis. **FBC** and **CRP** will likely reveal raised inflammatory markers and **blood cultures** should be taken as part of the sepsis 6 protocol. An urgent **MRI spine** is required to identify the site of the discitis or epidural abscess and assess the risk posed to the spinal cord.

## *Management*

Discitis often requires a very long course of **IV antibiotics** and an epidural abscess may require drainage.

# Diverticular Disease

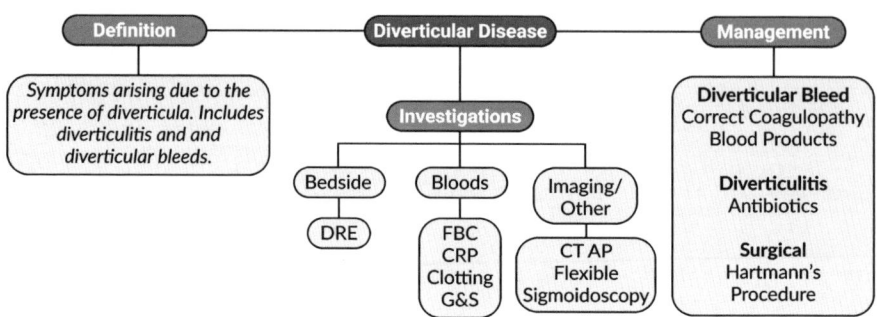

**Presentations**: Iliac Fossa Pain, Rectal Bleeding

## *Definition*

Colonic diverticula are outpouchings of the colon that are very common and often asymptomatic. They can, however, bleed or become infected.

## *Investigations*

A **DRE** may be performed in patients who report rectal bleeding to visualise the rectal bleeding (fresh red blood or melaenic stool). An **FBC** may reveal a drop in haemoglobin in patients with significant diverticular bleeding and will reveal a raised white cell count in diverticulitis (also associated with a raised **CRP**). If patients are bleeding significantly or are likely to require a surgical intervention, a **clotting screen** and **G&S** should be requested upon initial assessment. A **CT abdomen and pelvis with contrast** can confirm a diagnosis of diverticulitis and identify complications, such as abscesses and perforations. A **flexible sigmoidoscopy** may be performed to identify a diverticular bleed. This may be deferred by several weeks in the case of diverticulitis as an increased risk of complications is associated with performing endoscopic examinations when the colon is inflamed and friable.

## Management

Diverticular bleeds should be managed by **correcting coagulopathy** and administering **blood products** if indicated. Diverticulitis is often initially managed with **antibiotics**. In cases of severe diverticulitis, diverticular bleeds or perforations, a **Hartmann's procedure** (proctosigmoidectomy with an end colostomy and formation of a rectal stump) may be considered.

# Eating Disorders

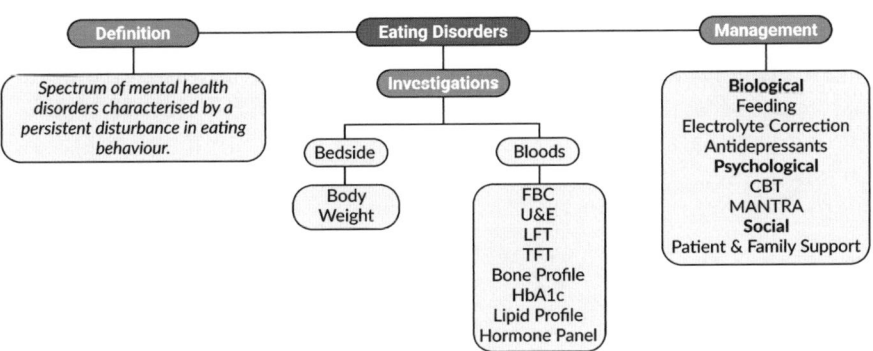

**Presentation**: Weight Loss

## Definition

Eating disorders are a subset of mental health conditions that are characterised by a disturbance in eating behaviour. They most commonly occur in teenagers and young adults.

## Investigations

The patient's **body weight** should be recorded at each health visit to track progress. Patients who are very underweight and malnourished can develop a pancytopaenia (**FBC**) and electrolyte derangements (**U&E** and **bone profile**). Patients can also develop malnutrition-induced hepatitis (**LFT**). **TFT** should be checked as hyperthyroidism is an alternative diagnosis that can cause significant weight loss. Anorexia nervosa can lead to abnormalities in lipid metabolism which would be identified in a **lipid profile** and patients can also develop hypopituitarism, so a **hormone panel** should be requested.

## *Management*

The management of eating disorders involves applying a bio-psycho-social model. Patients will need careful **feeding** to avoid worsening their relationship with food with close monitoring of their **electrolytes** as they are at risk of refeeding syndrome. **Antidepressants** are also often used in the management of eating disorders. Psychological approaches include **CBT** and **MANTRA**. Social **support** should also be offered to the patient and friends or relatives involved in their care.

# Ectopic Pregnancy

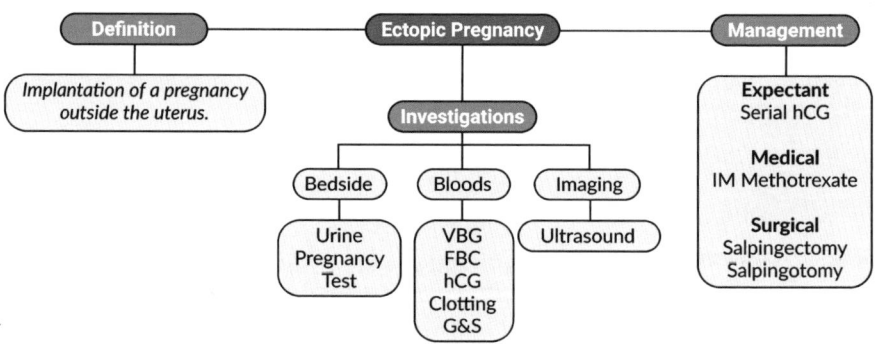

**Presentation**: Iliac Fossa Pain

## *Definition*

An ectopic pregnancy is a condition in which a pregnancy implants in a site other than the uterus (often the fallopian tubes).

## Investigations

Often, patients will not know that they are pregnant when presenting with an ectopic pregnancy as it usually manifests early in pregnancy. Therefore, a **urine pregnancy test** should be performed. A **VBG** will provide the haemoglobin and lactate results. A serum **hCG** should be requested with the blood as the level will help guide management. As the patient may require a surgical intervention, a **clotting screen** and **G&S** should be sent. A **transvaginal ultrasound** scan should be performed to locate the ectopic pregnancy and check for evidence of rupture (free fluid in the abdomen).

## Management

The management depends on the severity of the patient's symptoms, the size of the foetus and the serum hCG concentration. Expectant management involves allowing the ectopic pregnancy to miscarry spontaneously and measuring **serial hCG** concentrations to ensure that the levels are declining. Medical management involves administering **IM methotrexate** and surgical management may come in the form of a **salpingectomy** or **salpingotomy**.

# Epididymal Cyst

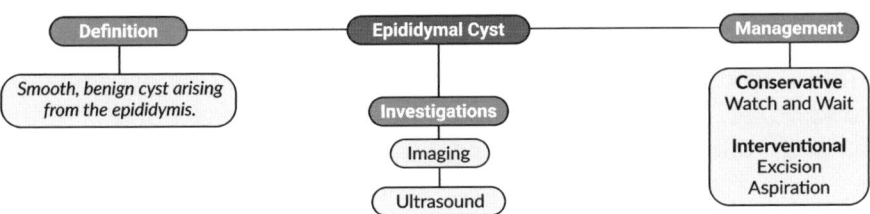

**Presentation**: Scrotal Mass

## Definition

An epididymal cyst is a collection of fluid that arises within the epididymis. It may cause some scrotal discomfort but rarely presents with acute pain.

## Investigations

It is primarily a clinical diagnosis based on examination findings but can be visualised with an **ultrasound**.

## Management

Epididymal cysts do not usually require intervention. If they are causing troublesome symptoms, they can be **aspirated** or **excised**.

# Food Bolus

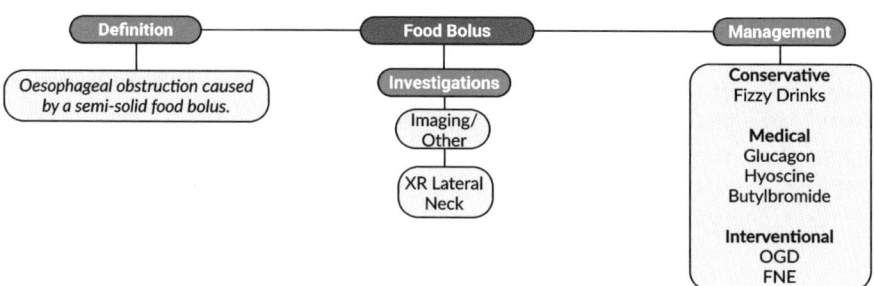

**Presentation**: Dysphagia

## Definition

Refers to oesophageal obstruction that is caused by a semi-solid food bolus. Patients usually present complaining that they felt the food get stuck down their throat as they were eating.

## Investigations

If the ingested food contains material that may be radio-opaque (e.g. cod fish bones), a **lateral neck X-ray** may be requested to identify its location.

## Management

Drinking **fizzy drinks** can help facilitate the passage of the food bolus. If ineffective, **glucagon** and **hyoscine butylbromide (Buscopan™)** may help relax the oesophageal sphincter. If conservative and medical treatment is ineffective, an **OGD** should be performed to identify and relieve the obstruction. A **flexible nasal endoscopy** may be performed by the ENT team if the obstruction is thought to lie above the level of the clavicle.

# Food Poisoning

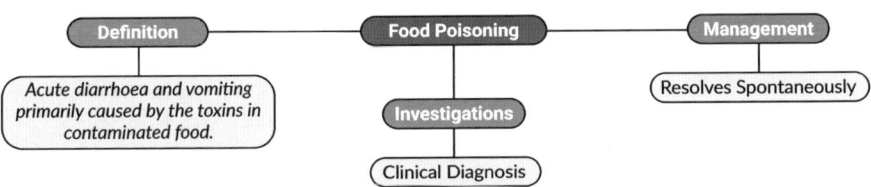

**Presentations**: Nausea and Vomiting, Diarrhoea

## Definition

Food poisoning refers to abrupt onset diarrhoea and vomiting that is caused by the toxins produced by bacteria found in contaminated food. *Staphylococcus aureus* is a common cause.

## Investigations

It is a clinical diagnosis.

## Management

Patients often manage symptoms at home, and they usually resolve spontaneously within days.

# Gastric Cancer

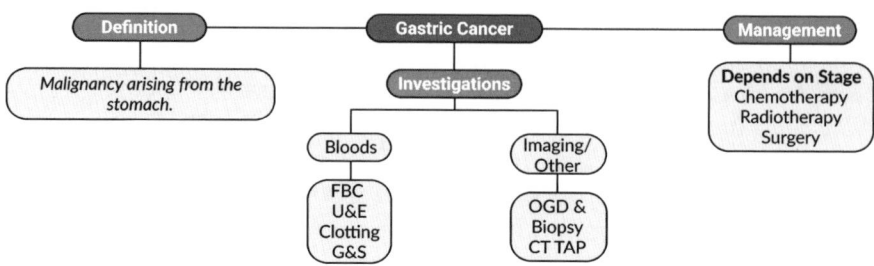

**Presentation**: Haematemesis

## *Definition*

Gastric cancer refers to a malignancy arising from the tissues of the stomach. Adenocarcinoma is the most common histological type of gastric cancer — others include carcinoid tumours, lymphoma and gastrointestinal stromal tumours.

## *Investigations*

An **FBC** may reveal a microcytic anaemia from chronic, insidious blood loss. **U&E** may reveal a raised urea due to the digestion of blood within the stomach. To identify coagulopathies that may worsen bleeding and as part of the work-up for surgical intervention, a **clotting screen** and **G&S** should be requested. If presenting acutely with haematemesis, a **VBG** will provide an early indication of the haemoglobin and lactate. The patients will need an **OGD and biopsy** to visualise the tumour and obtain a sample to establish a histological diagnosis. A **CT thorax, abdomen and pelvis** will allow the tumour to be staged.

## *Management*

The management depends on the type and stage of the tumour but will likely involve a combination of chemotherapy, radiotherapy and surgery.

# Gastritis and Peptic Ulcer Disease

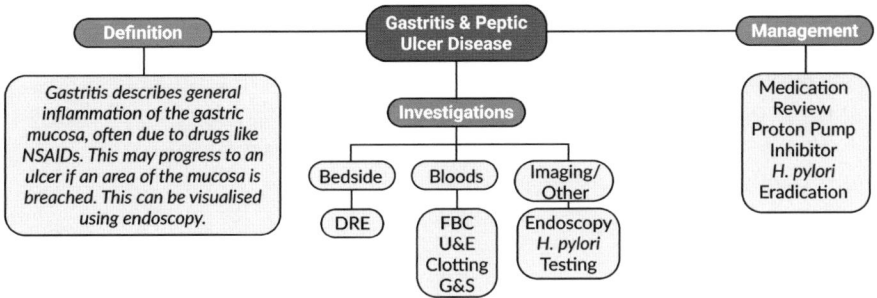

**Presentations**: Haematemesis, Epigastric Pain, RUQ Pain

## *Definition*

Gastritis refers to inflammation of the lining of the stomach which can cause epigastric discomfort and may be precipitated by certain common medications, such as NSAIDs. This can lead to erosions and, eventually, ulcers that can bleed or perforate.

## *Investigations*

If patients are presenting with reports of a change in the colour of their stool, a **DRE** could be performed to check for evidence of melaena. An **FBC** may reveal a decrease in haemoglobin and **U&E** may reveal a raised urea due to the digestion of blood in the stomach. A **clotting screen** and **G&S** should be requested as the patient may require blood transfusions and surgical intervention. Patients presenting with an upper gastrointestinal bleed should be triaged using a scoring system (e.g. Glasgow–Blatchford) which helps determine how urgently they should undergo **endoscopy**. Patients should also undergo *Helicobacter pylori* **testing** (either via a CLO test, urease breath test or stool antigen).

## Management

**Drugs** that contribute to the development of gastritis and peptic ulcer disease, such as NSAIDs and bisphosphonates, should be reviewed and withdrawn if appropriate. Patients should also be started on a **proton pump inhibitor** (e.g. omeprazole) and, if *H. pylori* is detected, they should undergo **eradication therapy** (two antibiotics and a PPI).

# Gastrointestinal Angiodysplasia

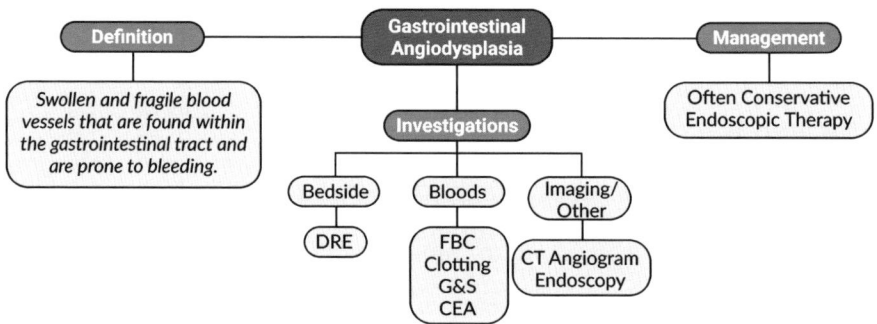

**Presentation**: Rectal Bleeding

## Definition

Gastrointestinal angiodysplasia is a condition that is characterised by the development of vascular abnormalities within the gastrointestinal tract that are prone to bleeding.

## Investigations

A **DRE** may allow visualisation of the rectal bleeding, and this can provide an important indication of where the bleed is likely to be (e.g. melaenic in upper gastrointestinal bleeds). An **FBC** may demonstrate a drop in haemoglobin. A **clotting screen** and **G&S** should be requested as the patient may require blood transfusions or an intervention. As colorectal cancer can present similarly, a

**carcinoembryonic antigen (CEA)** may also be requested. If ongoing bleeding is suspected, a **CT angiogram** can help pinpoint the location of the bleeding and identify a target for embolisation. An **endoscopy** can also help visualise the site of the bleeding.

## Management

If the bleeding is minimal, it is often managed conservatively. Endoscopy can also be used to try and stem the bleeding (e.g. using cautery).

# Giant Cell Arteritis

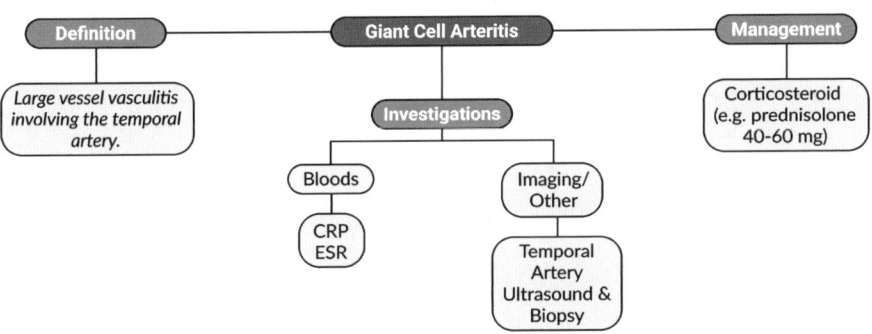

**Presentation**: Headache

## Definition

Giant cell arteritis (also known as temporal arteritis) is a large vessel vasculitis that primarily affects the temporal artery. It classically presents with a unilateral headache, scalp tenderness, jaw claudication and, in some cases, visual impairment. It is strongly associated with polymyalgia rheumatica.

## Investigations

As it is an inflammatory condition, the **CRP** and **ESR** are likely to be raised. The diagnosis can be confirmed by performing a

**temporal artery ultrasound and biopsy**, however, this cannot be used to definitively rule out the diagnosis as the sample may not necessarily have been taken from the affected area of the temporal artery.

## Management

As it is an inflammatory condition, it is treated with high-dose **steroids** (e.g. prednisolone).

# Gilbert Syndrome

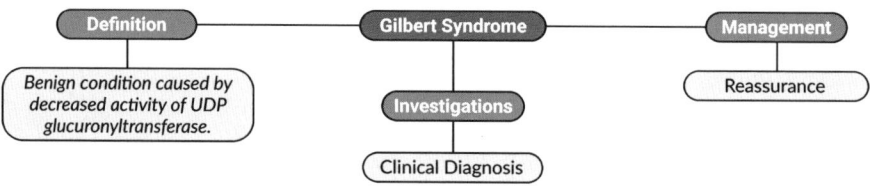

**Presentation**: Jaundice

## Definition

Gilbert syndrome is a common, benign condition that is characterised by mild jaundice that is precipitated by fatigue and recent illness. It occurs due to reduced activity of UGP glucuronyltransferase which is responsible for the conjugation of bilirubin in the liver.

## Investigations

It is usually noted incidentally when well patients are noted to have a mildly elevated bilirubin level. Patients may describe their eyes becoming mildly jaundiced whenever they are tired or unwell.

## Management

It is a benign condition that does not require active treatment.

# Gastro-Oesophageal Reflux Disease (GORD)

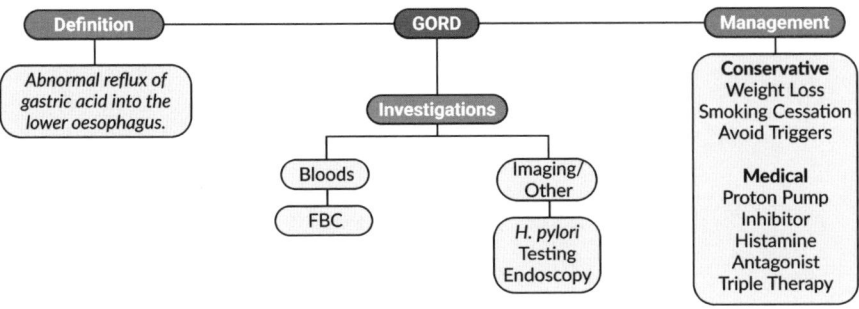

**Presentations**: Chest Pain, Epigastric Pain

## *Definition*

GORD is a very common condition that occurs due to the reflux of stomach acid into the oesophagus. It manifests with epigastric and retrosternal chest pain that is worse after eating and when lying down.

## *Investigations*

Patients presenting with epigastric pain may have developed a peptic ulcer which can bleed and cause an iron deficiency anaemia, so an **FBC** should be considered in patients presenting in this manner. If the symptoms are persistent, *H. pylori* testing (CLO test, urease breath test or stool antigen) should be considered. If there are any red flag features associated with dyspepsia, the patient should be referred for an **endoscopy** via the 2-week wait pathway.

## *Management*

Conservative measures that can help improve symptoms include **weight loss**, **smoking cessation** and the **avoidance of triggers** (e.g. spicy food). Medical treatments that reduce the acidity of the stomach contents, such as **proton pump inhibitors** and

**histamine antagonists**, are the mainstay of treatment. If *H. pylori* is detected, **eradication therapy** should be offered.

# Gout

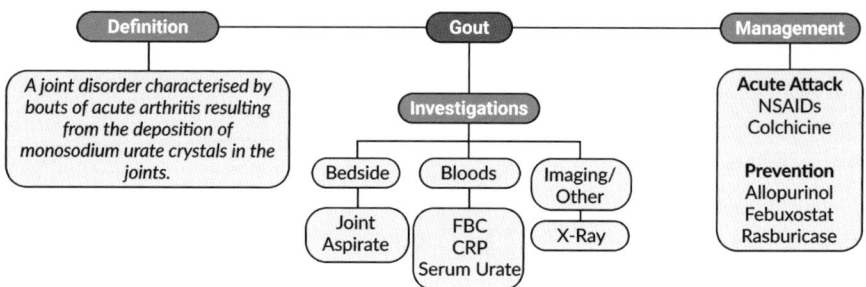

**Presentation**: Joint Pain

## *Definition*

Gout is a common crystal arthropathy that typically presents with acute pain affecting a single joint (most commonly the first metatarsophalangeal joint). It is caused by the deposition of monosodium urate crystals within the joint space.

## *Investigations*

At the bedside, a **joint aspirate** should be performed by a suitably trained individual to obtain a sample of synovial fluid to send for analysis. This will reveal negatively birefringent needle-shaped crystals and also allows septic arthritis to be ruled out. The patient's inflammatory markers are likely to be raised (**FBC** and **CRP**). Furthermore, a **serum urate** level is usually measured after an acute gout attack as this may be elevated in patients who are predisposed to developing gout.

## *Management*

The acute management of gout involves using **NSAIDs** and **colchicine**. Urate-lowering therapy (**allopurinol**, **febuxostat** and **rasburicase**) may be offered to some subsets of patients.

# Haemolytic Disorders

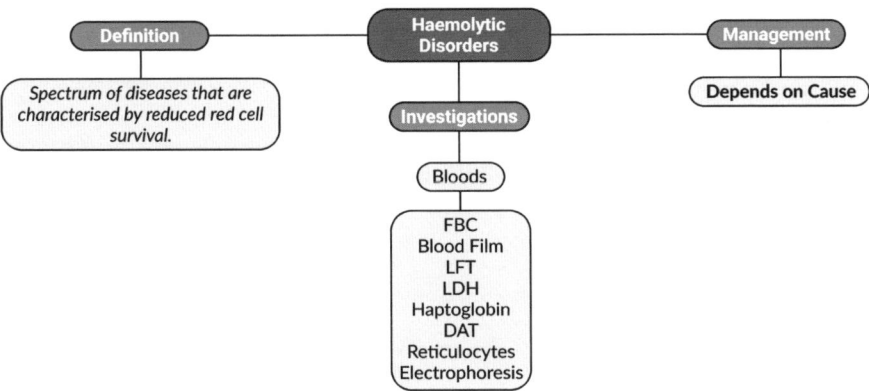

**Presentation**: Jaundice

## *Definition*

Haemolytic conditions are characterised by reduced survival of red cells. It can happen due to intrinsic red cell abnormalities (e.g. haemoglobinopathies, G6PD deficiency and pyruvate kinase deficiency) or due to extrinsic insults (e.g. malaria and hypersplenism). It can manifest with jaundice, shortness of breath and fatigue.

## *Investigations*

An **FBC** will show a low haemoglobin concentration and a **blood film** may reveal evidence of intravascular breakdown of red cells (e.g. schistocytes) or abnormal red cell morphology (e.g. spherocytosis). An **LFT** will reveal a raised bilirubin concentration and the **LDH** will be raised as it is a ubiquitous intracellular enzyme that is released into the serum when the red cells lyse. **Haptoglobins** are proteins that sequester free heme, so their level will be decreased in cases of haemolysis. A **direct antiglobulin test (DAT)** is used to identify autoimmune haemolytic anaemia. A raised **reticulocyte count** is seen in patients with haemolysis as the bone marrow attempts to respond to the anaemia by increasing its output of immature red cells. **Haemoglobin electrophoresis** is used to diagnose haemoglobinopathies, such as sickle cell disease and thalassemia.

### *Management*

The management of haemolytic anaemia depends largely on the cause.

# Haemorrhoids

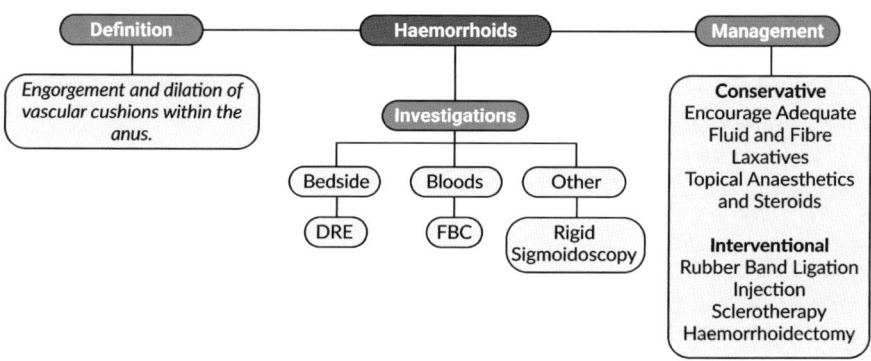

**Presentation**: Rectal Bleeding

### *Definition*

Haemorrhoids are very common dilations of the vascular cushions around the anus that result in mild rectal bleeding and are often managed in primary care.

## Investigations

External or prolapsed haemorrhoids may be visualised during a **DRE**. An **FBC** is useful to check for a drop in haemoglobin in case there has been significant blood loss from the haemorrhoids. The haemorrhoids may be visualised using **rigid sigmoidoscopy**.

## Management

Conservative measures that can help resolve haemorrhoids include maintaining a balanced diet with adequate **fluid and fibre**, **laxatives** and **topical preparations** of local anaesthetics and steroids. If persistent or severe, interventions such as **rubber band ligation**, **sclerotherapy** and **haemorrhoidectomy** may be considered.

# Hepatitis

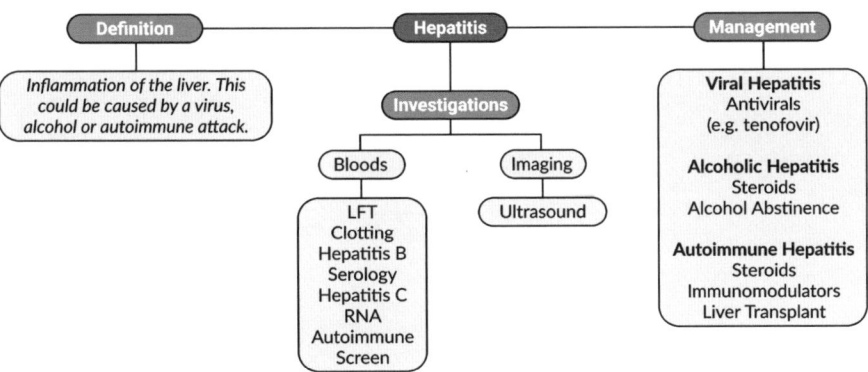

**Presentations**: Jaundice, RUQ Pain

## Definition

Hepatitis refers to inflammation of the liver that usually occurs due to alcohol excess, viral infection, visceral fat deposition and autoimmune attack. It may present with jaundice and RUQ discomfort or be incidentally noted on a blood test.

## Investigations

**LFTs** will reveal a transaminitis (raised ALT and AST). If the liver's synthetic function is impaired, abnormalities will be noted on the **clotting screen**. In undifferentiated hepatitis, a screen will include **hepatitis B and C serology** and an **autoimmune screen**. An **ultrasound** scan may provide evidence that is in keeping with hepatitis and can be used to assess for features of cirrhosis (e.g. surface nodularity).

## Management

The management depends on the cause. Hepatitis B and C may be managed with **antivirals**. Alcoholic hepatitis may be treated with **steroids** and supporting the patient to remain abstinent. Autoimmune hepatitis is generally managed with **steroids** and **immunomodulators**. Some patients may be considered for **liver transplantation**.

# Hepatocellular Carcinoma

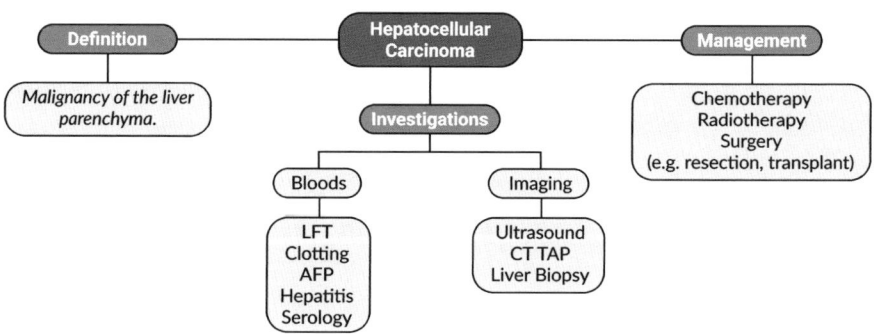

**Presentation**: Jaundice

## Definition

Hepatocellular carcinoma (HCC) is a cancer of the liver paren-chyma. Patients with a background of chronic liver disease are at increased risk.

## Investigations

Patients may be suspected of having an HCC upon noting a derangement in their **LFT**. A **clotting screen** should also be requested as there may be an impairment in the liver's synthetic function. **Alpha-Fetoprotein (AFP)** is a tumour marker that is associated with HCC. As HCC usually arises in the context of pre-existing liver disease, **hepatitis serology** should also be requested. An **ultrasound** scan may allow identification of suspicious masses within the liver which could then be **biopsied** under imaging guid-ance. Once diagnosed, a **CT thorax, abdomen and pelvis** will likely be performed to stage the cancer.

## Management

The management will depend on the stage of the tumour but will likely involve a combination of chemotherapy, radiotherapy and surgery.

# Hiatus Hernia

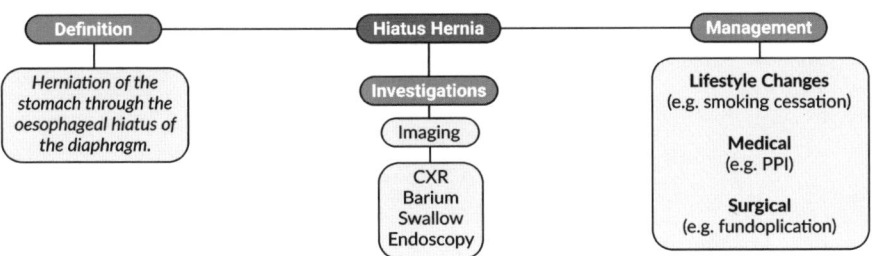

**Presentation**: Dysphagia

## Definition

A hiatus hernia is an anatomical abnormality in which part of the stomach herniates through the oesophageal hiatus into the thorax. This can cause symptoms of persistent dyspepsia and, sometimes, dysphagia.

## Investigations

Many hiatus hernias are asymptomatic and may be incidentally noted on a **chest X-ray** which reveals a gastric air bubble within the thorax. It can also be visualised using a **barium swallow** or an **endoscopy**.

## Management

If the symptoms are of mild dyspepsia, **lifestyle changes** such as smoking cessation advice may suffice. Patients may also be started on medical treatments to reduce the acidity of the stomach (e.g. **proton pump inhibitors**). If the symptoms are particularly persistent or bothersome, patients may be considered for surgical intervention (e.g. **Nissen fundoplication**).

# Human Immunodeficiency Virus (HIV)

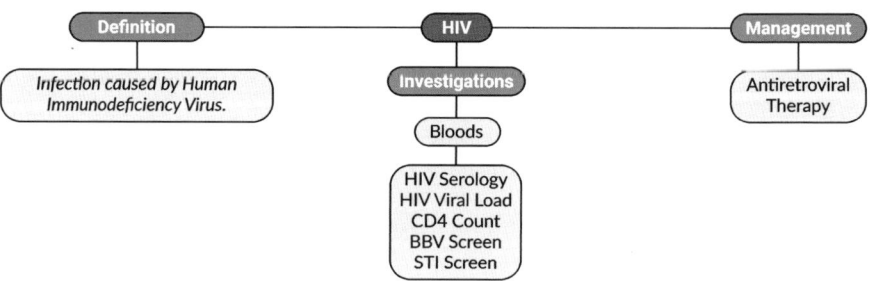

**Presentation**: Fatigue

## Definition

HIV is a virus that causes a chronic infection that can manifest with immunodeficiency, resulting in increased susceptibility to opportunistic infections and the development of acquired immunodeficiency syndrome (AIDS).

## Investigations

**HIV serology** allows a diagnosis to be made. The **HIV viral load** and **CD4 count** are used to monitor response to treatment. Patients who acquired HIV through sexual contact may be at risk of other sexually transmitted infections and bloodborne viruses, so an **STI screen** and **BBV screen** should be performed.

## Management

With good compliance, HIV can be very well controlled with **antiretroviral therapy**. Some patients may be started on prophylactic antibiotics (e.g. co-trimoxazole) to reduce the risk of developing opportunistic infections.

# Hypothyroidism

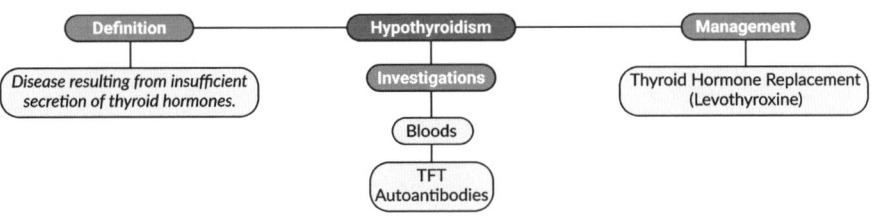

**Presentations**: Constipation, Fatigue

## Definition

Hypothyroidism is a common condition that is characterised by insufficient output of thyroid hormones by the thyroid gland. It most commonly occurs due to autoimmune destruction of the thyroid gland (Hashimoto's thyroiditis).

## Investigations

**TFTs** will reveal a raised TSH and a low $T_4$. Hashimoto's thyroiditis is associated with a raised **anti-thyroid peroxidase antibody** and, sometimes, an **anti-thyroglobulin antibody**.

## Management

Treatment involves providing exogenous thyroid hormone (**levo-thyroxine**) and titrating the dose based on the serum TSH concentration.

# Idiopathic Intracranial Hypertension (IIH)

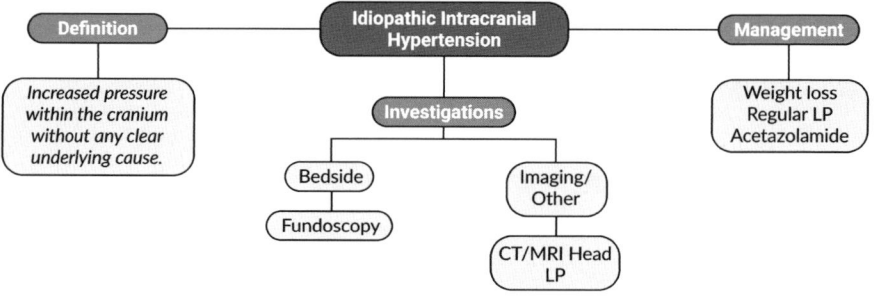

**Presentation**: Headache

## Definition

IIH is a condition in which raised intracranial pressure without a clear underlying cause leads to persistent headaches that do not usually respond to simple analgesia.

## Investigations

At the bedside, **fundoscopy** may reveal papilloedema. A **CT/MRI head** scan is usually requested to check for other causes of elevated CSF pressure, such as a brain tumour or a dural sinus thrombus. A **lumbar puncture** will reveal a raised opening pressure.

## Management

Being overweight is a significant risk factor for IIH, so patients should be advised to aim for a **healthy weight**. Some patients may have **regular lumbar punctures** to temporarily relieve the intracranial pressure. **Acetazolamide** is a carbonic anhydrase inhibitor that has been shown to reduce CSF secretion in the choroid plexus.

# Infectious Colitis

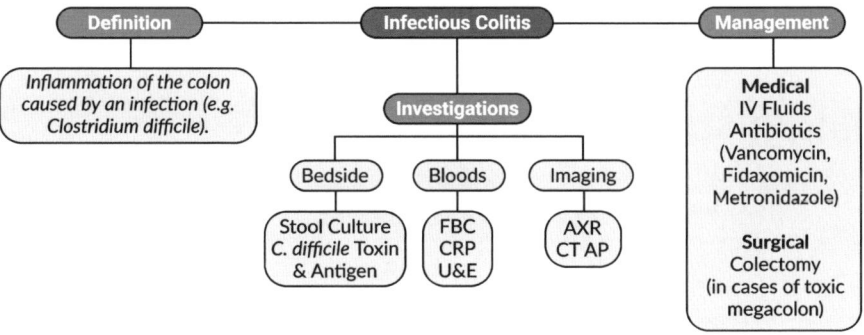

**Presentations**: Diarrhoea, Rectal Bleeding

## Definition

Infectious colitis refers to inflammation of the colon caused by an infection (e.g. *C. difficile* and *Salmonella*). *C. difficile* colitis is particularly common in elderly hospital inpatients and typically occurs after a course of antibiotics that alters the gut microbiome leading to the overgrowth of *C. difficile*. Common causative antibiotics include co-amoxiclav, ciprofloxacin, cephalosporins and ciprofloxacin.

## Investigations

At the bedside, a **stool sample** should be taken for culture and to test for ***C. difficile* toxin and antigen**. The **FBC** and **CRP** may reveal raised inflammatory markers and a drop in haemoglobin. The diarrhoea can cause electrolyte derangement, so the patient's **U&E** should be monitored. In severe cases, infectious colitis can progress to cause toxic megacolon which can be identified on an **abdominal X-ray** or **CT abdomen and pelvis with contrast**.

## Management

Medical treatment involves **IV fluid resuscitation** and **antibiotics** (e.g. vancomycin, metronidazole and fidaxomicin). In cases of toxic megacolon, **emergency surgery** may be required to remove the colon.

# Interstitial Lung Disease

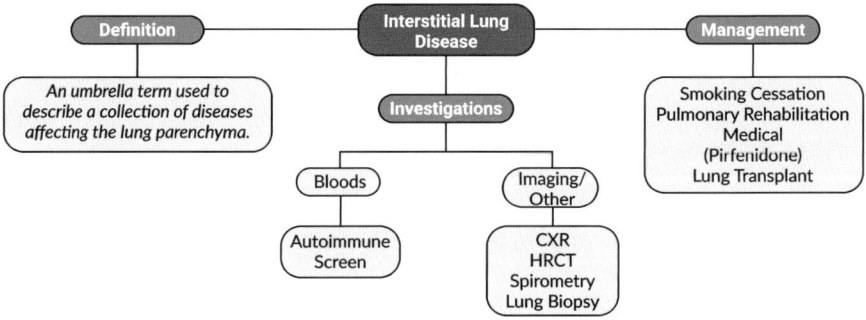

**Presentations**: Shortness of Breath, Cough

## Definition

Interstitial lung disease is an umbrella term that encompasses several diseases that affect the lung parenchyma (e.g. idiopathic pulmonary fibrosis and pneumoconiosis). Systemic autoimmune diseases (e.g. rheumatoid arthritis) can also lead to interstitial lung disease.

## Investigations

If an underlying autoimmune cause of interstitial lung disease is suspected, an **autoimmune screen** should be requested. Widespread reticulonodular shadowing may be noted on a **chest X-ray** but this can be better visualised with an **HRCT**. **Spirometry** will reveal a restrictive defect and a **lung biopsy** will facilitate a histological diagnosis.

## Management

It is often very difficult to treat but conservative measures that can provide symptomatic relief and limit progression include **smoking cessation** and **pulmonary rehabilitation**. Idiopathic pulmonary fibrosis can be treated with **pirfenidone** which has been shown to provide a survival benefit. **Steroids** may be considered in cases of interstitial lung disease that is caused by an underlying inflammatory or autoimmune condition. Some patients may be considered for **lung transplantation**.

# Intestinal Ischaemia

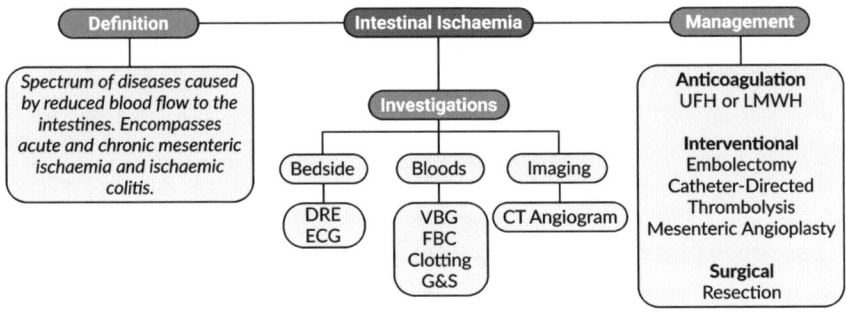

**Presentations**: Iliac Fossa Pain, Rectal Bleeding

## Definition

Intestinal ischaemia refers to a spectrum of diseases that arise due to a reduction in the blood flow to the intestines.

## Investigations

At the bedside, a **DRE** may reveal fresh blood upon withdrawal of the finger. An **ECG** may reveal atrial fibrillation which is a major risk factor for intestinal ischaemia as it increases the risk of a cardiogenic embolism. A **VBG** provides an early result for the lactate which will be raised due to tissue ischaemia. An **FBC** may reveal low haemoglobin. As the patient is likely to require an intervention, a **clotting screen** and **G&S** should be sent. Patients should undergo a **CT angiogram** to identify the occluded blood vessel.

## Management

Patients should be started on **anticoagulation** and the case should be urgently discussed with the on-call general surgical team. Interventions that can be used to re-establish perfusion to the bowel include **embolectomy**, **catheter-directed thrombolysis** and **mesenteric angioplasty**. If the bowel is no longer viable, it may be **surgically resected**.

# Intoxication

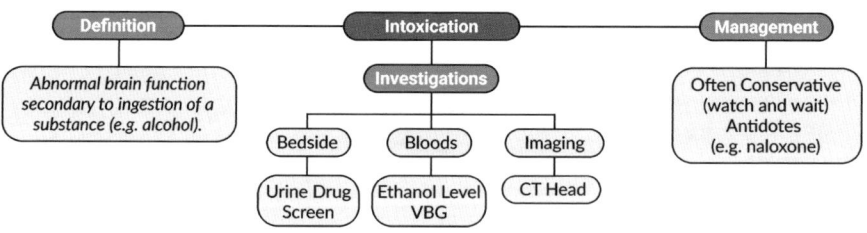

**Presentations**: Collapse, Confusion, Nausea and Vomiting

## Definition

Intoxication refers to a state of abnormal brain function due to the effects of an ingested substance (e.g. alcohol and illicit drugs). The manifestations vary greatly depending on the drug(s) involved.

## Investigations

A **urine drug screen** and an **ethanol level** can help identify the causative agent if the patient is unable or unwilling to provide any details. Patients who are intoxicated or have overdosed can also develop a metabolic acidosis, so a **VBG** should be taken and various drug levels (e.g. paracetamol and salicylates) may be requested based on the history. If there is an unclear history of trauma, there should be a low threshold for a **CT head** scan as the patient may have sustained a serious head injury that is contributing to their clinical state.

## Management

Most cases of intoxication are managed conservatively until the substances are excreted from their system. This involves the symptomatic management of toxidromes. **Antidotes** may be used in some cases (e.g. naloxone in opioid overdose).

# Intracranial Bleed

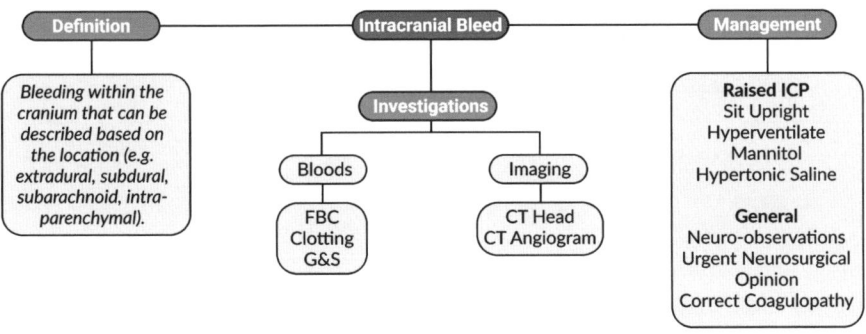

**Presentations**: Headache, Confusion

## Definition

An intracranial bleed is a bleed within the cranium that can be categorised based on the location and the aetiology (e.g. traumatic).

## Investigations

An **FBC** may reveal a low platelet count that is worsening the bleed and needs correcting. Similarly, a **clotting screen** should be sent in case there is a coagulopathy that needs correction. The patient may also need neurosurgical intervention, so a **G&S** should be sent. A **CT head** scan is often the initial imaging modality that is requested, and this may be followed by a **CT angiogram** to identify the source of the bleed.

## Management

If the patient has features of raised intracranial pressure (such as hypertension, bradycardia and irregular breathing), the on-call neurosurgical team should be informed immediately and carry out measures to reduce the pressure, such as **sitting the patient upright**, intubating and **hyperventilating** the patient and administering **mannitol** or **hypertonic saline**. Following a neurosurgical review, an intervention may be planned (e.g. decompressive craniectomy).

# Irritable Bowel Syndrome (IBS)

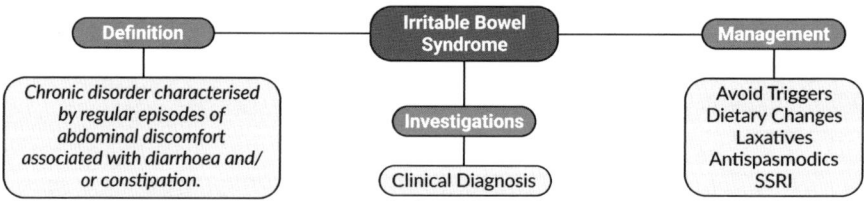

**Presentations**: Diarrhoea, Constipation

## Definition

IBS is a common condition that is characterised by intermittent episodes of constipation and diarrhoea associated with abdominal pain and bloating.

## Investigations

It is largely a clinical diagnosis though patients may undergo stool and blood tests to rule out other causes (e.g. inflammatory bowel disease and hyperthyroidism).

## Management

IBS may have clear triggers, so counselling the patient on **avoiding triggers** as well as certain **dietary changes** (e.g. FODMAP) may help improve the symptoms. **Antispasmodics** and **laxatives** can help relieve symptoms of cramping and constipation. IBS can be triggered by stress and low mood, so **SSRIs** may also make up part of the management.

# Joint Trauma

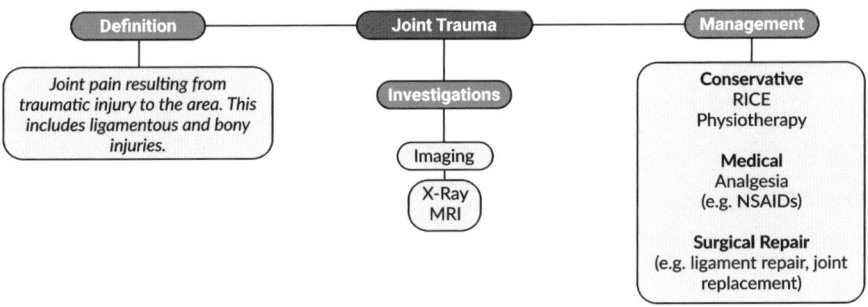

**Presentation**: Joint Pain

## *Definition*

Joint trauma, quite simply, refers to trauma sustained to a joint that can result in ligamentous and bony injuries.

## *Investigations*

Bony injury may be seen on an **X-ray**, whereas ligamentous injuries are better visualised on **MRI**.

## *Management*

Conservative management of soft tissue injuries involves **RICE** and **physiotherapy**. This can be facilitated by **simple analgesia**, such as NSAIDs. In some cases, **surgical intervention** may be considered (e.g. anterior cruciate ligament rupture).

# Mallory–Weiss Tear

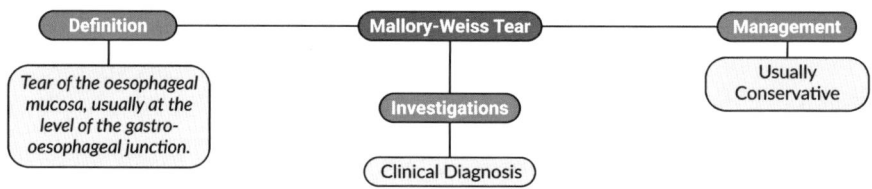

**Presentation**: Haematemesis

## *Definition*

A Mallory–Weiss tear is a superficial tear in the lining of the oesophagus that usually occurs following forceful vomiting or retching. Patients may describe the vomits as initially containing stomach acid and food contents and, later, becoming blood-stained.

## *Investigations*

It is a clinical diagnosis.

## *Management*

Mallory–Weiss tears resolve spontaneously once the vomiting subsides and rarely require intervention.

# Mechanical Back Pain

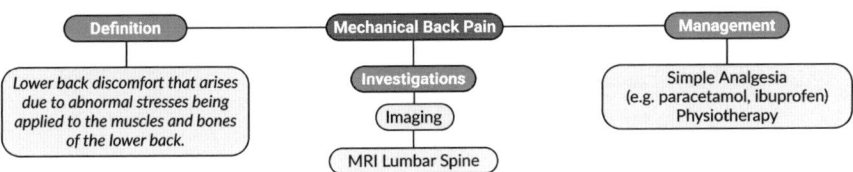

**Presentation**: Back Pain

## *Definition*

Mechanical back pain is a generic term used to describe lower back pain that arises due to abnormal stresses being placed on the muscles and bones of the lower back. It is an extremely common presentation in primary care.

## *Investigations*

Dangerous causes of back pain can often be excluded clinically. If the symptoms persist, patients may be referred for an **MRI lumbar spine** to check for evidence of disc herniation.

## *Management*

Mechanical back pain is generally managed in primary care with **simple analgesia** and **physiotherapy**.

# Medication Overuse Headaches

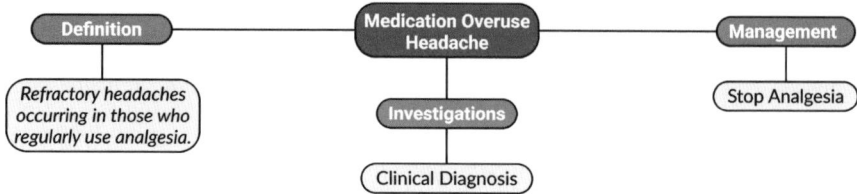

**Presentation**: Headache

## *Definition*

Medication overuse headaches are persistent headaches that develop in patients who regularly use analgesia.

## *Investigations*

It is a clinical diagnosis.

## *Management*

Patients should be advised to limit their use of analgesia.

# Metabolic Disturbance

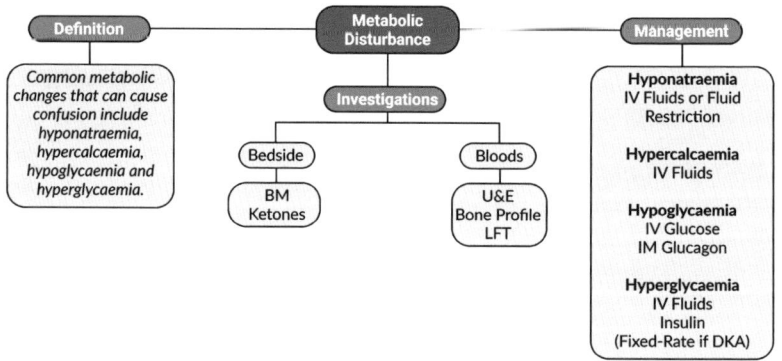

**Presentation**: Confusion

## Definition

There are several metabolic disturbances that can result in confusion which should be screened for in patients presenting with confusion without a clear cause.

## Investigations

Simple bedside investigations include a **BM** and **capillary ketones**. **U&E** and **bone profile** can demonstrate hyponatraemia and hypercalcaemia. Abnormal **LFTs** may indicate that the patient may have developed hepatic encephalopathy which can be directly measured by checking their serum ammonia concentration.

## Management

The management depends on the cause but often includes giving IV fluids. In cases of euvolaemic or hypervolaemic hyponatraemia, patients will be fluid-restricted. Hypoglycaemia may be managed with oral or IV glucose, or IM glucagon. DKA is managed with a fixed-rate insulin infusion. In some cases of hyperosmolar hyperglycaemic state, an insulin infusion may also be used.

# Multiple Sclerosis

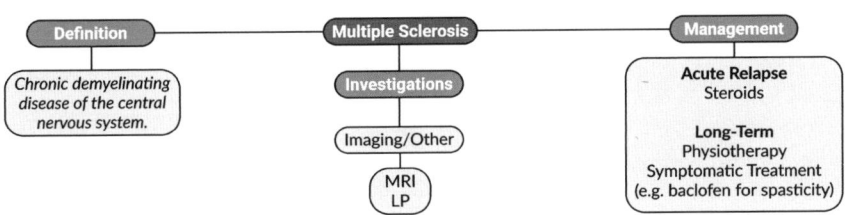

**Presentations**: Dysphagia, Constipation

## Definition

Multiple sclerosis (MS) is a chronic progressive demyelinating neuropathy.

## Investigations

MS is diagnosed after a patient has two or more episodes of neurological symptoms that are separated in time and space (i.e. occurring on different occasions and affecting different parts of the nervous system). Plaques can be visualised on an **MRI**. A **lumbar puncture** may show an elevated protein concentration and helps rule out other diagnoses (e.g. infection).

## Management

In relapsing–remitting MS, **steroids** may be used in patients presenting with a relapse. The long-term management focuses on maintaining the patient's functionality as best as possible. This usually involves **physiotherapy** and medications that help manage symptoms (e.g. baclofen for spasticity).

# Obstructed Venous Drainage

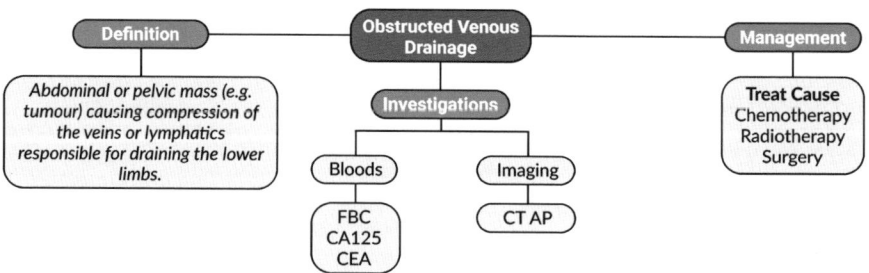

**Presentation**: Leg Pain

## Definition

Abdominal and pelvis masses (e.g. ovarian tumour) can compress the veins or lymphatics that come from the lower limbs resulting in bilateral lower limb swelling. This should be considered in patients with leg swelling without a clear alternative cause (e.g. heart failure).

## Investigations

In cases of occult malignancy, an **FBC** may reveal a microcytic anaemia. **CA125** and **CEA** are tumour markers that are associated with ovarian cancer and colorectal cancer, respectively. A **CT abdomen and pelvis** will allow a mass to be identified.

## Management

Treatment depends on the cause by may include a combination of chemotherapy, radiotherapy and surgery.

# Occult Malignancy

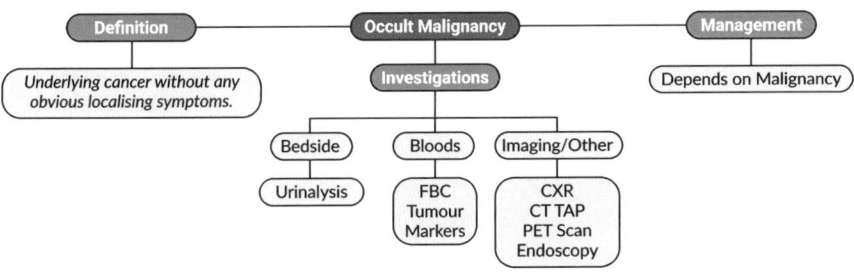

**Presentations**: Weight Loss, Fatigue

## Definition

An occult malignancy refers to a state in which an underlying malignant process is suspected but its location is unclear.

## Investigations

Renal or bladder cancer is likely to cause haematuria that may be microscopic and only detected when performing **urinalysis**. An **FBC** may reveal a microcytic anaemia or elevated white cell counts in leukaemia. Various tumour markers can also be detected in the blood (e.g. CA19-9, CA125 and CEA). A **chest X-ray** may reveal a lung tumour but a **CT thorax, abdomen and pelvis** acts as a more thorough screen. If a CT scan is inconclusive, a **PET scan** can be arranged to identify any abnormal areas of increased metabolic activity. If gastrointestinal tumours (e.g. oesophageal, stomach or colorectal cancer) are suspected, a faecal immunochemical test (FIT) is usually performed as a screening test, followed by an **endoscopy**.

## Management

The management depends on the cause.

# Oesophageal Varices

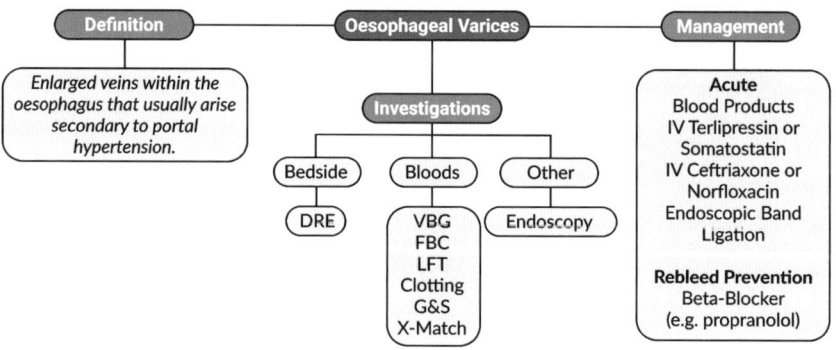

**Presentation**: Haematemesis

## Definition

Oesophageal varices are dilations of the veins within the oesophagus that are prone to bleeding and can present with massive haematemesis.

## Investigations

If the patient presents complaining of a change in their stool, a **DRE** can be performed to check for melaenic stools. If presenting with haematemesis, a **VBG** provides an early measure of haemoglobin which can be confirmed on an **FBC**. The **LFT** may reveal deranged liver function as oesophageal varices usually occur secondary to portal hypertension in patients with chronic liver disease. A **clotting screen** should be sent to identify any coagulopathies that could be corrected and a **G&S** and **X-match** should also be requested as the patient may require blood products. Oesophageal varices can be visualised and banded using **endoscopy**.

## Management

Patients presenting with large volume haematemesis should be resuscitated using blood products as indicated. **Terlipressin** or **somatostatin** can cause splanchnic vasoconstriction and reduce flow to the bleeding varices. IV **antibiotics** have also been shown to improve outcomes in patients with variceal bleeds. The case should be discussed with the on-call **endoscopist** to plan an intervention.

# Oesophagitis

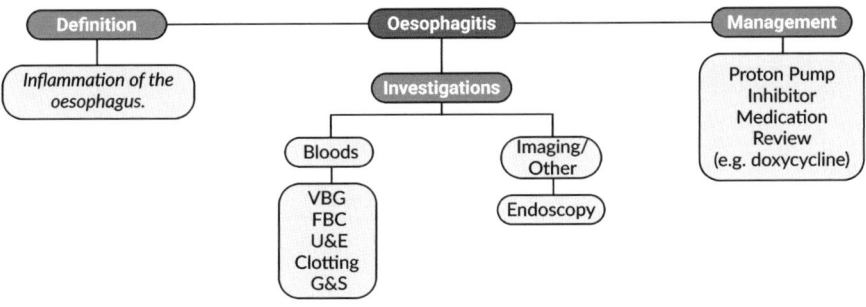

**Presentations**: Dysphagia, Haematemesis

## Definition

Oesophagitis refers to inflammation of the oesophagus that can occur due to reflux of stomach acid but may also be precipitated by certain medications (e.g. doxycycline).

## Investigations

If the patient is thought to have bled significantly, a **VBG** should be taken to check the haemoglobin. This can then be confirmed on the **FBC**. **U&E** may reveal a raised urea if the oesophagitis is causing a bleed. A **clotting screen** and **G&S** should be requested as, if there is significant bleeding, blood products may be required. The affected area can be visualised using **endoscopy**.

## Management

Oesophagitis can often be managed with **proton pump inhibitors** and by conducting a **medication review** to identify any medications that could precipitate or worsen oesophagitis.

# Orthostatic Hypotension

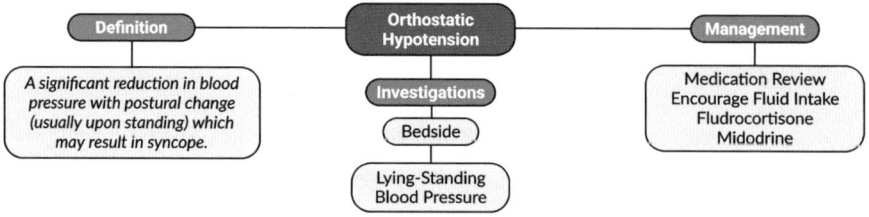

**Presentation**: Collapse

## Definition

Orthostatic hypotension (also known as postural hypotension) refers to a drop in blood pressure that occurs when changing position (e.g. lying or sitting to standing).

## *Investigations*

The patient should have **lying-standing blood pressure** checked — this involves measuring the blood pressure when lying flat and then at 1 minute and 3 minutes after standing. A systolic drop of more than 20 mm Hg or a diastolic drop of more than 10 mm Hg is considered significant.

## *Management*

Orthostatic hypotension is usually caused by **medications** (e.g. antihypertensives) that can affect the body's ability to adjust its blood pressure to tolerate postural changes. Patients should also be advised to increase their **fluid intake**. Medications such as **fludrocortisone** and **midodrine** may be used in cases that do not respond to conservative measures.

# Osteoarthritis

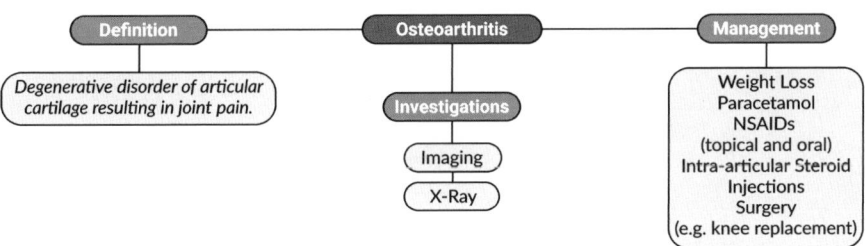

**Presentation**: Joint Pain

## *Definition*

Osteoarthritis is a condition in which erosion of the articular cartilage leads to joint pain. This can occur either due to constitutionally weak cartilage or due to excessive or abnormal forces being exerted on the cartilage.

## Investigations

The **X-ray** changes that are seen in osteoarthritis include loss of joint space, osteophytes, subchondral cysts and subchondral sclerosis.

## Management

Osteoarthritis affecting large weight-bearing joints can be improved by **losing weight**. Patients should be advised to use **simple analgesia** and escalate in accordance with the WHO analgesic ladder. Some patients may benefit from **intra-articular steroid injections**. If the symptoms are particularly debilitating and not responding to medical treatment, **surgery** should be considered (e.g. joint replacement).

# Ovarian Cyst Accident

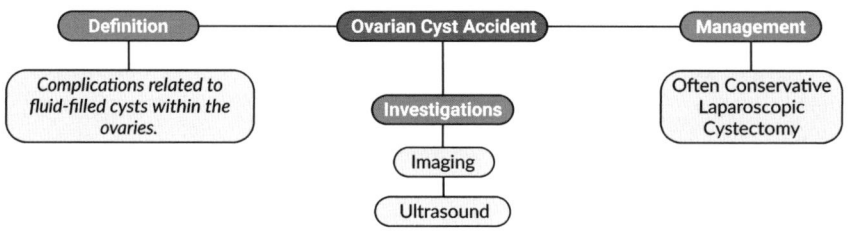

**Presentation**: Iliac Fossa Pain

## Definition

Ovarian cysts are very common fluid-filled sacs that can cause acute lower abdominal pain if they rupture.

## Investigations

It is largely a clinical diagnosis, however, patients may undergo an **ultrasound** scan to rule out other differentials (e.g. ovarian torsion).

## *Management*

The pain from ovarian cyst accidents normally resolves spontaneously. If the cysts are causing persistent issues, patients may be considered for a **laparoscopic cystectomy**.

# Pancreatic Cancer

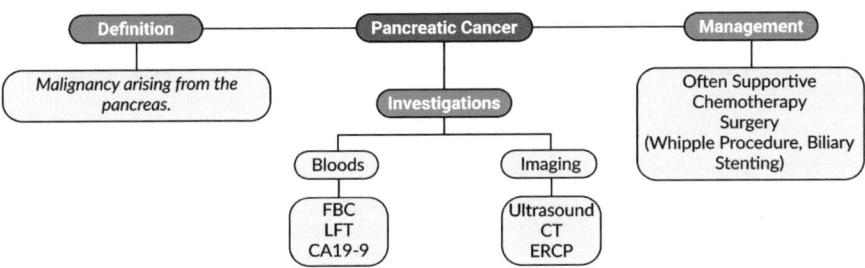

**Presentation**: Jaundice

## *Definition*

Pancreatic cancer refers to a malignancy arising from the pancreas that often presents late and, therefore, carries a poor prognosis.

## *Investigations*

An **FBC** may reveal anaemia and the **LFTs** may demonstrate an obstructive pattern (raised ALP and GGT) if the pancreatic mass is obstructing biliary outflow. **CA19-9** is a tumour marker that is associated with pancreatic cancer. Biliary tree dilation can be visualised on an **ultrasound scan**. The pancreatic mass, itself, can be visualised using **CT** and an **ERCP** may be performed to take a biopsy.

## *Management*

If localised, patients may be considered for a **Whipple's procedure**. Treatment may also involve **chemotherapy**. Much of the time, the disease is no longer curable and the management is largely **supportive**.

# Parkinson's Disease

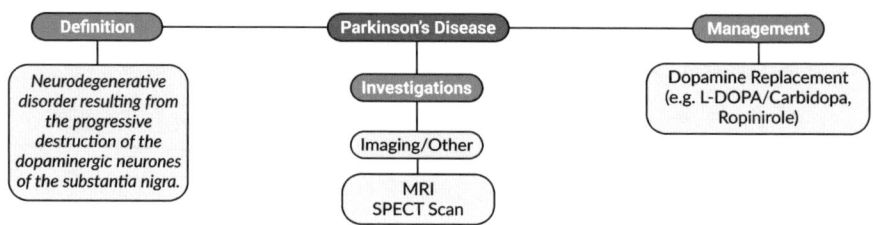

**Presentations**: Dysphagia, Constipation

## *Definition*

Parkinson's disease is a neurodegenerative condition resulting from the destruction of the dopaminergic neurones of the substantia nigra. It is characterised by a pill-rolling tremor, postural instability, rigidity and bradykinesia.

## *Investigations*

An **MRI SPECT scan** can demonstrate reduced dopaminergic activity within the substantia nigra.

## *Management*

The mainstay of managing Parkinson's disease involves **dopamine replacement**. This often involves administering L-DOPA with a peripheral DOPA-decarboxylase inhibitor (e.g. Carbidopa).

# Pelvic Inflammatory Disease (PID)

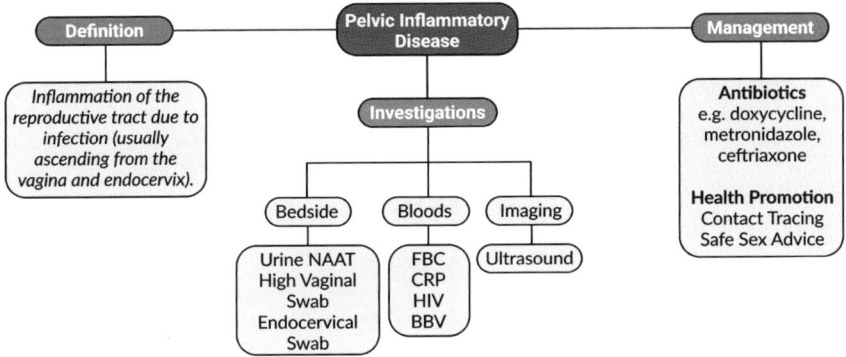

**Presentation**: Iliac Fossa Pain

## *Definition*

PID refers to inflammation of the female reproductive tract due to an infection.

## *Investigations*

At the bedside, a urine sample can be taken for **NAAT** and a **high vaginal** and **endocervical swab** should be taken to try and identify the causative organism. **FBC** and **CRP** may reveal raised inflammatory markers and blood cultures should be considered if the patient is septic. As PID is likely caused by an STI, the patient may be at risk of contracting bloodborne viral infections, such as HIV and hepatitis B, so a **bloodborne viral screen** and **HIV test** should be sent.

## *Management*

Patients are usually treated empirically with a combination of **antibiotics** (e.g. ceftriaxone, doxycycline and metronidazole). Patients should also be provided with advice about practising **safe sex** and offered **contact tracing**.

# Pericarditis

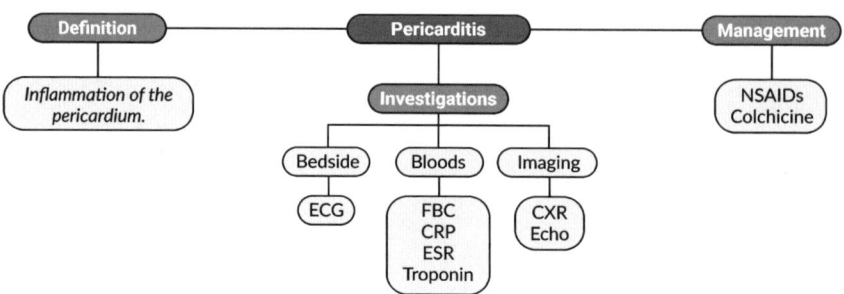

**Presentation**: Chest Pain

## *Definition*

Pericarditis refers to inflammation of the pericardium that usually occurs due to a viral infection.

## *Investigations*

An **ECG** may reveal widespread, saddle-shaped ST elevation or PR depression. The patient's inflammatory markers are likely to be raised (**FBC**, **CRP** and **ESR**) and, in the case of myocarditis, the serum **troponin** concentration is likely to be significantly elevated. A **chest X-ray** is usually performed to rule out other causes of chest pain (e.g. pneumonia and pneumothorax) and may reveal a globular heart in patients who have developed a pericardial effusion. An **echocardiogram** can also be performed to check for a pericardial effusion.

## *Management*

**NSAIDs** and **colchicine** are the main anti-inflammatory agents used in the management of pericarditis. If a significant pericardial effusion has developed, it may need to be drained.

# Pharyngeal Pouch

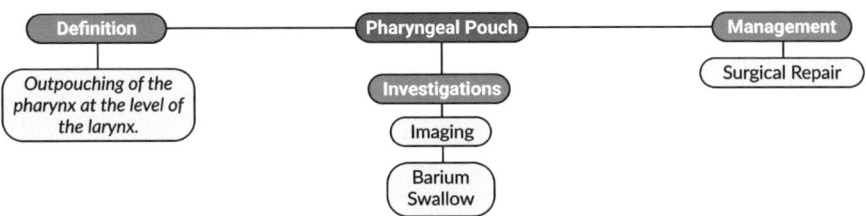

**Presentation**: Dysphagia

## *Definition*

A pharyngeal pouch is an outpouching of the pharynx that can cause dysphagia, regurgitation and halitosis.

## *Investigations*

The pouch can be visualised using a **barium swallow**.

## *Management*

If causing persistent or troublesome symptoms, the pouch can be **surgically repaired**.

# Pneumonia

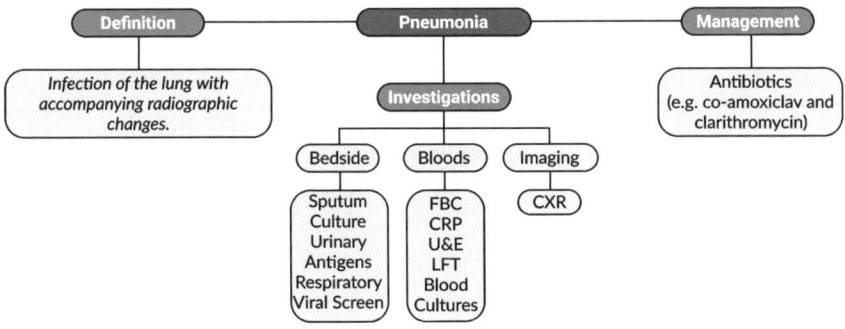

**Presentations**: Chest Pain, Cough, Shortness of Breath, RUQ Pain

## Definition

A pneumonia is an infection of the lung which has accompanying radiographic changes (e.g. consolidation).

## Investigations

At the bedside, the patient should be asked to provide a **sputum sample** to send for microscopy, culture and sensitivities. A urine sample should also be taken to check for **urinary antigens** (*Legionella pneumophila* and *Streptococcus pneumoniae*). Several common viruses can cause pneumonia, such as influenza, so a **respiratory viral screen** should be performed upon initial assessment. The patient's inflammatory markers (**FBC** and **CRP**) are likely to be raised. Atypical pneumonias can sometimes cause hyponatraemia, AKI and deranged liver function which would be defective on the **U&E** and **LFT**. If the patient is septic, **blood cultures** should also be taken. A **chest X-ray** will allow confirmation of the diagnosis.

## Management

The setting in which pneumonia is managed depends on the severity of the symptoms and can be aided by scoring tools, such as CURB-65. It is treated with **antibiotics**: co-amoxiclav and clarithromycin is a commonly used combination. A follow-up chest X-ray should be arranged for around 4–6 weeks after the initial presentation to ensure that there is no underlying malignancy that may have predisposed the patient to develop pneumonia.

# Pneumothorax

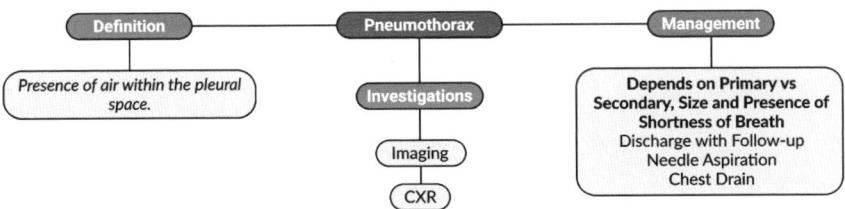

**Presentations**: Chest Pain, Shortness of Breath

## *Definition*

A pneumothorax refers to the presence of air within the pleural place. It can either be spontaneous, traumatic or occur in the context of pre-existing lung disease (e.g. COPD).

## *Investigations*

A pleural edge may be visible on a **chest X-ray** and the size of the pneumothorax can also be measured.

## *Management*

The management depends on the presence of pre-existing lung disease, the size of the pneumothorax and whether the patient is short of breath. It may be managed conservatively, or with needle aspiration or chest drain insertion.

# Postnasal Drip

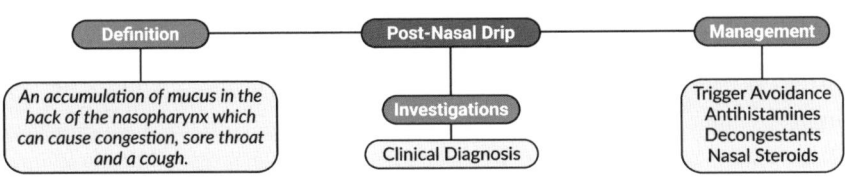

**Presentation**: Cough

## Definition

Postnasal drip is a very common condition that is characterised by a nocturnal cough that occurs due to mucus accumulating at the back of the nasopharynx.

## Investigations

It is a clinical diagnosis.

## Management

The symptoms can be managed using **antihistamines, decongestants** and **intranasal steroids**.

# Primary Sclerosing Cholangitis (PSC) and Primary Biliary Cholangitis (PBC)

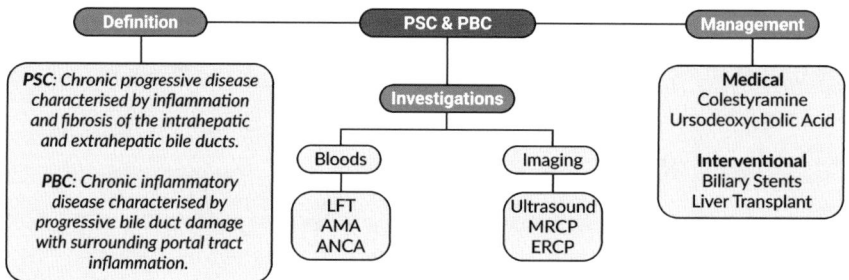

**Presentation**: Jaundice

## Definition

PSC and PBC are inflammatory conditions that lead to progressive bile duct destruction.

## Investigations

Both conditions will give rise to an obstructive pattern (raised ALP and GGT) on the **LFTs**. PSC is associated with a raised **pANCA**, whereas PBC is associated with an **anti-mitochondrial antibody (AMA)**. An **ultrasound** scan may reveal dilation of the biliary tree. An **MRCP** and **ERCP** will demonstrate the involvement of both the intra- and extrahepatic bile ducts in PSC, whereas primarily the intrahepatic ducts are affected in PBC.

## Management

**Ursodeoxycholic acid** is of prognostic benefit in PBC, whereas the management of PSC is largely supportive. **Colestyramine** can help reduce pruritus. Some patients may be considered for interventions, such as **biliary stents** and **liver transplants**.

# Pseudogout

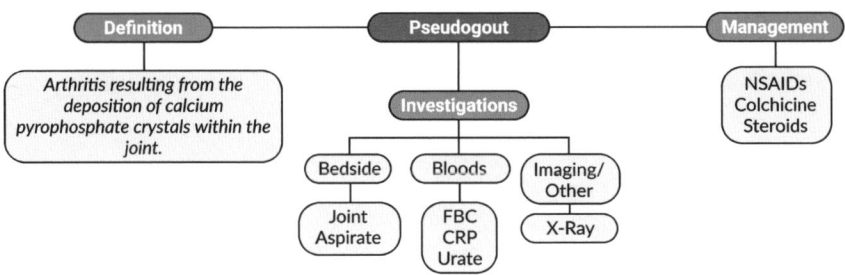

**Presentation**: Joint Pain

## Definition

Pseudogout is a crystal arthropathy that arises due to the deposition of calcium pyrophosphate crystals within a joint. It usually affects large joints.

## Investigations

At the bedside, a **joint aspirate** should be performed and sent for analysis. Microscopy will reveal positively birefringent rhomboid-shaped crystals. The patient's inflammatory markers are likely to be raised (**FBC** and **CRP**) and as it can be difficult to distinguish from gout, serum **urate** concentration should also be checked. An **X-ray** of the affected joint may reveal chondrocalcinosis.

## Management

The mainstay of managing pseudogout involves **NSAIDs** and **colchicine**. In some cases, **steroids** are used.

# Psoriatic Arthritis

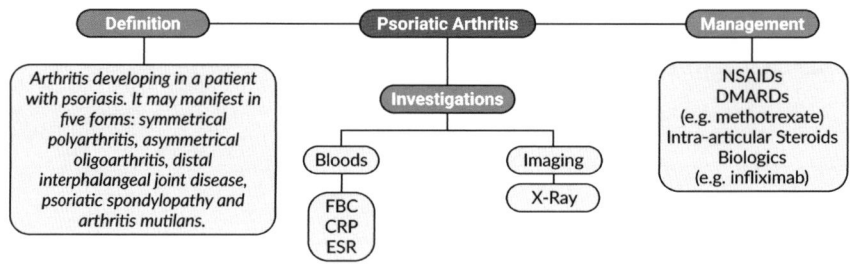

**Presentation**: Joint Pain

## Definition

Psoriatic arthritis refers to arthritis that arises in patients with psoriasis.

## Investigations

As it is an inflammatory condition, the patient's white cell count (**FBC**), **CRP** and **ESR** are likely to be raised. An **X-ray** may be used to check for erosive changes.

## Management

Psoriatic arthritis is usually managed by rheumatologists and involves using **NSAIDs**, **DMARDs**, **intra-articular steroids** and **biologics**.

# Psychosis

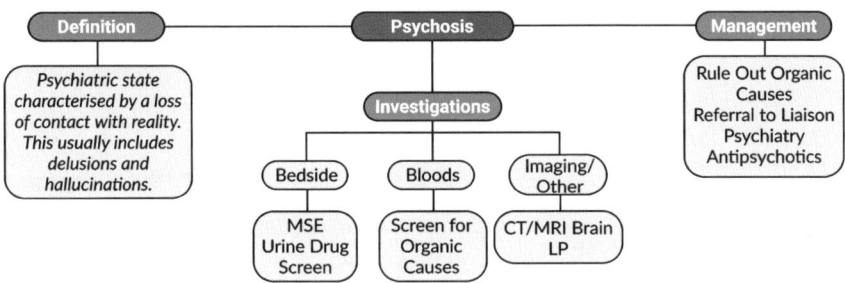

**Presentation**: Confusion

## Definition

Psychosis is a mental state that is characterised by a loss of contact with reality, which usually manifests with delusions (false, fixed beliefs that are held despite the presence of evidence to the contrary) and hallucinations (abnormal perceptions in the absence of stimuli).

## Investigations

If patients are presenting for the first time with psychosis, investigations should be requested to rule out organic causes. A **mental state examination (MSE)** provides a structure for assessing the patient and a **urine drug screen** should be requested if there is any concern about intoxication. Various blood tests, such as inflammatory markers and autoimmune screens, may be performed to check for organic causes. Patients will likely undergo some form of cross-sectional brain imaging (e.g. **CT/MRI brain**) to check for structural abnormalities that may give rise to confusion and personality changes (e.g. brain tumour). A **lumbar puncture** may be considered if encephalitis is a plausible differential.

## Management

Once organic causes have been ruled out, the patient should be referred to **liaison psychiatry** services for further assessment and coordination of care. Treatment often involves the use of **antipsychotic** medications.

# Pulmonary Oedema

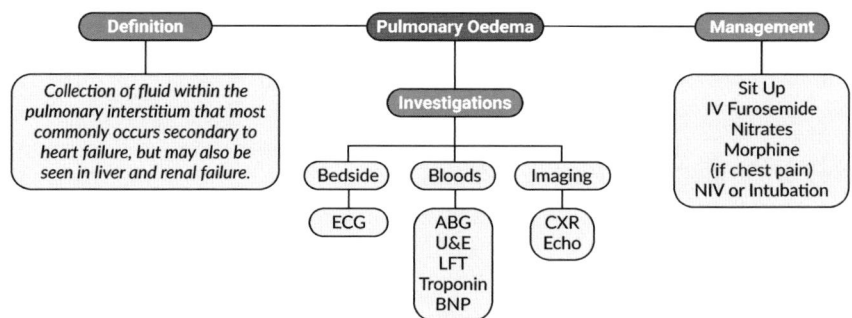

**Presentations**: Cough, Shortness of Breath

## Definition

Pulmonary oedema refers to the accumulation of fluid within the interstitium of the lungs.

## Investigations

At the bedside, an **ECG** should be performed as pulmonary oedema may be triggered by arrhythmias and ischaemic events. An **ABG** will allow identification of respiratory failure. As renal failure and liver failure are potential causes of pulmonary oedema, **U&E** and **LFT** should be requested. A **troponin** will allow identification of ischaemic events that can precipitate pulmonary oedema and **BNP** is likely to be raised in patients with heart failure. A **chest X-ray** may reveal alveolar shadowing, Kerley B lines, cardiomegaly, upper lobe diversion and pleural effusions. An **echocardiogram** allows assessment of left ventricular ejection fraction and the identification of valvular disease and regional wall motion abnormalities.

## Management

In acute pulmonary oedema, the patient should be **sat up** and started on **high-flow oxygen**. IV **furosemide** will help offload fluid and lessen the preload on the struggling heart. The patient should also be catheterised to allow close fluid balance monitoring. If the patient's blood pressure is stable, **nitrates** may be given to achieve further venodilation and reduce preload. **Morphine** may be used in patients complaining of chest pain. If patients fail to respond to initial treatment, they may need **NIV** or **intubation and ventilation**.

# Rheumatoid Arthritis

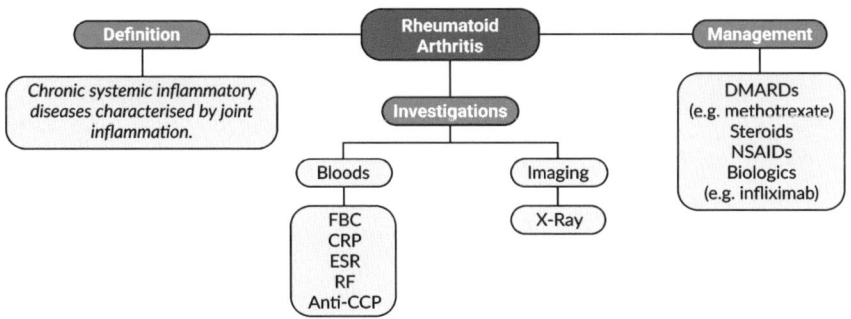

**Presentation**: Joint Pain

## Definition

Rheumatoid arthritis is a systemic inflammatory condition that is most commonly associated with joint inflammation but can also cause a range of extra-articular phenomena, such as interstitial lung disease, pericarditis and neuropathy.

## Investigations

As it is an inflammatory condition, the patient's inflammatory markers are likely to be raised (**FBC**, **CRP** and **ESR**). **Rheumatoid factor (RF)** is detected in about 60% of cases and high titres are associated with increased disease activity. **Anti-cyclic citrullinated peptic (anti-CCP) antibodies** have a high specificity in rheumatoid arthritis. An **X-ray** of the affected joints may reveal joint space narrowing, erosions and soft tissue swelling.

## Management

Rheumatoid arthritis is managed by rheumatologists and often involves using **NSAIDs**, **steroids**, **DMARDs** and, in some cases, **biologics**.

# Ruptured Baker's Cyst

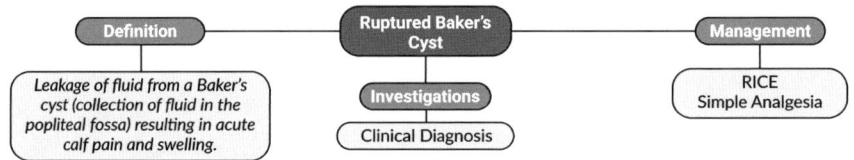

**Presentation**: Leg Pain

## Definition

A Baker's cyst is a collection of fluid behind the knee that can rupture causing sudden onset leg pain and swelling.

## *Investigations*

It is largely a clinical diagnosis, but investigations may be requested to rule out other diagnoses (e.g. an ultrasound scan to check for a DVT).

## *Management*

Patients should be advised about **RICE** and to manage their pain using **simple analgesia**.

# Seizure

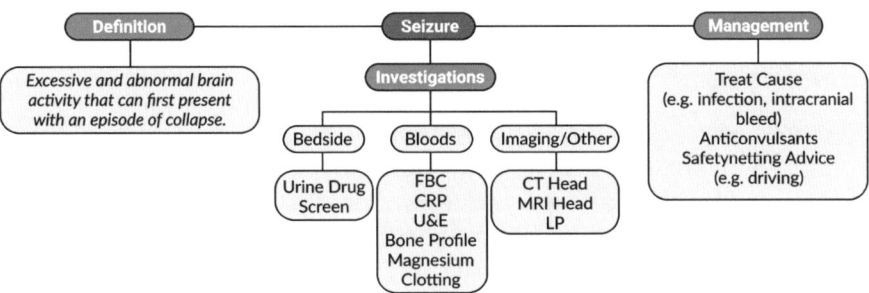

**Presentation**: Collapse

## *Definition*

A seizure is an episode of excessive and abnormal brain activity that can present with collapse. An important distinction to make is that a seizure does not necessarily mean that a patient has epilepsy. Epilepsy refers to a tendency to develop recurrent unprovoked seizures.

## *Investigations*

Seizures can be precipitated by several illicit drugs, so a **urine drug screen** should be considered in patients presenting with a seizure for the first time. Intracranial infections can also cause seizures, in which case the inflammatory markers (**FBC** and **CRP**) are likely to be raised. Electrolyte derangements, such as hyponatraemia and hypercalcaemia, can cause seizures, so **U&E**, **bone profile** and **magnesium** level should be checked. Intracranial bleeds can also lead to seizures so a **CT head** scan should be considered, and a **clotting screen** should be sent. If the CT head scan is inconclusive, an **MRI scan** may be requested to check for structural abnormalities that can give rise to seizures (e.g. brain tumour). To check for evidence of intracranial infection or inflammation, a **lumbar puncture** may be performed. It is important to thoroughly assess the patient for evidence of other injuries that may have been sustained during the seizure (e.g. shoulder dislocation) and request imaging appropriately (e.g. X-ray).

### Management

Seizures often terminate spontaneously, and the mainstay of treatment involves identifying and treating any reversible causes. **Anticonvulsants** can be used to prevent further seizures. Patients should also be provided with clear safety netting advice about high-risk activities (e.g. swimming and driving).

## Sexually Transmitted Infections (STI)

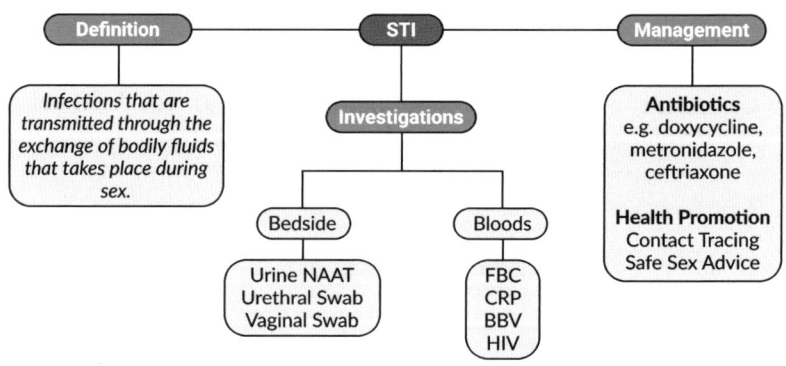

**Presentation**: Dysuria

## Definition

STIs are infections that are transmitted through sexual contact. Common causes include chlamydia and gonorrhoea. They may be asymptomatic but may also present with dysuria and abnormal discharge.

## Investigations

A **urine NAAT** is a non-invasive screen that is often performed in asymptomatic patients. **Urethral** and **vaginal swabs** can help identify the causative organism. The patient may be at risk of developing bloodborne viral infections, so a **bloodborne viral screen** and **HIV test** should be requested. Patients may also have raised inflammatory markers (**FBC** and **CRP**).

## Management

The treatment of STIs usually involves a combination of **antibiotics** (e.g. ceftriaxone, metronidazole and doxycycline). Patients should also be provided with advice about **safe sex** and offered **contact tracing**.

# Sinusitis

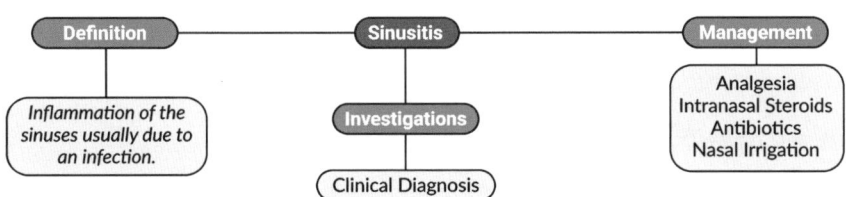

**Presentation**: Headache

## Definition

Sinusitis refers to inflammation of the sinuses usually due to infection. It is very common and often resolves spontaneously.

## Investigations

It is a clinical diagnosis.

## Management

Symptoms often resolve over time and can be managed using **simple analgesia**. If symptoms persist, **intranasal steroids, antibiotics** (e.g. penicillin V) and **nasal irrigation** may be considered.

# Spinal Stenosis

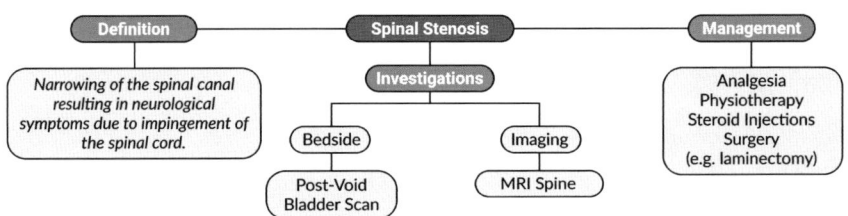

**Presentation**: Back Pain

## Definition

Spinal stenosis refers to narrowing of the spinal cord that results in impingement of the spinal cord. It is usually caused by osteoarthritis and herniated discs.

## Investigations

Impingement of the spinal cord can result in urinary retention which can be objectively measured with a **post-void bladder scan**. If suspected, an urgent **MRI spine** should be requested.

## Management

If the symptoms are mild, patients could be managed with **analgesia** and **physiotherapy**. In some cases, **steroid injections** and **surgery** may be considered.

# Stroke

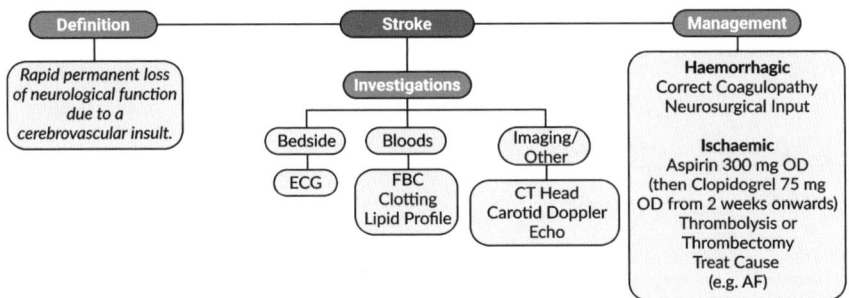

**Presentation**: Dysphagia

## Definition

A stroke refers to a rapid, permanent loss of neurological function that occurs due to a thrombus or haemorrhage in the brain.

## Investigations

At the bedside, an **ECG** may reveal AF, which is a major risk factor for the development of stroke. An **FBC** (to check the platelets) and a **clotting screen** will allow identification of issues with blood clotting which may require reversal in patients with haemorrhagic strokes. A **lipid profile** is involved in the assessment of the patient's risk factors. An urgent **CT head** scan is essential in ruling out a haemorrhagic stroke. After the acute situation has been attended to, a **carotid Doppler** (to check for carotid atherosclerosis) and an **echocardiogram** (to check for valvular abnormalities) should be arranged.

## Management

Haemorrhagic strokes are the minority of strokes and are generally managed by correcting coagulopathy and getting a neurosurgical opinion. Once a haemorrhagic stroke has been ruled out, the patient should be started on **aspirin 300 mg OD**. This will be changed to **clopidogrel 75 mg OD** after 2 weeks. Depending on how soon the patient presents after the onset of symptoms, they may be considered for **thrombolysis** (<4.5 hours) and/or **thrombectomy** (up to 24 hours).

# Systemic Lupus Erythematosus (SLE)

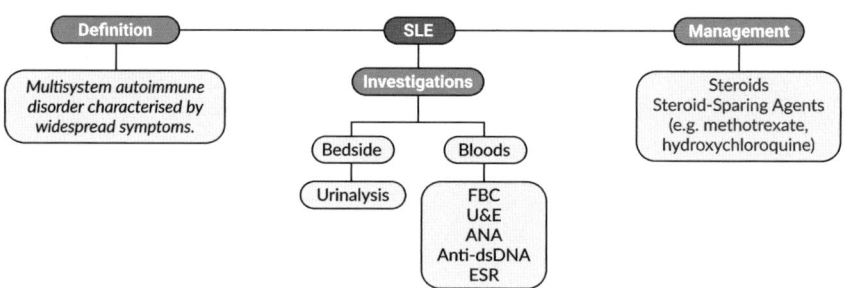

**Presentation**: Fatigue

## Definition

SLE is a multisystem autoimmune condition that is characterised by a variety of manifestations that can be remembered using the mnemonic '**SOAP BRAIN MD**' (**S**erositis, **O**ral ulcers, **A**rthritis, **P**hotosensitivity, **B**lood abnormalities (pancytopaenia), **R**enal impairment, **A**NA, **I**mmunological (anti-dsDNA) and **N**europsychiatric features (psychosis and seizures)).

## Investigations

**Urinalysis** may reveal blood and protein, suggestive of glomerulonephritis. An **FBC** may reveal low cell counts and **U&E** may reveal renal impairment. **Anti-Nuclear Antibody (ANA)** has a high sensitivity for SLE, whereas **Anti-dsDNA Antibody** has a high specificity. The **ESR** is likely to be raised.

## *Management*

SLE is generally managed by rheumatologists and usually involves a combination of **steroids** and **steroid-sparing agents**.

# Tension Headache

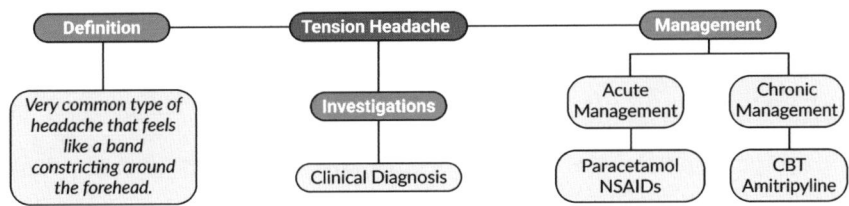

**Presentation**: Headache

## *Definition*

Tension headaches are common headaches that present with pain across the forehead.

## *Investigations*

It is a clinical diagnosis.

## *Management*

Tension headaches usually respond well to **simple analgesia** (paracetamol and NSAIDs). If chronic or recurrent, patients may benefit from **CBT** and **amitriptyline**.

# Testicular Cancer

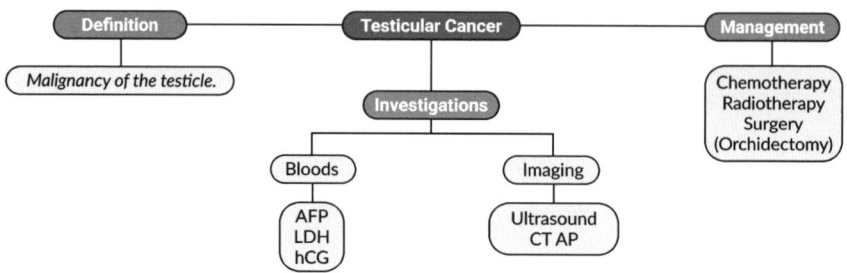

**Presentation**: Scrotal Mass

## *Definition*

Testicular cancer is a malignancy of the testicle that most commonly occurs in children and young adults.

## *Investigations*

Tumour markers that are associated with testicular cancer include **AFP**, **LDH** and **hCG**. The testicular mass can be visualised with an **ultrasound** scan. A **CT abdomen and pelvis** may be requested to help stage the tumour.

## *Management*

Testicular cancer is generally very responsive to **chemotherapy**. **Radiotherapy** may be used for affected lymph nodes. An **orchidectomy** involves removing the affected testicle.

# Testicular Torsion

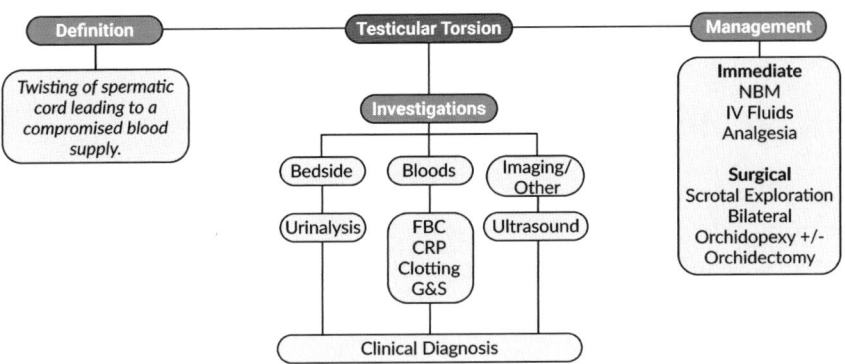

**Presentation**: Scrotal Mass

## *Definition*

Testicular torsion is a urological emergency that occurs when the testicle twists on the spermatic cord resulting in a compromised blood supply. If left untreated, it can lead to testicular necrosis.

## *Investigations*

Testicular torsion is a clinical diagnosis and patients should be urgently referred to a urologist based on clinical suspicion alone. **Urinalysis** may demonstrate leucocytes, nitrites and blood in cases of epididymitis that can present similarly to testicular torsion. An **FBC** and a **CRP** may reveal raised inflammatory markers in epididymitis. As the patient will likely need to go for exploratory surgery, a **clotting screen** and **G&S** should be sent. An **ultrasound** scan may reveal a swollen testicle with a compromised blood supply.

## *Management*

The initial management involves keeping the patient **nil-by-mouth**, **IV fluids** and **analgesia**. Following urgent referral to urology, patients are likely to undergo **scrotal exploration with bilateral orchidopexy**. If the testicle is found to no longer be viable, it will be removed (**orchidectomy**).

# Tuberculosis

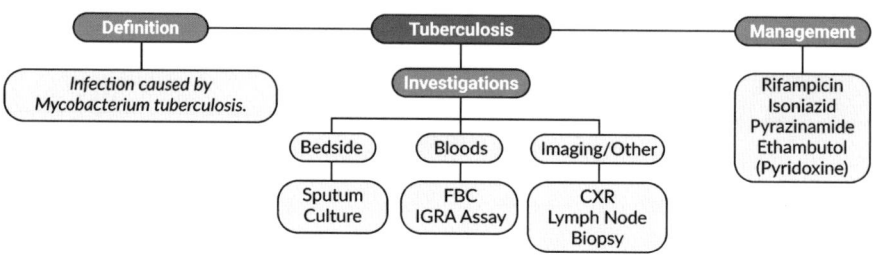

**Presentation**: Fatigue

## *Definition*

Tuberculosis (TB) is a chronic infection caused by *Mycobacterium tuberculosis*. The infection can affect multiple organ systems and manifest in many different ways.

## *Investigations*

Patients with suspected TB should be asked to provide three **sputum samples** for microscopy and culture to identify acid-fast bacilli. An **FBC** may reveal raised inflammatory markers. An **interferon gamma release assay (IGRA)** is a blood test that is used to identify TB, though it cannot distinguish between latent and active TB. As the lungs are the usual primary site in which TB becomes established, a **chest X-ray** should be requested and may reveal changes, such as cavitation and bilateral hilar lymphadenopathy. A **lymph node biopsy** should be performed if enlarged lymph nodes are identified clinically or radiographically.

## Management

The mainstay of managing TB involves a combination of four anti-TB medications: **rifampicin** and **isoniazid** (for 6 months), and **pyrazinamide** and **ethambutol** (for the first 2 months). Isoniazid can cause vitamin B6 deficiency resulting in peripheral neuropathy, so patients should also be started on pyridoxine. In cases of drug-resistant TB, other agents such as moxifloxacin, bedaquiline and cycloserine may be used.

# Urinary Tract Calculi

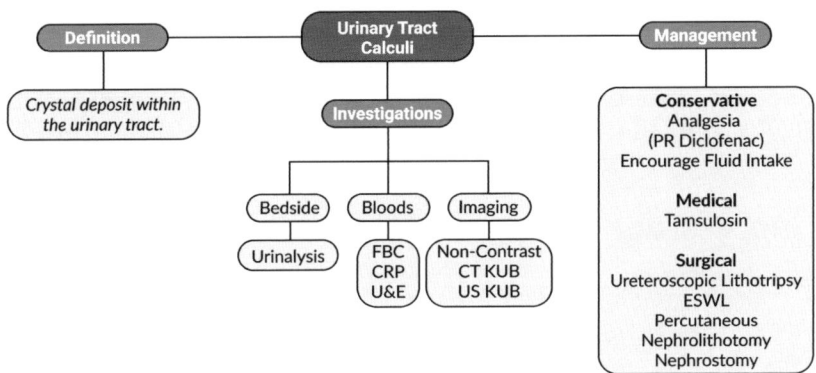

**Presentations**: RUQ Pain, Iliac Fossa Pain, Dysuria

## Definition

Urinary tract calculi are crystal deposits within the urinary tract that present with acute onset severe flank pain that radiates to the groin.

## Investigations

**Urinalysis** will likely reveal microscopic haematuria. An **FBC** and a **CRP** may reveal raised inflammatory markers in cases of infected and obstructed urinary tracts. Hydronephrosis secondary to an obstructing stone can lead to a derangement in renal function (**U&E**).

The first-line imaging modality in suspected urinary tract calculi is a **non-contrast CT KUB** to visualise the stone and check for evidence of obstruction. An **ultrasound KUB** avoids ionising radiation and can help identify hydronephrosis, however, it does not have a high sensitivity for visualising stones.

## Management

The management depends largely on the size of the stone and whether it is causing an obstruction. Small, non-obstructing calculi can be managed with **analgesia** (e.g. PR diclofenac) and by **encouraging fluid intake**. **Tamsulosin** is an alpha-blocker that can relax the smooth muscle around the ureters to facilitate passage of the stone. Interventions to remove the stone include **ureteroscopic lithotripsy, extracorporeal shockwave lithotripsy (ESWL), percutaneous nephrolithotomy** and **nephrostomy**.

# Urinary Tract Infection (UTI)

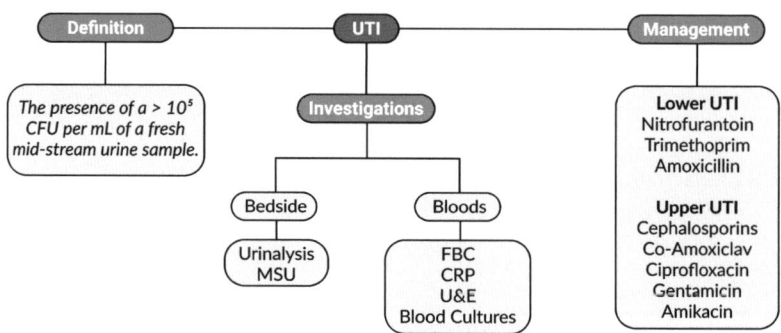

**Presentations**: RUQ Pain, Dysuria, Polyuria

## Definition

A UTI refers to an infection of the urinary system that is technically defined by the presence of over $10^5$ colony-forming units per mL of urine. It is most commonly caused by *Escherichia coli* and can affect both the lower (cystitis) and upper (pyelonephritis) urinary tract.

## Investigations

At the bedside, **urinalysis** may reveal leucocytes and nitrites. In some cases, it may also be positive for blood and protein (especially in cases of pyelonephritis). An **FBC** and a **CRP** may reveal raised inflammatory markers. **U&E** may reveal deranged renal function in cases of pyelonephritis or in cases of urosepsis. If patients appear septic, **blood cultures** should be taken.

## Management

Uncomplicated UTIs can generally be managed in primary care with antibiotics, such as **nitrofurantoin**, **trimethoprim** and **amoxicillin**. Patients who are unwell with a UTI should be treated in accordance with the sepsis 6 protocol and IV antibiotics. Commonly used agents include cephalosporins and aminoglycosides (e.g. amikacin).

# Varicocele

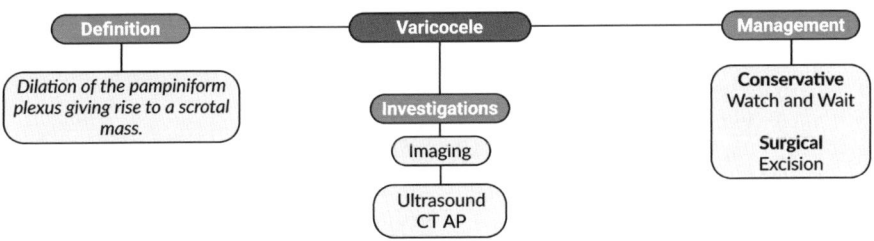

**Presentation**: Scrotal Mass

## Definition

A varicocele is a dilation of the pampiniform plexus (venous plexus within the spermatic cord) that can present with scrotal discomfort and is associated with subfertility.

## Investigations

An **ultrasound** scan can help distinguish varicoceles from other causes of scrotal masses (e.g. hydrocele and epididymal cyst). Varicoceles, especially if left-sided, may be suggestive of an underlying malignancy (e.g. renal cell carcinoma) which can be identified with a **CT abdomen and pelvis**.

## Management

In some cases, varicoceles may be managed conservatively, however, it is associated with subfertility, so patients may benefit from surgical **excision**.

# Vasovagal Syncope

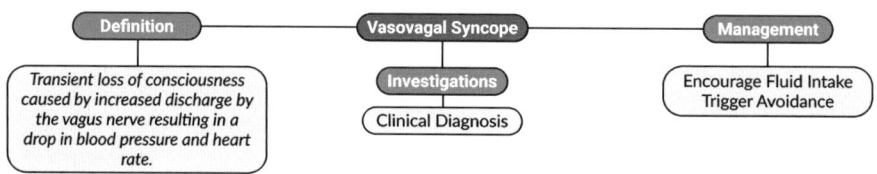

**Presentation**: Collapse

## Definition

Vasovagal syncope is a very common cause of collapse that is caused by increased vagal discharge resulting in a short-lived syncopal episode with rapid recovery.

## Investigations

It is a clinical diagnosis, however, patients may undergo investigations to rule out more sinister causes of collapse (e.g. ECG and echocardiogram).

## Management

Vasovagal syncope can generally be managed conservatively with advice regarding fluid intake and avoiding triggers.

# Venous Sinus Thrombosis

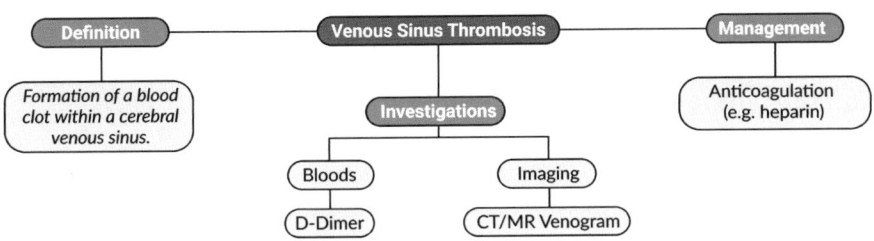

**Presentation**: Headache

## Definition

A venous sinus thrombosis is a clot within the cerebral venous sinuses that can present with a sudden onset, intense headache with focal neurology. It is associated with risk factors for hypercoagulability such as pregnancy and the combined oral contraceptive pill.

## Investigations

A **D-Dimer** can help assess the risk of venous sinus thrombosis in low-risk patients. Patients will usually initially undergo a CT head scan, but a **CT or MR Venogram** will better allow identification of a venous sinus thrombosis.

## Management

The mainstay of treatment involves **anticoagulation**. In some cases, catheter-directed thrombolysis may be performed by neuroradiologists.

# Vertebral Fracture

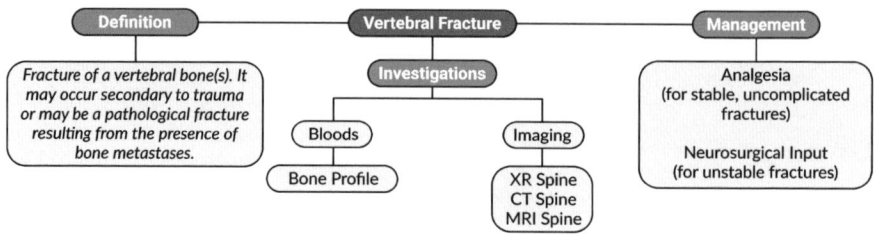

**Presentation**: Back Pain

## *Definition*

A vertebral fracture refers to a fracture of the vertebra that may occur in the context of trauma, malignancy and osteoporosis.

## *Investigations*

If a pathological fracture is suspected, a **bone profile** may reveal hyperkalaemia caused by bone metastases. An **X-ray** may reveal obvious fractures, though **CT** has a higher sensitivity for detecting vertebral fractures. If there is any concern about compression of the spinal cord or cauda equina, an **MRI** scan should be arranged.

## *Management*

If the fracture is stable and uncomplicated, patients may be managed with **analgesia** alone. In cases of unstable fractures that may be threatening the spinal cord or cauda equina, an **urgent neurosurgical opinion** should be sought.

# Vestibular Disorders

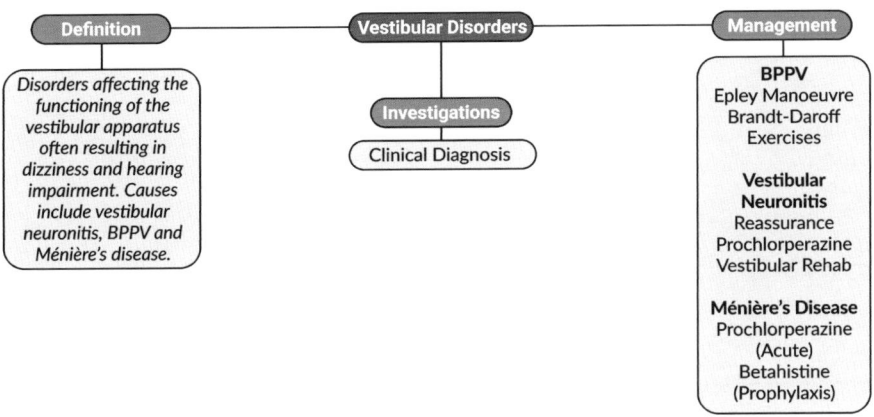

**Presentations**: Nausea and Vomiting

## *Definition*

The vestibular apparatus plays a crucial role in balance. Common diseases that affect the vestibular apparatus include benign paroxysmal positional vertigo (BPPV), vestibular neuronitis and Ménière's disease.

## *Investigations*

They are largely clinical diagnoses based on the history and the findings of certain special examinations (e.g. Dix–Hallpike manoeuvre).

## *Management*

BPPV can be treated acutely by performing an **Epley manoeuvre**. Patients can also be provided with advice about **Brandt–Daroff exercises** that can help manage their symptoms at home. Certain medications are used in the management of vestibular neuronitis and Ménière's disease, such as **prochlorperazine** and **betahistine**.

# Index